Study Guide

Pharmacology

A Patient-Centered Nursing Process Approach

Study Guide

Pharmacology

A Patient-Centered Nursing Process Approach

9th Edition

Linda E. McCuistion, PhD, MSN
NCLEX Live Review Presenter
Mandeville, Louisiana

Kathleen Vuljoin-DiMaggio, RN, MSN
Assistant Professor of Nursing
The University of Holy Cross
New Orleans, Louisiana

Mary B. Winton, PhD, RN, ACANP-BC
Assistant Professor
Tarleton State University
Stephenville, Texas

Jennifer J. Yeager, PhD, RN, AGNP
Assistant Professor and Director of the Graduate Nursing Program
Tarleton State University
Stephenville, Texas

Study Guide prepared by
Mary B. Winton, PhD, RN, ACANP-BC
Assistant Professor, Nursing
Tarleton State University
Stephenville, Texas

ELSEVIER

ELSEVIER

3251 Riverport Lane
St. Louis, Missouri 63043

Notices

Knowledge and best practice in this field are constantly changing. As new research and experience broaden our
understanding, changes in research methods, professional practices, or medical treatment may become necessary.

   Practitioners and researchers must always rely on their own experience and knowledge in evaluating and
using any information, methods, compounds, or experiments described herein. In using such information or
methods they should be mindful of their own safety and the safety of others, including parties for whom they
have a professional responsibility.

   With respect to any drug or pharmaceutical products identified, readers are advised to check the most
current information provided (i) on procedures featured or (ii) by the manufacturer of each product to be
administered, to verify the recommended dose or formula, the method and duration of administration, and
contraindications. It is the responsibility of practitioners, relying on their own experience and knowledge of
their patients, to make diagnoses, to determine dosages and the best treatment for each individual patient, and
to take all appropriate safety precautions.

   To the fullest extent of the law, neither the Publisher nor the authors, contributors, or editors assume any
liability for any injury and/or damage to persons or property as a matter of products liability, negligence or
otherwise, or from any use or operation of any methods, products, instructions, or ideas contained in the
material herein.

Content Strategist: Sonya Seigafuse
Content Development Manager: Lisa P. Newton
Senior Content Development Specialist: Charlene Ketchum/Tina Kaemmerer
Publishing Services Manager: Deepthi Unni
Project Manager: Manchu Mohan
Cover Designer: Muthukumaran Thangaraj

Printed in the United States of America

Last digit is the print number: 9   8   7   6   5   4   3   2   1

Working together
to grow libraries in
developing countries

www.elsevier.com • www.bookaid.org

Preface

This comprehensive *Study Guide* is designed to provide the learner with clinically based situation practice problems and questions. This book accompanies the text *Pharmacology: A Patient-Centered Nursing Process Approach,* Ninth Edition, and may also be used independently of the text.

Opportunities abound for the enhancement of critical thinking and decision-making abilities. Hundreds of study questions and answers are presented on nursing responsibilities in therapeutic pharmacology. Each chapter follows a format that includes NCLEX-style study questions (including multiple choice, matching, labeling, prioritizing, and completion exercises), and case studies.

This new edition provides more than 160 drug calculation problems and questions, many relating to actual patient care situations and enhanced with updated, real drug labels. The learner is also expected to recognize safe dosage parameters for the situation. The combination of the instructional material in the text and the multiplicity of a variety of practice problems in this *Study Guide* precludes the need for an additional drug dosage calculation book.

New to the ninth edition includes a step-by-step approach to using dimensional analysis on selected drug calculation problems, including critical care drugs. Multiple practice opportunities are provided in the areas of measurement, reading of drug labels, and calculation of oral and injectable dosages (including pediatric and critical care drugs), and flow rates of intravenous fluids.

The nursing process is used throughout the patient situation–based questions and case studies. Chapters have questions that relate to assessment data, including laboratory data and side effects, planning and implementing care, patient/family teaching, cultural and nutritional considerations, and effectiveness of the drug therapy regimen.

Because of the ever-expanding number of drugs available, pharmacology can be an overwhelming subject. To help learners grasp essential content without becoming overwhelmed, chapters have been divided into multiple smaller sections. The result is a layout that is user-friendly.

To underscore the importance of the nurse's role in patient safety, a new safety icon has been added to call attention to questions concerning safe patient care. As one of the six core competencies of the Quality and Safety Education for Nurses (QSEN) initiative, patient safety has never been more at the forefront of nursing education.

Answers to all questions are presented in the Answer Key to make studying easier. The ninth edition provides are rationales for selected application-level questions and case study questions.

The *Study Guide* is part of a comprehensive pharmacology package, including the textbook and Instructor and Student Resources available on the companion Evolve website. This package and each of its components were designed to promote critical thinking and learning. We are excited about this edition of the *Study Guide* because it offers the learner a variety of modalities for mastering the content.

Contents

1 Drug Development and Ethical Considerations

STUDY QUESTIONS

Match the act or amendment in Column I with the description in Column II.

Column I

_____ 1.   Kefauver-Harris Amendment

_____ 2.   Food, Drug, and Cosmetic Act

_____ 3.   The Orphan Drug Act

_____ 4.   Durham-Humphrey Amendment

_____ 5.   Harrison Narcotic Act

Column II

a.   Determines which drugs can be sold with or without a prescription

b.   Tightened controls on drug safety and testing

c.   Mandated physicians and pharmacists in keeping records of prescribed narcotics

d.   Promotes the development of drugs used to treat rare illnesses

e.   Empowered the FDA to monitor and regulate the manufacturing and marketing of drugs

Complete the following.

6.   The _____ name is owned by the manufacturer.

7.   Schedule _____ drugs are not approved for medical use.

8.   The Health Insurance Portability and Accountability Act (HIPAA) allows patients more control over their

_____ _____.

9.   The Food and Drug Administration Safety and Innovation Act (FDASIA) strengthens the _____

to safeguard and advance public _____ by expediting development of _____,

_____, and _____ products.

10.   Practicing nurses should be knowledgeable about the _____ _____ _____
to safely administer drugs.

Answer the following questions as true or false.

_____ 11.   Substance examples of Schedule II drugs include peyote, heroin, and *Cannabis*.

_____ 12.   Examples of Schedule IV substances include the category of benzodiazepines.

_____ 13.   All drugs become less effective over time.

_____ 14.   There is no difference on a drug's effect between children and older adults.

_____ 15.   A nurse advances the health care profession through research and scholarly inquiry.

NCLEX STYLE QUESTIONS

Select the best response.

16. Before administering controlled drugs to a patient, a nurse should:
    a. verify orders before drug administration.
    b. not document all wasted drugs.
    c. keep controlled drugs accessible for patient's convenience.
    d. have a witness for wastage of only Scheduled III drugs.

17. What resource provides the basis for standards in drug strength and composition throughout the world?
    a. *United States Pharmacopeia/National Formulary*
    b. *American Hospital Formulary Service (AHFS) Drug Information*
    c. *MedlinePlus*
    d. *International Pharmacopeia*

18. What is the current authoritative source for drug standards?
    a. Controlled Substances Act
    b. *MedlinePlus*
    c. The *Medical Letter*
    d. *United States Pharmacopeia/National Formulary*

19. What is the primary purpose of federal legislation related to drug standards?
    a. Provide consistency
    b. Establish cost controls
    c. Ensure safety
    d. Promote competition

20. Which legislation identified those drugs that require a new prescription for a refill?
    a. Controlled Substances Act
    b. Durham-Humphrey Amendment
    c. Food, Drug, and Cosmetic Act of 1938
    d. Kefauver-Harris Amendment

21. The Kefauver-Harris Amendment was passed to improve safety by requiring which information to be included in the drug's literature?
    a. Recommended dose
    b. Pregnancy category
    c. Side effects and contraindications
    d. Adverse reactions and contraindications

22. The patient presents to the emergency department with hallucinations. The patient's friend states he has been using lysergic acid diethylamide (LSD) and mescaline. To which schedule do these drugs belong?
    a. Schedule IV
    b. Schedule III
    c. Schedule II
    d. Schedule I

23. In which schedule would the nurse find codeine, an ingredient found in many cough syrup?
    a. II
    b. III
    c. IV
    d. V

24. Where must controlled substances be stored in an institution/agency?
    a. In a double-wrapped and labeled container
    b. In the patient's drug bin
    c. Near the nurse's station
    d. In a locked, secured area

25. A 35-year-old male diagnosed with advanced pancreatic cancer agrees to participate in a clinical research for a new chemotherapy regimen to treat pancreatic cancer. The patient asks the nurse which group he will be in. The nurse answers, knowing that:
    a. he will receive information about the study through the mail.
    b. the nurse has the role in explaining the study to the patient.
    c. the patient must be alert and comprehend the information being provided.
    d. information should be vague because the patient does not need to know the study protocol.

26. The nurse must be alert for counterfeit prescription drugs. What are clues to the identification of counterfeit products? *(Select all that apply.)*
    a. Different color
    b. Different dose
    c. Different taste
    d. Different labeling
    e. Different shape

CASE STUDY

Read the scenario, and answer the following question on a separate sheet of paper.

L.L. has received a prescription for a drug to treat hypertension and is preparing for discharge from the emergency department. He says to the nurse, "I don't understand all of this paperwork that I have to sign. I sign this same form every time. What is HIPAA, and why should I even care?"

1. How will the nurse explain HIPAA to the patient as it pertains to his medications?

2. What should the nurse tell the patient about the boundaries on the use and release of his health records?

2 Pharmacokinetics, Pharmacodynamics, and Pharmacogenetics

STUDY QUESTIONS

Complete the following.

1. The pharmacokinetic phase is composed of _____, _____, _____, and _____.

2. The $t_{1/2}$ or the _____ is when 50% of the drug concentration is eliminated.

3. _____ is the effect of drug action on cells.

4. Drug absorption is the movement of the drug into the _____ after _____.

5. Drugs that are _____ block responses.

6. Cell membranes contain _____ that enhance drug actions.

Match the terms in Column I with their descriptions in Column II.

Column I

_____ 7. Dissolution

_____ 8. Hepatic first pass

_____ 9. Nonselective receptors

_____ 10. Passive absorption

_____ 11. Protein-bound drug

_____ 12. Unbound drug

_____ 13. Facilitated diffusion

Column II

a. Drug absorbed by diffusion
b. Causes inactive drug action/response
c. Drugs that affect various receptors
d. Free active drug causing a pharmacologic response
e. Proceeds directly from intestine to the liver
f. Breakdown of a drug into smaller particles
g. Drug requiring a carrier for absorption

Match the terms in Column I with their descriptions in Column II.

Column I

_____ 14. Duration of action

_____ 15. Onset

_____ 16. Peak action

_____ 17. Therapeutic index

Column II

a. Length of time a drug has a pharmacologic effect
b. The margin of safety of a drug
c. Occurs when a drug has reached its highest plasma concentration
d. Time it takes a drug to reach minimum effective concentration

NCLEX REVIEW QUESTIONS

Select the best response.

18. Which drug form is most rapidly absorbed from the gastrointestinal (GI) tract?
    a. Capsule
    b. Sublingual
    c. Suspension
    d. Tablet

19. Disintegration of enteric-coated tablets occurs in the:
    a. colon.
    b. liver.
    c. small intestine.
    d. stomach.

20. Usually food _____ dissolution and absorption of drug.
    a. increases
    b. decreases
    c. has no effect on
    d. prevents

21. Which statement places the four processes of pharmacokinetics in the correct sequence?
    a. Absorption, metabolism, distribution, excretion
    b. Distribution, absorption, metabolism, excretion
    c. Distribution, metabolism, absorption, excretion
    d. Absorption, distribution, metabolism, excretion

22. Which type of drug passes rapidly through the GI membrane?
    a. Lipid-soluble and ionized
    b. Lipid-soluble and nonionized
    c. Water-soluble and ionized
    d. Water-soluble and nonionized

23. Which factor(s) most commonly affect(s) a drug's absorption? (Select all that apply.)
    a. Body mass index
    b. Hypotension
    c. Pain
    d. Sleep
    e. Stress

24. The patient is taking diazepam for anxiety. Two days later she is started on ampicillin with sulbactam for an infection. What does the nurse know will happen to the diazepam in the patient's body?
    a. The diazepam remains highly protein bound.
    b. The diazepam is deactivated.
    c. Most of the diazepam is released, and it becomes more active.
    d. The diazepam is excreted in the urine unchanged.

25. Which body organ is the major site of drug metabolism?
    a. Kidney
    b. Liver
    c. Lung
    d. Skin

26. Which route of drug absorption has the greatest bioavailability?
    a. Intramuscular
    b. Intravenous
    c. Oral
    d. Subcutaneous

27. Which is the best description of a drug's serum half-life?
    a. The time required for half of a drug dose to be absorbed
    b. The time required after absorption for half of the drug to be eliminated
    c. The time required for a drug to be totally effective
    d. The time required for half of the drug dose to be completely distributed

28. The patient is taking a drug that has a half-life of 24 to 30 hours. In preparing discharge teaching, what is the dosing schedule the nurse anticipates will be prescribed for this drug?
    a. Daily
    b. Every other day
    c. Twice per day
    d. Three times per day

29. Which type of drug metabolite can be eliminated through the kidneys?
    a. Enteric-coated
    b. Lipid-soluble
    c. Protein-bound
    d. Water-soluble

30. The older adult patient has a decreased estimated glomerular filtration rate (eGFR) of less than 30. The patient has been prescribed trimethoprim for a urinary tract infection. If the normal dose is 200 mg per day, what does the nurse anticipate will occur with the dosing regimen?
    a. The dose will double.
    b. The dose will decrease by one-half.
    c. The dose will stay the same.
    d. The dose will increase to three times per day.

31. Which is the best determinant of the biologic activity of a drug?
    a. The fit of the drug at the receptor site
    b. The misfit of the drug at the receptor site
    c. The inability of the drug to bind to a specific receptor
    d. The ability of the drug to be rapidly excreted

32. Which type of drug prevents or inhibits a cellular response?
    a. Agonist
    b. Antagonist
    c. Cholinergic
    d. Nonspecific drug

33. A receptor located in different parts of the body may initiate a variety of responses depending on the anatomic site. Which type of receptor responds in this manner?
    a. Ligand-gated
    b. Nonselective
    c. Nonspecific
    d. Placebo

34. _____ measures the margin of safety of a drug.
    a. Therapeutic range
    b. Therapeutic index
    c. Duration of action
    d. Biologic half-life

35. The nurse has just given the patient her prescribed antibiotic. Which measurement checks for the highest plasma/serum concentration of the drug?
    a. Peak level
    b. Minimal effective concentration
    c. Half-life
    d. Trough level

36. Before administering a medication, the nurse checks a drug reference book or pamphlet to obtain pertinent data. Which data should the nurse note? *(Select all that apply.)*
    a. Contraindications
    b. Half-life
    c. Maximum effective concentration
    d. Protein-binding effect
    e. Therapeutic range

37. Which types of physiologic effects are predictable or associated with the use of a specific drug?
    a. Severe adverse reactions
    b. Side effects
    c. Synergistic effects
    d. Toxic effects

38. The nurse is giving a large initial dose of a drug to rapidly achieve minimum effective concentration in the plasma. What is this type of dosage called?
    a. Therapeutic dose
    b. Toxic dose
    c. Loading dose
    d. Peak dose

39. A time-response curve evaluates parameters of a drug's action. Which parameter(s) is/are part of the time-response curve? *(Select all that apply.)*
    a. Duration of action
    b. Onset of action
    c. Peak action
    d. Therapeutic range
    e. Minimum effective concentration

40. Which intervention(s) regarding drug therapy should the nurse implement? *(Select all that apply.)*
    a. Assess for side effects, with a focus on undesirable side effects.
    b. Check reference books or drug inserts before administering the medication.
    c. Teach the patient to wait 1 week after the appearance of side effects to see if they disappear.
    d. Check the patient's serum therapeutic range of drugs that have a narrow therapeutic range.
    e. Evaluate peak and trough levels before administering drugs with a narrow therapeutic range.

CASE STUDY

Read the scenario, and answer the following questions on a separate sheet of paper.

M.E. has been prescribed verapamil for angina. The nurse knows that this drug is part of the ligand-gated ion channel receptor family.

1. Explain the receptor theory and the four receptor families. What class of drug is verapamil, and how does it work?

2. What key teaching points will the nurse provide to M.E. regarding this drug?

3 Cultural Considerations

Match the term in Column I with its definition in Column II.

Column I

_____ 1. Assimilation

_____ 2. Complementary health therapies

_____ 3. Pharmacogenetics

_____ 4. Ethnopharmacology

_____ 5. Culture

_____ 6. Alternative health therapies

_____ 7. Ethnomedicine

Column II

a. Ways different cultures conceptualize health and illness
b. Learned beliefs shared by a group of people
c. Occurs when a less powerful group changes its ways and practices to blend with the dominant group
d. Study of drug responses unique to an individual as a result of social, cultural, and biologic phenomena
e. Combines traditional beliefs with mainstream practices
f. The effect of a drug varies from the predicted response because of genetic factors
g. The use of new therapies in place of mainstream therapies to treat an illness

Complete the following.

8. Verbal and nonverbal _____ helps nurses provide culturally competent care.

9. Traditional healers may perform rituals to seek _____ and _____ in health practices.

10. Polymorphisms are _____ _____ that occur within a specific _____.

NCLEX REVIEW QUESTIONS

Select the best response.

11. Which statement reflects the physiologic response of individuals of African descent to a drug?
    a. They are less responsive to beta blockers than are individuals of European descent and Hispanics.
    b. They are more responsive to beta blockers than are individuals of European descent and Hispanics.
    c. They experience fewer toxic side effects with psychotropic drugs than do individuals of European descent.
    d. They experience fewer toxic side effects with antidepressant drugs than do individuals of European descent.

12. Which ethnic or cultural group may experience decreased effects from codeine?
    a. African descent
    b. Latin American descent
    c. Asian descent
    d. Native American descent

13. What communication style is characteristic of people of European descent?
    a. Comfortable with periods of silence
    b. Maintenance of eye contact
    c. Use of a soft voice
    d. Use of few words

14. The patient, who is Jamaican, is currently 4 months pregnant and informs the nurse during a prenatal visit that she eats red clay to provide nutrients to the fetus. She states that this is a practice her grandmother told her would ensure a healthy pregnancy. What is the best action by the nurse?
    a. Contact Child Protective Services.
    b. Insist that the patient stop the practice immediately.
    c. Determine the amount of clay she eats daily.
    d. Discuss the research about dietary intake of clay.

15. The older adult patient is newly diagnosed with diabetes and has been prescribed metformin. The patient's healer has recommended that the patient drink sabila tea three times per day to improve nutrition and help control blood sugar level. What is the nurse's best action?
    a. Encourage the patient to drink the tea four times per day instead.
    b. Discourage the practice because sabila tea potentiates metformin.
    c. Tell the patient to stop the tea immediately.
    d. Advise the patient he can continue to drink the tea, but he also needs to continue his drugs.

16. Which factor(s) may affect a patient's physiologic responses to drugs? *(Select all that apply.)*
    a. Age
    b. Diet
    c. Language
    d. Genetics
    e. Values

17. Which factor(s) may affect a patient's adherence to drug regimens? *(Select all that apply.)*
    a. Access to health care
    b. Heredity
    c. Poverty
    d. Trust in provider
    e. Use of same language

CASE STUDY

Read the scenario, and answer the following questions on a separate sheet of paper.

A Chinese couple brings their 4-year-old, 19-kg daughter to the emergency department (ED). She was seen in the same ED 2 days earlier and was diagnosed with a pulmonary infection. During her previous visit, she was prescribed erythromycin 200 mg, 1 teaspoon every 6 hours for 10 days. The parents are concerned that their daughter is not well yet. They bring the bottle of liquid erythromycin with them in a plastic bag, along with a porcelain soup spoon that is the size of a tablespoon. The bottle is almost half empty.

1. What is the nurse's first concern?

2. How will the nurse approach the family and child to provide culturally competent care?

4 Complementary and Alternative Therapies

STUDY QUESTIONS

Match the description in Column I with the letter of the reference in Column II.

Column I

_____ 1. Therapeutic value of plants

_____ 2. Clarified marketing regulations for dietary supplements

_____ 3. Assures manufacturing quality controls

_____ 4. Reviews global literature on herbal studies by clinicians and researchers

_____ 5. Supports study of alternative therapies

Column II

a. Current Good Manufacturing Practices

b. Dietary Supplement Health and Education Act of 1994

c. National Center for Complementary and Integrative Health

d. Natural Standard Research Collaboration

e. Phytomedicine

Complete the following.

6. Pouring boiling water over _____ is called _____.

7. A(n) _____ is derived from soaking fresh or dried herbs in a solvent.

8. _____ of a plant added to a solvent and applied topically is called a(n) _____.

9. Tea made from boiling plants, such as bark, rhizomes, and roots, is called a(n)_____.

10. Aromatic _____ oils from plants are called _____ _____ _____.

Match the herb in Column I with the letter of its description in Column II. Some herbs may have more than one description.

Column I

_____ 11. *Ginkgo biloba*

_____ 12. Peppermint oil

_____ 13. Dong quai

_____ 14. Garlic

_____ 15. Cinnamon

_____ 16. Chamomile

_____ 17. Hawthorn

_____ 18. Echinacea

_____ 19. Ginger

_____ 20. St. John's wort

Column II

a. May be used to treat bronchitis and diabetes

b. May be used to treat kidney disease

c. Immune enhancer

d. May be helpful in intermittent claudication and Alzheimer's disease

e. Relief from stiffness and pain of osteoarthritis and rheumatoid arthritis

f. May be used to induce sleep

g. May be effective treatment for tension headache

h. May interfere with anticoagulants

i. "Herbal Prozac"

j. May help lower cholesterol and prevent stomach cancer

9

Select the best response.

21. The patient presents to the clinic with complaints of abdominal discomfort and nausea. When obtaining the health history, the nurse inquires about herbal preparations. Which herb would the nurse recognize as one that provides relief of digestive and gastrointestinal distress?
    a. Chamomile
    b. Milk thistle
    c. *Echinacea*
    d. St. John's wort

22. The nurse is assisting a patient with Alzheimer's disease. The daughter asks about a complementary therapy that can improve memory. The nurse provides information knowing that _____ has been used in patients with Alzheimer"s disease.
    a. *echinacea*
    b. ginger
    c. *Ginkgo biloba*
    d. peppermint

23. The patient has just started taking warfarin for atrial fibrillation. Health teaching for this patient would include information on which herbal product(s)? *(Select all that apply.)*
    a. Bilberry
    b. Garlic
    c. Ginseng
    d. Licorice
    e. Turmeric

24. A patient with a recent diagnosis of deep vein thrombosis was prescribed an anticoagulant. The nurse noticed the patient has been taking ginseng. Which of the following would be appropriate interventions by the nurse? *(Select all that apply.)*
    a. Discuss with the patient the potential interactions of ginseng with anticoagulants.
    b. Tell the patient to stop taking the anticoagulant.
    c. Advise the patient to continue taking the same brand of herbal therapy.
    d. Advise the patient to report signs and symptoms of bleeding.
    e. Discuss with the patient foods to avoid.

25. Which statement(s) by the patient reflect(s) prudent use of herbs? *(Select all that apply.)*
    a. "Herbs are fine to use when breastfeeding."
    b. "Do not take a large quantity of any one herbal product."
    c. "Give the herb time to work for a persistent symptom before seeking care from a health care provider."
    d. "Do not give herbs to infants or young children."
    e. "Brands of herbal products are interchangeable."

26. The nurse is caring for a patient who takes a variety of herbal products and is starting a prescription antidiabetic drug. Which herb(s) will change the effect of the antidiabetic drug? *(Select all that apply.)*
    a. *Astragalus*
    b. *Echinacea*
    c. Ginseng
    d. Milk thistle
    e. Peppermint

27. The patient tells the nurse he is taking St. John's wort. Which drug(s) has/have negative interactions with St. John's wort? *(Select all that apply.)*
    a. Anticoagulants
    b. Anticonvulsants
    c. Antidepressants
    d. Birth control drugs
    e. Paralytic drugs

28. The patient has a history of hypertension, atrial fibrillation, chronic obstructive pulmonary disease, and insomnia. She tells the nurse at discharge, "I really love the taste of licorice. It motivates me to walk every day." What drug-herb interactions are seen when given in combination with licorice? *(Select all that apply.)*
    a. Antihypertensive drug effects are decreased.
    b. Corticosteroid effects are increased.
    c. CNS depressant drug effects are decreased.
    d. Digoxin effects are increased.
    e. Rifampin effects are decreased.

CASE STUDY

Read the scenario, and answer the following questions on a separate sheet of paper.

K.E., 21 years old, has a history of nausea and vomiting and severe migraine headaches. She has started missing classes and tells the nurse, "I really can't stand feeling terrible all the time." K.E. tells the nurse she has started trying "a bunch" of herbal remedies to attempt to get her symptoms under control. She does not know the names of any of them. She has presented to the student health clinic with a headache.

1. Which drugs would the nurse suspect this patient is taking for these symptoms, and what is their presumed mechanism of action?

2. With which drugs do these herbals interact?

3. What health teaching will the nurse provide for K.E. regarding the use of herbal preparations?

5 Pediatric Considerations

Complete the following.

1. Infants have _____ protein sites than adults, resulting in _____ risk of toxicity.

2. The degree and rate of absorption of drugs in a pediatric patient are based on _____,
    _____, _____, and _____.

3. Gastric pH does not reach adult acidity until between _____ and _____ year(s) of age.

4. Distribution of a drug throughout the body is affected by _____,
    _____, _____, and effectiveness of various barriers to drug transport.

5. Until about the age of _____, the pediatric patient requires a(n) _____ dose of water-soluble drugs to achieve therapeutic levels.

Match the child's age group in Column I with a cognitive element to consider when administering drugs in Column II.

Column I

_____ 6.   Infant

_____ 7.   Toddler

_____ 8.   Preschool

_____ 9.   School-age

_____ 10. Adolescent

Column II

a. Allow some choice
b. Involve in administration process
c. Collaborate regarding plan of care
d. Provide simple explanation
e. Use minimum restraint necessary

NCLEX REVIEW QUESTIONS

Select the best response.

11. The nurse is administering an oral drug with a low pH to the 2-week-old infant. What is the impact of the patient's age on the absorption of this drug? (*Select all that apply.*)
    a. Absorption may be slower in this patient.
    b. Absorption may be quicker in this patient.
    c. This drug will be absorbed at the same rate as an older patient.
    d. Oral drugs should not be administered to this age group.

12. The 18-month-old child has been prescribed an oral drug that is water-soluble. Based on the nurse's knowledge of drug distribution, how may the dosage need to be modified for the patient in order to reach therapeutic levels?
    a. Alternate route
    b. Decreased
    c. Increased
    d. No change

13. The blood-brain barrier in infants is immature. Which outcome is more likely in infants?
    a. Increased effect of drug
    b. More side effects from drug
    c. Quicker results of drug
    d. Higher toxicity risk

14. The 3-year-old patient requires a topical drug. What does the nurse know about the rate of absorption for topical drugs in this age group?
    a. The drug will absorb faster.
    b. The drug will absorb slower.
    c. There will be no difference.
    d. It depends on the sex of the child.

15. What are the components of pharmacokinetics? *(Select all that apply.)*
    a. Absorption
    b. Distribution
    c. Excretion
    d. Metabolism
    e. Onset

16. The 12-year-old patient has been admitted for nausea, vomiting, and diarrhea, and the health care provider has prescribed several drugs. What concern(s) will the nurse have regarding drug administration? *(Select all that apply.)*
    a. Renal tubular function is decreased.
    b. Dehydration may lead to toxicity.
    c. The drugs should not be administered by the oral route.
    d. Rectal administration will promote quick absorption.
    e. Developmental levels must be considered.

17. The nurse is teaching a group of parents how to administer drugs to their children. Which element(s) of drug administration will be included in the teaching? *(Select all that apply.)*
    a. Allow the child to determine the time of drug administration.
    b. Lightly restrain the child as needed.
    c. Praise the child after successful administration.
    d. Never threaten the child into taking the drug.
    e. Never tell the child what to expect; just give the drug.
    f. Herbal preparations should not, in general, be given to children.

CASE STUDY

Read the scenario, and answer the following questions on a separate sheet of paper.

A.M., 4 years old, fell from a tree branch and fractured her forearm. An IV needs to be established and analgesia administered.

1. What strategies may the nurse implement to provide developmentally appropriate care for this patient?

2. Discuss the utilization of topical anesthetics before inserting an IV.

3. How may the caregiver be involved in the patient's care while the IV is established?

6 Geriatric Considerations

Complete the following.

1. Age-related factors among older adults influence drug _____, _____, _____, and excretion.

2. Drugs for older adults are prescribed at _____ dosages and _____ increase in dosage based on therapeutic _____.

3. Some of the characteristics in older adults that increase the risk for problems related to drugs include _____ and _____ changes associated with _____.

4. Pharmacodynamic responses to drugs are altered with aging as a result of changes in the number of _____ sites, which affects the _____ of certain drugs.

5. Identify at least five drugs that nurses should avoid administering to older adults with stage 4 or 5 chronic kidney disease.

Match the physiologic changes in Column II with the pharmacokinetic responses in Column I.

Column I

6. Absorption

7. Distribution

8. Metabolism

9. Excretion

Column II

a. Altered by the decline in renal function
b. Altered by a decline in muscle mass and an increase in fat
c. Altered by decreased small-bowel surface area, decreased gastric emptying, and reduced gastric blood flow
d. Altered by the decline in hepatic circulation, liver atrophy, and a reduction in hepatic enzyme activity

Identify the drug class for each group of drugs.

_____ 10. Lisinopril, benazepril, enalapril, quinapril

_____ 11. Acebutolol, atenolol, sotolol

_____ 12. Lithium, gabapentin, duloxetine, bupropion, venlafaxine, pregabalin

_____ 13. Irbesartan, losartan, valsartan

13

Answer the following questions as true or false.

_____ 14. Risk factors associated with polypharmacy do not include advanced age.

_____ 15. Risk factors associated with polypharmacy include being female.

_____ 16. Risk factors associated with polypharmacy include having more than one health care provider.

_____ 17. Risk factors associated with polypharmacy do not include the use of OTC drugs.

_____ 18. Risk factors associated with polypharmacy include having no less than six chronic diseases.

_____ 19. Risk factors associated with polypharmacy include the use of vitamin and mineral supplements.

_____ 20. Polypharmacy increases the risk of falls among older adults.

NCLEX REVIEW QUESTIONS

Select the best response.

21. What is an indicator of the glomerular filtration rate and the normal value for an adult?
    a. Creatinine clearance: 100–125 mL/min
    b. SGOT: 4–12 mL/min
    c. Troponin: 80–120 mL/min
    d. Urea: 1.2–4.5

22. The safest antihypertensive agents for older adults have a low incidence of what side effect?
    a. Constipation
    b. Electrolyte imbalance
    c. Loss of appetite
    d. Vision disturbances

23. The older adult patient presents to the provider's office for a follow-up visit and also with complaints of sneezing, runny nose, headache, and scratchy eyes after working out in the garden. The patient states he takes digoxin, fluoxetine, and a multivitamin regularly and has started taking diphenhydramine for the current symptoms. What statement by the patient indicates that further teaching is needed?
    a. "I cannot work outside anymore because of the digoxin."
    b. "I think I need to find a different allergy drug to take."
    c. "I take fluoxetine because I have depression."
    d. "I should not take my wife's headache drug."

24. Which drug would have fewer adverse and toxic effects?
    a. Fat-soluble, half-life of 50 hours
    b. Fat-soluble, 90% protein bound
    c. Half-life of 4 hours, 50% protein bound
    d. Fat-soluble, 60% protein bound

25. Which specific lab value(s) should be monitored in a geriatric patient to assess kidney function? _(Select all that apply.)_
    a. BUN
    b. Creatinine clearance
    c. CBC
    d. Lipase
    e. Triglycerides

26. The patient, who is 75 years old, reports feeling dizzy every morning when he gets outs of bed. What effect does the nurse recognize the patient is probably experiencing?
    a. Bradycardia
    b. Intermittent claudication
    c. Hyperventilation
    d. Orthostatic hypotension

27. What changes will the nurse recommend to a patient who experiences dizziness when arising from bed?
    a. Change positions slowly.
    b. Move a chair close to the bed.
    c. Take deep breaths.
    d. Take his pulse before standing.

28. Following hospitalization, the older adult patient receives a home visit from the nurse. The patient asks if she should continue to take the drugs she took before hospitalization. What is the most appropriate response?
    a. "Yes, you should continue to take the drugs that you took before going to the hospital."
    b. "You should take one-half the dosage of each drug that you took prior to hospitalization."
    c. "You should take only the drugs that have been prescribed on discharge and not drugs that you took prior to hospitalization unless otherwise indicated."
    d. "You should continue to take those drugs that have been helpful to you."

14

29. The older adult patient states he has difficulties opening his bottle of celecoxib. What is the nurse's best response?
   a. "Please ask your pharmacist to place your drug in a bottle with a non-childproof cap."
   b. "You can keep your drug in a glass cup in the medicine cabinet."
   c. "You could place your drug in an envelope."
   d. "A family member could help you with your daily drug regimen."

30. An older adult patient is to take newly prescribed drugs at different times. What will the nurse suggest so that the patient can comply with the drug regimen?
   a. "Line up the bottles of medications on a table and take them in that order."
   b. "Obtain a weekly pill container with multiple time slots from the drugstore and fill the container the day or week before with the drugs."
   c. "Ask a neighbor to give the daily drugs."
   d. "Write down the drugs that you have taken each day."

31. In older adults, drug dosages are adjusted based on which factor(s)? (Select all that apply.)
   a. Amount of adipose tissue
   b. Height
   c. Nutritional status
   d. Laboratory results
   e. Response to drug

32. Before administering drugs to the older adult, what should the nurse know? (Select all that apply.)
   a. Whether the drug is highly protein bound
   b. Half-life of the drug
   c. Patient's last bowel movement
   d. Serum levels of drugs with a narrow therapeutic range
   e. Baseline vital signs

CASE STUDY

Read the scenario and answer the following questions on a separate sheet of paper.

M.Z., 80 years old, presents to her health care provider for her annual checkup. She has a medical history of diabetes, insomnia, and hypertension. Vital signs are temperature 37.2° C, heart rate 83 beats/minute, respiratory rate 16 breaths/minute, blood pressure 142/90 mm Hg, and blood glucose 96 mg/dL. During the health history, M.Z. complains of having trouble falling asleep and staying asleep, and having to get up several times per night to go to the bathroom. M.Z. says her current drugs include hydrochlorothiazide, triazolam, and chamomile tea. "I try to remember to take my drugs, and sometimes I take an extra one, just in case I forgot one," she says.

1. What laboratory tests would the nurse anticipate for this patient?

2. What suggestions can the nurse make to help with M.Z.'s sleeping difficulties?

3. What further teaching will the nurse provide to the patient about her drug regimen?

7 Drugs for Substance Use Disorder

Match the therapy in Column I to its description in Column II.

Column I

_____ 1. Cognitive behavioral therapy

_____ 2. Motivational enhancement therapy

_____ 3. Contingency management

Column II

a. Based on frequent behavior monitoring and removal of rewards for substance use

b. Recognize and stop negative patterns and enhance self-control

c. Develop motivation internally to commit to specific plan

Complete the following.

4. Misused drugs typically increase _____ and other _____ in the limbic system of the brain.

5. The _____ _____ is a structure within the brain that regulates the body's ability to feel pleasure.

6. The study of environmental influences on genetics is called _____.

7. Disulfiram _____ the enzyme involved in metabolizing alcohol.

8. Heroin addiction may be treated with _____.

9. Benzodiazepines are FDA approved to treat addiction to _____.

10. Opioids provide a sense of _____ and _____; methadone _____ these feelings.

11. _____ questionnaire can be used to screen for alcohol misuse.

12. Substance use disorder among nurses can be recognized by changes in _____, _____, _____, and _____.

Answer the following questions as true or false.

If the statement is false, reword the sentence to make it true.

_____ 13. Electronic cigarettes are safer than tobacco products.

_____

_____ 14. Dehydroepiandrosterone (DHEA) is found in many dietary supplements and is approved to slow aging.

_____

_____ 15. Discrepancies in controlled-drug handling and records among health care professionals may indicate drug diversion.

_____

17

Match the term in Column I with the definition in Column II.

Column I

_____ 16. Craving

_____ 17. Impaired control

_____ 18. Tolerance

_____ 19. Withdrawal syndrome

Column II

a. Diminished ability to control the use of a drug in terms of onset, level, or termination

b. A strong desire for the drug effects

c. A group of signs and symptoms of physiologic disturbance upon cessation or reduction of a drug

d. Requiring a significantly increased amount of a drug to achieve the desired effect

NCLEX REVIEW QUESTIONS

Select the best response.

20. The patient presents to the emergency department (ED) under the custody of local law enforcement. The patient reportedly swallowed a small balloon full of cocaine. What clinical manifestations would the nurse expect to see if the balloon ruptured?
    a. Dilated pupils and restlessness
    b. Hypotension and tachycardia
    c. Insomnia and fine tremors
    d. Respiratory depression and pinpoint pupils

21. Which drug can be given to aid a patient with opioid withdrawal?
    a. Disulfiram
    b. Lorazepam
    c. Methadone
    d. Naloxone

22. The patient has decided to quit smoking. What key point(s) must the nurse include in the teaching plan? *(Select all that apply.)*
    a. Assess that the patient is motivated to quit.
    b. Set a quit date of 1 month.
    c. Help the patient identify the cultural context that increases the desire to smoke.
    d. Advise the patient he may use chewing tobacco as a substitute.
    e. Provide the patient with a list of over-the-counter and prescription options for smoking cessation aids.
    f. Advise that the patient must use an aid to quit.

23. What percentage of nurses abuse drugs and demonstrate impaired practice attributable to that abuse?
    a. 1–2%
    b. 3–6%
    c. 7–10%
    d. 10–15%

24. A mother brings her 13-year-old daughter to the ED because she is "acting strange." The mother states she found a package of "bath salts" in her daughter's bedroom. "Bath salts" are classified as which type of drug?
    a. Amphetamine
    b. Benzodiazepine
    c. Hallucinogenic
    d. Synthetic cathinone

CASE STUDY

Read the scenario and answer the following questions on a separate sheet of paper.

C.L., 57 years old, presents to the ED. He is unresponsive to verbal and painful stimuli and smells strongly of alcohol. Vital signs include temperature of 96.8° F, heart rate of 104 beats/minute, respiratory rate of 6 breaths/minute, blood pressure of 90/68 mm Hg, and oxygen saturation of 88% on room air.

1. What is the initial treatment for C.L.?

2. What are the potential complications for alcohol toxicity?

3. Describe the pharmacokinetics for disulfiram and the side effects if taken with any alcohol.

4. Identify the drug–drug interactions that can occur when taken concomitantly with disulfiram.

8 The Nursing Process and Patient-Centered Care

Complete the following.

1. The Quality Safety Education for Nurses (QSEN) guides nurses in the practice of _____, _____ care.

2. _____-_____ practice integrates best current evidence with clinical expertise and patient preferences.

3. _____ assist in communication, knowledge management, mitigating errors, and supporting decision making.

4. Patient- and _____-_____ care recognizes the patient as the source of control and full partner.

5. Collaboration and teamwork function effectively to achieve _____ patient care.

Arrange the following actions of the nursing process in correct order.

6. a. Implementation
   b. Planning
   c. Evaluation
   d. Assessment
   e. Nursing diagnosis

Match the step of the nursing process in Column II with the phrases in Column I. The nursing process in Column II will be used more than once.

Column I

_____ 7. Nonadherence related to forgetfulness

_____ 8. Current health history

_____ 9. Goal setting

_____ 10. Patient's environment

_____ 11. Action to accomplish goals

_____ 12. Drug allergies and reactions

_____ 13. Referral

_____ 14. Patient/significant other education

_____ 15. Use of teaching drug cards

_____ 16. Laboratory test results

_____ 17. Effectiveness of health teaching and drug therapy

Column II

a. Assessment
b. Nursing diagnosis
c. Planning
d. Implementation/intervention
e. Evaluation

Match the clinical manifestations in Column I with the data type in Column II. The data type in Column II will be used more than once.

Column I

_____ 18. Productive cough

_____ 19. Pain in left ear

_____ 20. Lab values

_____ 21. Nausea

_____ 22. Heart rate

_____ 23. Patient perception of drug's effectiveness

_____ 24. Reported allergies

Column II

a. Subjective
b. Objective

NCLEX REVIEW QUESTIONS

Select the best response.

25. *Risk for injury* would be included in which phase of the nursing process for a patient who is taking a sedative-hypnotic?
    a. Assessment
    b. Implementation
    c. Planning
    d. Nursing diagnosis

26. The patient has congestive heart failure and has been prescribed a diuretic. *Obtain patient's weight to be used for future comparison* is included in which phase of the nursing process?
    a. Assessment
    b. Evaluation
    c. Planning
    d. Nursing diagnosis

27. *The patient will receive adequate nutritional support through enteral feedings* is included in which phase of the nursing process?
    a. Assessment
    b. Implementation
    c. Planning
    d. Nursing diagnosis

28. *The patient will be free from hyperactivity* is included in which phase of the nursing process?
    a. Assessment
    b. Evaluation
    c. Planning
    d. Nursing diagnosis

29. The patient has been diagnosed with angina and hypertension and has been started on a drug. *Instruct patient to avoid caffeine-containing beverages* is included in which phase of the nursing process?
    a. Evaluation
    b. Implementation
    c. Nursing diagnosis
    d. Planning

30. Revision of goals is included in which phase of the nursing process?
    a. Assessment
    b. Evaluation
    c. Implementation
    d. Planning

31. The patient has been prescribed a diuretic to treat hypertension. *Sleep pattern disturbance* is included in which phase of the nursing process?
    a. Assessment
    b. Evaluation
    c. Implementation
    d. Nursing diagnosis

32. The pediatric patient has been started on antibiotics for strep throat. *Advise the child's parents to report adverse reactions such as nausea and vomiting to the health care provider* is included in which phase of the nursing process?
    a. Assessment
    b. Implementation
    c. Planning
    d. Potential nursing diagnosis

33. The patient has been prescribed an opioid pain drug after hip surgery. *Acute confusion* is included in which phase of the nursing process?
   a. Implementation
   b. Evaluation
   c. Nursing diagnosis
   d. Planning

34. *Instruct patient not to discontinue drugs abruptly* is included in which part of the nursing process for a patient with epilepsy who is taking phenytoin?
   a. Assessment
   b. Evaluation
   c. Implementation
   d. Planning

Read the scenario, and answer the following question on a separate sheet of paper.

O.Y., 53 years old, has been diagnosed with diabetes and has been prescribed insulin. In speaking to the nurse, O.Y. says, "I don't think I can give myself shots. I can't stick myself with a needle."

1. Utilizing the nursing process, how will the nurse develop a teaching plan for O.Y.?

2. How will the nurse determine the effectiveness of the teaching plan?

9 Safety and Quality

Match the statement in Column I with the nursing implication of drug administration in Column II.

Column I

_____ 1. Right route

_____ 2. Right patient

_____ 3. Right time

_____ 4. Right documentation

_____ 5. Right assessment

_____ 6. Right drug

_____ 7. Right dose

_____ 8. Right education

_____ 9. Right to refuse

_____ 10. Right to evaluation

Column II

a. Measurement of a patient's apical pulse
b. Amount of drug given as prescribed
c. Drug given IM as prescribed
d. Teaching a patient about possible side effects of the drug
e. The patient refuses to take drug
f. Verification of patient ID
g. Nurse charts that patient pain was decreased after drug administration
h. Patient receives the prescribed drug
i. Nurse checks blood pressure following blood pressure drug administration
j. Drug given at the time prescribed

Match the instructions in Column II with the situation in Column I.

Column I

_____ 11. Drugs poured by others

_____ 12. Patient states that drug is different than usual

_____ 13. Bad-tasting drugs first, then pleasant-tasting drugs

_____ 14. Drugs transferred from a labeled container to an unlabeled container

_____ 15. Drugs with date and time opened and your initials on label

_____ 16. Drugs left with visitors

Column II

a. Do not administer
b. Do administer

17. Provide the meaning of each abbreviation, and determine if it is acceptable to use.
   a. ID
   b. MS
   c. q.o.d.
   d. gtt
   e. kg
   f. 1.0 mg
   g. mg
   h. qd
   i. KVO
   j. IVPB
   k. $\bar{c}$
   l. $\bar{a}$
   m. bid

18. Provide the meaning of the following abbreviations on the drug type.

Abbreviation	Meaning
CR	
ER	
IM	
XR	
XT	

NCLEX REVIEW QUESTIONS

Select the best response.

19. The patient has been prescribed antibiotics that are scheduled for every 8 hours. What statement by the patient indicates the need for more teaching regarding the drug regimen?
    a. "I take this drug every 8 hours around the clock."
    b. "I have to take the drug even if I feel better."
    c. "I just take it divided into three doses while I'm awake."
    d. "I cannot take it more often even if I don't feel better."

20. The patient has been prescribed a drug to be taken a.c. and h.s. What instructions should the nurse give the patient?
    a. "Take this drug every 6 hours."
    b. "Take this drug before meals and at bedtime."
    c. "Take this drug after meals and first thing in the morning."
    d. "Take this drug after meals and as needed."

21. What is the purpose of the "tall man" letters?
    a. To assist with drug reconciliation
    b. To aid in labeling drug allergies
    c. To promote safety between drugs with similar names
    d. To label differences in dosage strength of the same drug

22. The nurse is calculating an opioid dose for the patient. The dose seems "large." What is the best initial action for the nurse to take?
    a. Check the patient's name band and administer the drug.
    b. Call the health care provider.
    c. Recalculate the dose.
    d. Withhold the drug and document as not given.

23. The nurse working in a clinic will be administering flu shots from a multidose vial. What is/are the correct piece(s) of information that the nurse must use to label the bottle? *(Select all that apply.)*
    a. Nurse's full name
    b. Date vial opened
    c. Prescribing provider
    d. Time vial opened
    e. Expiration date

24. The older adult patient tells the nurse, "I'm not taking that pill. I don't want it, and I won't take it!" What is the nurse's first action?
    a. Document the patient's refusal.
    b. Force the patient to take the drug.
    c. Educate the patient on the importance of the drug.
    d. Call the health care provider.

25. What abbreviation(s) is/are not allowed by The Joint Commission? *(Select all that apply.)*
    a. IM
    b. U
    c. IU
    d. q.d.
    e. MS

26. The "right to education" includes which action(s)? *(Select all that apply.)*
    a. Drug trial information collected before administration of the drug
    b. Education about the drug and why it has been prescribed
    c. Evaluation of the patient's response
    d. Laboratory monitoring of baseline values
    e. Possible side effects

Read the scenario, and answer the following question on a separate sheet of paper.

A nurse is preparing to administer three of RL's morning drugs. The nurse tells the patient the drugs are for his blood pressure, diabetes, and depression. When the patient looked at the drugs, he exclaims "these are not the pills I take."

1. What are the "five rights" in drug administration?

2. What methods can the nurse use to determine the "right patient" is receiving the drugs?

10 Drug Administration

Complete the following.

1. _____ and _____ capsules must be swallowed whole.

2. Handheld nebulizers deliver a very _____ _____ in a spray of drug.

3. When giving a patient a drug via a handheld nebulizer, the patient should be placed in _____ position.

4. A nasogastric tube should be flushed with _____ mL of water (or the prescribed amount) following drug administration.

5. Following insertion of a rectal suppository, the patient should remain in a side-lying position for atleast _____ minutes.

Match the route in Column I with the correct length of needle in Column II.

Column I

_____ 6. Subcutaneous (subcut)

_____ 7. Intradermal (ID)

_____ 8. Intramuscular (IM)

Column II

a. $\frac{1}{4}$ to $\frac{1}{2}$ inch in length

b. $\frac{5}{8}$ to $1\frac{1}{2}$ inches in length

c. $\frac{3}{8}$ to $\frac{5}{8}$ inch in length

Complete the following.

9. The injection site that is away from major nerves and is a preferred site for Z-track injections is _____.

10. The preferred site for intramuscular injections for infants and children is _____.

11. The site that is easily accessible but is suitable for only small-volume doses is _____.

12. The preferred site for the Z-track technique is _____.

13. The site that is no longer use because of possible adverse outcome from hitting the sciatic nerve is _____.

14. Label the landmarks for ventrogluteal injection.

27

Select the best response.

15. The patient is vomiting and has been prescribed an antiemetic. Which route does the nurse know is contraindicated for this patient?
    a. Intradermal
    b. Intravenous
    c. Oral
    d. Rectal suppository

16. The 2-year-old patient has been prescribed antibiotic eardrops. The nurse is providing education to the parents. Which is the correct direction in which to pull the auricle?
    a. Down and back
    b. Forward and back
    c. Forward and up
    d. Up and back

17. The patient has been prescribed an intramuscular injection. The drug is thick and must be administered deep IM. Which does the nurse choose for the injection site?
    a. Deltoid
    b. Dorsolateral
    c. Vastus lateralis
    d. Ventrogluteal

18. What is the preferred site for an IM injection for an 8-week-old infant?
    a. Deltoid
    b. Dorsogluteal
    c. Vastus lateralis
    d. Ventrogluteal

19. The patient is being discharged on new drugs. Which statement made by the patient would indicate that more teaching is required?
    a. "I can take any over-the-counter drug or herbal preparation that I think would be helpful."
    b. "I need to make sure I keep appointments with my health care provider."
    c. "I need to report any side effects to my health care provider."
    d. "I will contact my pharmacy if I am going out of town to ensure that I have enough drug."

20. The patient has been started on a new oral drug. What information will the nurse include in the patient teaching? *(Select all that apply.)*
    a. Desired effect of the drug
    b. Dietary considerations
    c. Storage of all drug in the refrigerator
    d. Research testing and development
    e. Written instructions on how to administer the drug

21. The patient has been prescribed a steroid metered-dose inhaler (MDI) for asthma. What statement by the patient indicates understanding of how to use this drug?
    a. "I can use it as often as I need it."
    b. "I need to rinse out my mouth after I use it."
    c. "I should put my mouth tightly over the end."
    d. "I can administer multiple puffs at one time."

CASE STUDY

Read the scenario and answer the following question on a separate sheet of paper.

AJ, 20-year-old male, is prescribed promethazine 12.5 mg intramuscular (IM) for intractable nausea. The nurse prepares to administer the drug.

1. List the supplies needed for IM injection.

2. What are the potential IM injection sites for this patient?

3. What method should the nurse use for this IM injection? Why?

11 Drug Calculations

INTRODUCTION

The Drug Calculations chapter in this Study Guide is subdivided into five sections: (11A) Systems of Measurement With Conversion Factors; (11B) Calculation Methods: Enteral and Parenteral Drug Dosages; (11C) Calculating Dosages: Drugs That Require Reconstitution; (11D) Calculation Methods: Insulin Dosages; and (11E) Calculation Methods: Intravenous Flow Rates.

Numerous drug labels appear in the drug calculation problems. The purpose is to become familiar with reading drug labels and calculating drug dosages from the information provided on the drug labels.

Drug calculation practice problems provide an opportunity gain skill and competence in collecting and organizing the required data. Practice problems have examples of the administration of drugs via a variety of routes, including both oral and parenteral (subcutaneous, intramuscular, and intravenous). Practice problems also include calculating dosages based on body weight and body surface area and intravenous heparin infusions and critical care drugs.

When calculating dosages, select one of the three methods (basic formula, ratio and proportion/fractional equation, or dimensional analysis) presented in the accompanying textbook. After completing the required calculations, determine if the calculated answer is reasonable. In the event of a discrepancy, review both the thought process used in answering the problem and the actual mathematical calculation. It may be necessary to review the related section in Chapter 11 of the textbook. Practice problems provide reinforcement to gain expertise in the process of actually calculating drug dosages.

For all calculations, round to the nearest *tenth* for the following: milliliters, milligrams, and units; round to the nearest *whole number* for kilograms, pounds, and drops; round to the nearest hundredths for body surface areas (m²); and round to the nearest *minute* for time.

The answers are located in the back of the Study Guide. Some of the calculations will be illustrated in the Answer Key using dimensional analysis.

SECTION 11A—SYSTEMS OF MEASUREMENT WITH CONVERSION FACTORS

Metric and Household Systems

Match the term in Column I with the appropriate abbreviation in Column II.

Column I

_____ 1. Gram

_____ 2. Milligram

_____ 3. Liter

_____ 4. Milliliter

_____ 5. Kilogram

_____ 6. Microgram

_____ 7. Meter

_____ 8. Fluid ounce

_____ 9. Quart

_____ 10. Pint

_____ 11. Pound

_____ 12. Cup

_____ 13. Tablespoon

_____ 14. Teaspoon

_____ 15. Drops

Column II

a. T or tbsp
b. g
c. mL
d. lb
e. fl oz
f. mg
g. L or l
h. gtt
i. kg
j. mcg
k. t or tsp
l. c
m. pt
n. qt
o. m

Complete the following.

16. The most frequently used conversions within the metric system are:

    A. 1 g = _____ mg

    B. 1 L = _____ mL

    C. 1 mg = _____ mcg

Complete the unit equivalent for the following measurements.

17. 3 grams = _____ milligrams

18. 1.5 liters = _____ milliliters

19. 0.1 gram = _____ milligrams

20. 2500 milliliters = _____ liters

21. 250 milliliters = _____ liter

22. 500 milligrams = _____ gram

23. 2 quarts = _____ pints

24. 2 pints = _____ fluid ounces

25. 1½ quarts = _____ fluid ounces

26. 32 fluid ounces = _____ pints

27. 3000 micrograms = _____ milligrams

28. 3 teaspoons = _____ milliliters

29. 30 milliliters = _____ fluid ounce

30. 1 tablespoon = _____ teaspoon

Metric and Household Systems

Convert the following units of measurement to metric and household equivalents. Refer to Tables 11A.1 and 11A.2 in the textbook as needed.

31. 1 g = _____ mg

32. _____ g = 500 mg

33. 0.1 g = _____ mg

34. _____ L = 1000 mL, or _____ qt

35. 240 mL = _____ fl oz

36. 30 mL = _____ fl oz, or _____ T, or _____ t

37. 5 mL = _____ t

38. 3 T = _____ fl oz, or _____ t

39. 5 fl oz = _____ mL, or _____ T

Select the best response.

1. Before calculating drug dosages, all units of measurement must be converted to one system. Which system should the nurse use?
   a. Any system the nurse prefers
   b. A system that fits with how the nurse will administer the drug
   c. A system that is easy to convert to
   d. The system on the drug label

2. What are the methods for administering drugs by parenteral routes? *(Select all that apply.)*
   a. Via a nasogastric tube
   b. Subcutaneous
   c. Intramuscular
   d. Intradermal
   e. Intravenous
   f. Any liquid drug via all routes

3. What are the routes of administration for insulin and heparin? *(Select all that apply.)*
   a. Oral
   b. Intramuscular
   c. Subcutaneous
   d. Intravenous
   e. Intradermal

4. Vials are glass containers with (self-sealing rubber tops/tapered glass necks). Vials are usually (discarded/reusable if properly stored). *(Circle correct answers.)*

5. Before drug reconstitution, the nurse should check the drug circular and/or drug label for instructions. After a drug has been reconstituted and additional doses are available, what should the nurse write on the drug label? *(Select all that apply.)*
   a. Date to discard
   b. Initials
   c. The health care provider's order
   d. What it is reconstituted with

6. The nurse is preparing an IM injection for an average adult. What needle gauge and length could be used to administer the IM?
   a. 20, 21 gauge; ½, ⅝ inch in length
   b. 23, 25 gauge; ½, ⅝ inch in length
   c. 19, 20, 21 gauge; 1, 1½, 2 inches in length
   d. 25, 26 gauge; 1, 1½ inches in length

7. Which two parts of a syringe must remain sterile?
   a. Outside of syringe and plunger
   b. Tip of the syringe and plunger
   c. Both the tip and outside of the syringe
   d. Tip and outside of syringe and plunger

8. Subcutaneous injections can be administered at which degree angle(s)?
   a. 10-degree and 15-degree angles
   b. 45-degree, 60-degree, and 90-degree angles
   c. 45-degree angle only
   d. 90-degree angle only

9. The nurse calculates the drug dosage to be 0.25 milliliter. What type of syringe should be selected?
   a. 3-mL syringe
   b. Insulin syringe
   c. Tuberculin syringe
   d. 10-mL syringe

10. To mix 4 milliliters of sterile saline solution in a vial containing a powdered drug, which size syringe should be selected?
    a. Tuberculin syringe
    b. Insulin syringe
    c. 3-mL syringe
    d. 5-mL syringe

11. Solutions in drug A and drug B are compatible. To combine 5 milliliters of drug A with 8 milliliters of drug B to be administered via syringe pump, the nurse would use which syringe size(s)?
    a. One 5-mL syringe and one 10-mL syringe
    b. Two 10-mL syringes
    c. One 20-mL syringe
    d. Two 5-mL syringes and one 10-mL syringe

Interpreting Drug Labels

Note: When converting a unit of measurement from one system to another, convert to the unit on the *drug label*.

    Example:

Order: Penicillin V 0.5 g PO q8h

Available:

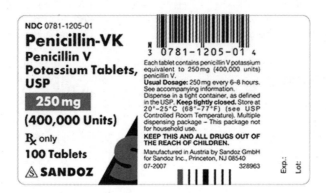

Convert _____ to _____ (unit of measurement to unit of measurement)

Answer: grams to milligrams

12.   Provide the information requested on the following drug label.

    A.   What is the brand name of this drug? _____

    B.   What is the generic name of this drug? _____

    C.   What is the dosage of this drug? _____

    D.   What is the form of this drug? _____

13. Provide the information requested on the following drug label.

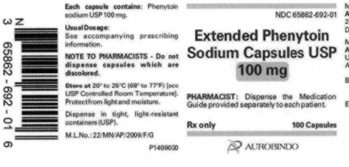

A. What is the name of the drug? _____

B. What is the dosage of this drug? _____

C. Is this drug a controlled substance? _____

D. Circle on the label the marking that indicates it is a controlled substance.

E. What is the form of the drug? _____

F. How should the drug be stored? _____

G. What company manufactured the drug? _____

14. Provide the information requested on the following drug label.

A. What is the generic name of the drug? _____

B. Is the drug a controlled substance? _____

C. What is the form of the drug? _____

D. How much of the drug is in each capsule? _____

E. Circle the marking on the label that indicates whether a prescription is required.

F. How should the drug be stored? _____

15. Provide the information requested on the following drug label.

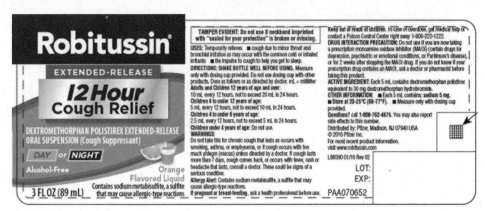

A. What is generic name of the drug? _____

B. What is the trade name? _____

C. Does this drug require a prescription? _____

D. What is the form of the drug? _____

E. What is the concentration of the drug? _____

F. What is the total volume in mL? _____

G. What is the usual dose for adults and children 12 years of age and over? _____

H. How many adult dosages are available? _____

16. Provide the information requested on the following drug label.

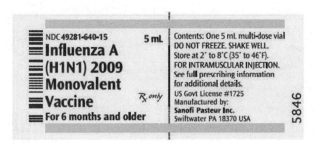

A. What is the name of the drug? _____

B. What is the form of the drug? _____

C. Is the vial a single dose vial or multi-dose vial? _____

D. How should the drug be stored? _____

E. How should this drug be administered? _____

17. Provide the information requested on the following drug label.

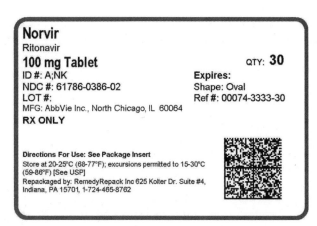

KEEP REFRIGERATED   NDC 42238-111-12

ACTIMMUNE®
(Interferon gamma-1b)

How supplied: Each carton contains 12 single-use vials of Interferon gamma-1b, ACTIMMUNE.

Contents: Each 0.5 mL vial of ACTIMMUNE contains 100 mcg (2 million IU) Interferon gamma-1b formulated in 20 mg mannitol, 0.37 mg disodium succinate hexahydrate, 0.14 mg succinic acid, 0.05 mg polysorbate 20 and Sterile Water for Injection for subcutaneous injection. ACTIMMUNE contains no preservatives.

Dosage and administration: See package insert for full prescribing information. ACTIMMUNE is suitable for single-use only. DO NOT SHAKE.

Storage: Refrigerate at 2° to 8°C/36° to 46°F. DO NOT FREEZE.

A. What is the generic name? _____

B. What is the trade name? _____

C. How should it be stored? _____

Drug Calculations

Use the basic formula, ratio and proportion/fractional equation, or dimensional analysis methods to calculate the following drug problems.

18. Order: ritonavir 0.5 g PO bid
    Available:

Norvir
Ritonavir
100 mg Tablet   QTY: **30**
ID #: A;NK
NDC #: 61786-0386-02   Expires:
LOT #:   Shape: Oval
MFG: AbbVie Inc., North Chicago, IL 60064   Ref #: 00074-3333-30
RX ONLY

Directions For Use: See Package Insert
Store at 20-25°C (68-77°F); excursions permitted to 15-30°C (59-86°F) [See USP]
Repackaged by: RemedyRepack Inc 625 Kolter Dr. Suite #4, Indiana, PA 15701, 1-724-465-8762

A. Is conversion needed to give this medication?
    a. No; it may be administered in grams.
    b. No; the pill may be broken if needed.
    c. Yes; it should be converted to grains.
    d. Yes; it should be converted to milligrams.

B. How much of this medication should the nurse administer?
    a. ½ tablet
    b. 1 tablet
    c. 3 tablets
    d. 5 tablets

19.   Order: diphenhydramine 25 mg PO q6h, PRN
       Available: diphenhydramine 12.5 mg/5 mL

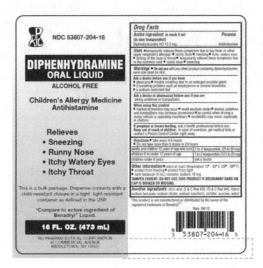

    A.   Is conversion needed to give this drug?
         a. No; it can be administered in milligrams as ordered.
         b. No; you cannot mix mg and mL.
         c. Yes; it should be converted to grains.
         d. Yes; it should be converted to grams.

    B.   How many mL should the nurse give?
         a. 5 mL
         b. 10 mL
         c. 15 mL
         d. 20 mL

20.   Order: clarithromycin 0.25 g PO bid
       Available:

    A.   Is conversion needed to give this medication?
         a. No; it may be administered in grams.
         b. No; you cannot mix mg and mL.
         c. Yes; it should be converted to grains.
         d. Yes; it should be converted to milligrams.

    B.   How many mL should be administered?
         a. 5 mL
         b. 10 mL
         c. 15 mL
         d. 20 mL

21. Order: hydroxyzine 25 mg PO q6h
    Available:

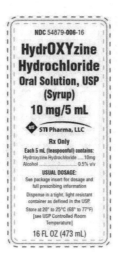

    How many mL should be administered?
    a. 5 mL
    b. 7.5 mL
    c. 10 mL
    d. 12.5 mL

22. Order: ceftriaxone 500 mg IM q8h
    Available:

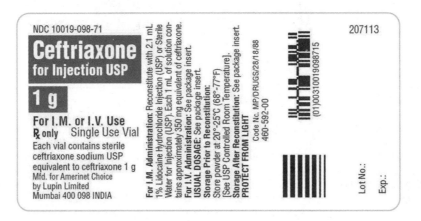

    How many mL should be administered?
    a. 1 mL
    b. 1.4 mL
    c. 2 mL
    d. 2.4 mL

23.   Order: acarbose 50 mg PO tid
       Available:

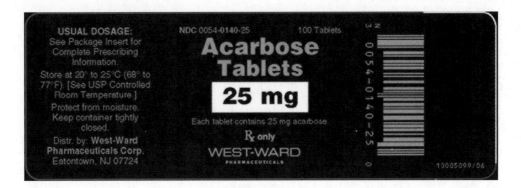

    A.   How many tablets should be administered per dose?
         a. 1 tablet
         b. 2 tablets
         c. 3 tablets
         d. 4 tablets

24.   Order: losartan potassium 100 mg daily
       Available:

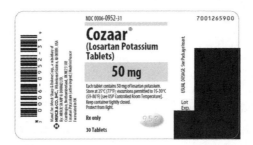

    A.   What is the generic name? _____

    B.   What is the trade name? _____

    C.   How many total tablets are in the container? _____

    D.   How many tablets should the patient receive per day?
         a. 1 tablet
         b. 2 tablets
         c. 3 tablets
         d. 4 tablets

25.   Order: propranolol 15 mg PO q6h
       Available: propranolol 10-mg and 20-mg scored tablets

    A.   Which tablet strength should be administered? Why?
         a. 10-mg tablets
         b. 20-mg tablets

    B.   How many tablets should be administered?
         a. 1 tablet
         b. 1½ tablets
         c. 2 tablets
         d. 2½ tablets

26. Order: furosemide 80 mg PO daily
Available:

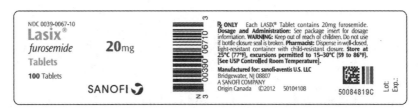

A. What is the generic name? _____

B. What is the trade name? _____

C. How should the medication be stored? _____

D. How many tablets should be administered?
   a. 2 tablets
   b. 3 tablets
   c. 4 tablets
   d. 5 tablets

27. Order: potassium ER 40 mEq PO daily
Available:

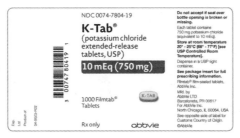
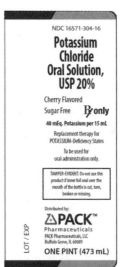

A. Which form should be used? Why?

B. Upon assessment, the nurse discovers the patient has a nasogastric tube (NGT) and is unable to swallow. What should the nurse do?
   a. Give the drug as ordered.
   b. Give the oral liquid.
   c. Call the physician.
   d. Give the drug IV.

C. After calling the physician, the order was changed to 20 mEq via a nasogastric tube bid.

   a. Which form should be used? Why? _____

   b. How many milliliters should the nurse give per dose? _____

Chapter **11** Drug Calculations

28. Order: verapamil 60 mg PO qid
     Available:

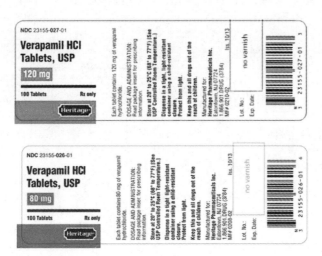

   A. Which strength of verapamil should be selected?
       a. 120-mg tablet
       b. 80-mg tablet

   B. How many tablets should be administered?
       a. ½ tablet
       b. 1 tablet
       c. 1½ tablets
       d. 2 tablets

29. Order: trihexyphenidyl 4 mg/d PO in two divided doses q12h
     Available:

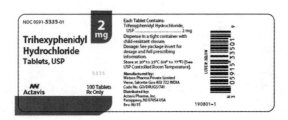

   A. How many tablets per dose? _____

   B. How many tablets per 24 hours? _____

30. Order: oxacillin 400 mg IM daily
    Available:

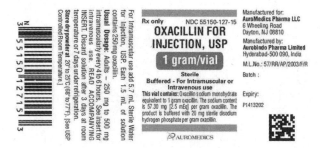

A. How much diluent should be added for an intramuscular injection? _____

B. How many milliliters should the patient receive?
   a. 0.5 mL
   b. 1.5 mL
   c. 2 mL
   d. 2.4 mL

31. Order: adalimumab 40 mg subcut every other week
    Available:

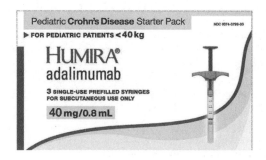

A. What is the route of administration?_____

B. What is the dosage strength? _____

C. How many milliliters should the patient receive? _____

D. What size syringe(s) should be used? *(Select all that apply.)*
   a. Tuberculin
   b. Insulin
   c. 1-mL syringe
   d. 3-mL syringe

32. Order: trazodone 150 mg PO daily
    Available: trazodone in 50-mg tablets and 100-mg tablets

A. How many tablets should be administered if the 50-mg tablet is used?
   a. 1 tablet
   b. 2 tablets
   c. 3 tablets
   d. 4 tablets

B. How many tablets should be administered if the 100-mg tablet is used?
   a. ½ tablet
   b. 1 tablet
   c. 1½ tablets
   d. 2 tablets

33. Order: warfarin 7.5 mg PO daily
    Available:

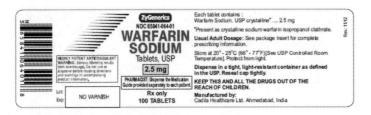

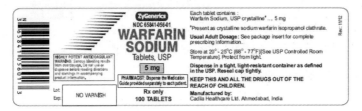

A. Which dosage strength should be selected?
   a. Warfarin 2.5 mg
   b. Warfarin 5 mg

B. How many tablet(s) should be administered? *(Consider all the possible combinations).*

34. Order: lithium carbonate 300 mg PO tid
    Available: lithium carbonate in 150- and 300-mg capsules and 300-mg tablets. The patient's lithium level is 1.8 mEq/L (normal value is 0.5–1.5 mEq/L).

    What is the best action by the nurse?
    a. Give 150 mg (half the dose).
    b. Give 300-mg tablet and not the capsule.
    c. Advise the patient not to take the dose for a week.
    d. Withhold the drug and contact the health care provider.

35. Order: carvedilol 6.25 mg PO bid
    Available:

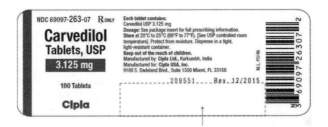

A. How many tablets should be administered per dose?
   a. 1 tablet
   b. 2 tablets
   c. 3 tablets
   d. Call the pharmacy to bring 6.25 tabs

B. How many tablets should the patient receive in 24 hours?
   a. 4 tablets
   b. 6 tablets
   c. 8 tablets
   d. 10 tablets

36. Order: azithromycin 500 mg PO on day 1, then 250 mg PO daily for next 4 days
Available:

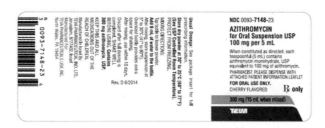

A. How many milliliters should be administered the first day?
   a. 2.5 mL
   b. 6.5 mL
   c. 12.5 mL
   d. 25 mL

B. How many milliliters should be administered per day for the next 4 days?
   a. 5 mL/day
   b. 6.25 mL/day
   c. 10 mL/day
   d. 12.5 mL/day

37. Order: trihexyphenidyl elixir 1 mg PO tid
Available: trihexyphenidyl 2 mg/5 mL

What amount should be administered per dose?
   a. 2 mL
   b. 2.5 mL
   c. 3 mL
   d. 5 mL

38. Order: trimethobenzamide 200 mg IM STAT
Available: trimethobenzamide ampule, 100 mg/1 mL

How many milliliters should be administered?
   a. 0.5 mL
   b. 0.8 mL
   c. 1 mL
   d. 2 mL

39.   Order: chlorpromazine 20 mg deep IM tid
        Available:

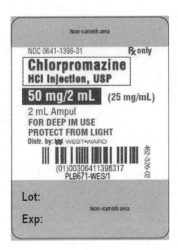

How many milliliters should be administered?
a. 0.3 mL
b. 0.5 mL
c. 0.8 mL
d. 1 mL

40.   A patient is scheduled to take digoxin 0.25 mg. The hospital is currently out of stock of digoxin 0.25 mg and only has 0.125-mg doses on hand. The patient is concerned when she receives the pills because they are a different color and a different amount from those she takes daily. When the patient questions the tablets, what is the nurse's best response?
a. "Please don't worry; it is because we use generic drugs."
b. "Please don't worry; I calculated this carefully and it is your regular dose."
c. "We don't have the 0.25-mg tablets available, so I brought you two pills of 0.125 mg to equal your 0.25 mg dose."
d. "You are right, this is the wrong dosage. I will be right back with the correct one."

41.   Order: carbidopa 12.5mg/levodopa 125 mg PO bid
        Available:

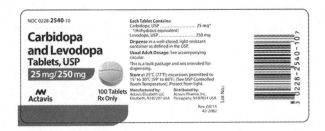

How many tablets should be administered per dose?
a. ½ tablet should be given.
b. 1 tablet should be given.
c. 1½ tablets should be given.
d. Do not administer the medication, and call the pharmacy for the correct dose.

42.   Order: lactulose 25 g PO q6h
        Available:

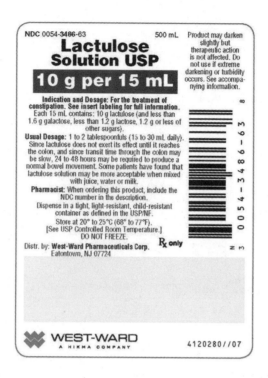

How many milliliters should the patient receive per dose?
a. 10 mL
b. 16.7 mL
c. 25 mL
d. 37.5 mL

43.   Order: hydromorphone 2 mg subcut q4h PRN for pain
        Available:

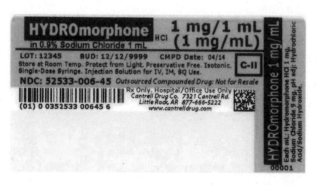 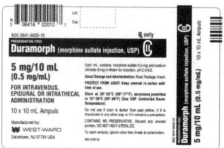

A.   Are the drugs on the label interchangeable?

B.   How many mL would you give of the correct drug?
        a. 0.5 mL
        b. 1 mL
        c. 1.5 mL
        d. 2 mL

44.	Order: cyanocobalamin 1000 mcg IM daily for 5 days
	Available: cyanocobalamin 10,000 mcg/10 mL

	How many milliliters should be administered?
	a.	0.4 mL
	b.	0.6 mL
	c.	0.8 mL
	d.	1 mL

45.	Order: heparin 3000 units subcut q6h
	Available:

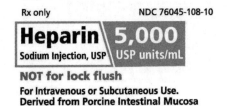

	How many milliliters should be administered?
	a.	0.2 mL
	b.	0.4 mL
	c.	0.6 mL
	d.	0.8 mL

46.	Order: insulin regular 15 units subcut before breakfast
	Available:

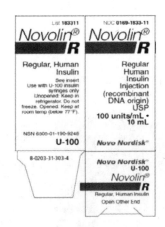

Shade in the dosage on the syringe.

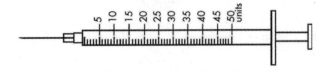

47. Order: topiramate 50 mg per day PO administered in 2 divided doses
    Available:

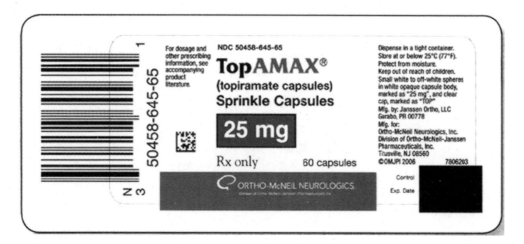

A.   What is the trade name? _____

B.   What is the generic name? _____

C.   What is the form? _____

D.   How many capsules per dose? _____

Body Weight and Body Surface Area

Use the basic formula, ratio and proportion/fractional equation, or dimensional analysis methods to calculate the following drug problems.

1.   Order: penicillin V potassium 200,000 units PO q6h
     Child weighs 46 pounds.
     Recommended child's drug dosage: 25,000–90,000 units/kg/day in 3–6 divided doses.
     Available: (NOTE: The dosage per 5 mL is in mg and units.)

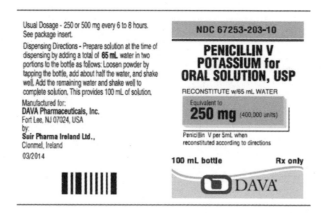

A.   Is the prescribed dose in a safe range?
     a. No
     b. Yes

B.   How many milliliters should the child receive for each dose?
     a. 1 mL
     b. 1.5 mL
     c. 2 mL
     d. 2.5 mL

2. Order: cefuroxime axetil 200 mg PO q12h
    Child's age: 8 years; weight: 75 pounds
    Recommended child's drug dosage (3 months–12 years): 10–15 mg/kg/day
    Available:

A. Is the prescribed dose appropriate?
    a. No
    b. Yes

B. If the 200-mg dose is given, how many milliliters should the child receive per dose?
    a. 2 mL
    b. 4 mL
    c. 6 mL
    d. 8 mL

3. Order: amoxicillin 75 mg PO q8h
    Child weighs 5 kg.
    Recommended child's drug dosage: 80–90 mg/kg/day in divided doses
    Available:

A. Is the prescribed dose appropriate?
    a. No
    b. Yes

B. According to the order, how many milligrams would the child receive per day (24 hours)?
    a. 225 mg
    b. 400 mg
    c. 450 mg
    d. 600 mg

4. Order: acetaminophen 250 mg PO q6h PRN
    Available: 160 mg/5 mL
    How many milliliters should be administered?
    a. 3.2 mL
    b. 6 mL
    c. 7.8 mL
    d. 10 mL
    e. 12 mL

5.   Order: ceftriaxone 50 mg/kg IM daily
      Child weighs 8 kg.
      Available:

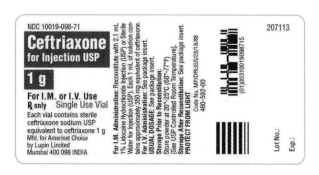

    A. How much diluent is needed? _____

    B. What is the final concentration? _____

    C. How many milliliters should the child receive per dose?
        a. 0.5 mL
        b. 1.1 mL
        c. 1.5 mL
        d. 2 mL
        e. 2.4 mL

6.   Order: erythromycin suspension 160 mg PO q6h
      Child weighs 25 kg.
      Recommended child's drug dosage: 30–50 mg/kg/day in divided doses q6h
      Available:

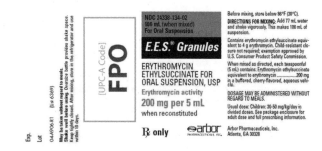

    A. Is the prescribed dosage within dose parameters?
        a. Yes, the dosage is safe.
        b. No, the dosage is too low.
        c. No, the dosage is too high.

    B. How many milliliters should the child receive for the ordered dosage?
        a. 0.25 mL
        b. 2 mL
        c. 3 mL
        d. 4 mL

7. Order: cefaclor 75 mg PO q8h
   Child weighs 22 pounds.
   Recommended child's drug dosage: 20–40 mg/kg/day in 3 divided doses.
   Available:

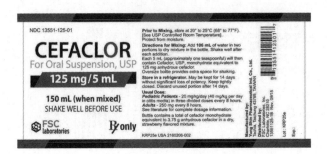

   A. Calculate the minimum and maximum recommended dosage range per dose. _____

   B. Is the ordered dosage appropriate? _____

   C. How many milliliters per dose should be given?
      a. 2 mL
      b. 3 mL
      c. 4 mL
      d. 5 mL
      e. 6 mL

8. Order: amoxicillin/clavulanate potassium 150 mg (amoxicillin component) PO q8h
   Child weighs 26 pounds.
   Recommended child's drug dosage: 45 mg/kg/day in 3 divided doses.
   Available:

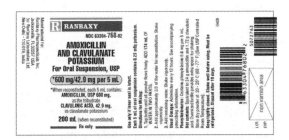

   A. How many kilograms does the child weigh?
      a. 10 kg
      b. 12 kg
      c. 14 kg
      d. 15 kg

   B. Is the prescribed dosage within dose parameters?
      a. Yes, the dosage is safe.
      b. No, the dosage is too low.
      c. No, the dosage is too high.

   C. How many milliliters of the ordered dosage should the child receive per dose?
      a. 1.3 mL
      b. 1.5 mL
      c. 2 mL
      d. 3.5 mL

9.   Order: acetaminophen 135 mg PO q6h PRN for fever
     Child weighs 25 pounds.
     Recommended dosage range is 10–15 mg/kg/dose q4–6h PRN.

   A.   What is the child's weight in kilograms? _____

   B.   What are the minimum and maximum safe dosage ranges? _____

   C.   Is the ordered dose safe? _____

10.   A 3-year-old is ordered ticarcillin/clavulanic acid 50 mg/kg (ticarcillin component) IV q6h. The child weighs 23 pounds. How many milligrams will the child receive per dose? _____

11.   A child with meningitis is ordered ceftriaxone 100 mg/kg/day IV divided q12h. The child weighs 65 pounds.

   A.   How many milligrams will the child receive per day? _____

   B.   How many milligrams will the child receive per dose? _____

Use the West nomogram as indicated in the following drug calculations.

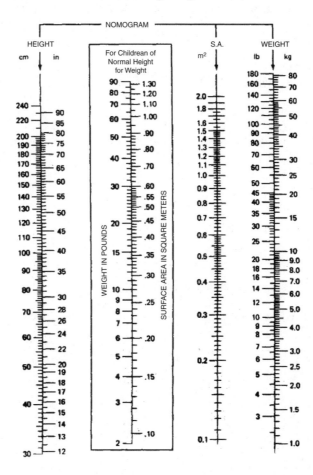

12.   Refer to the West nomogram and determine the BSA for the following children of normal height and weight.

   A.   Child weighs 5 pounds. _____

   B.   Child weighs 25 pounds. _____

   C.   Child weighs 53 pounds. _____

13. Refer to the West nomogram to determine the following BSAs.

   A. A child who is 43 inches tall and weighs 54 pounds _____

   B. A child who is 39 inches tall and weighs 60 pounds _____

   C. A child who is 56 centimeters tall and weighs 15 kilograms _____

14. Calculate the following BSA using the square root method for inches and pounds.

   A. A child weighs 25 pounds and is 32 inches tall. _____

   B. A child weighs 58 pounds and is 48 inches tall. _____

   C. A child is 40 inches tall and weighs 34 pounds. _____

15. Calculate the following BSAs using the square root method for centimeters and kilograms.

   A. A child weighs 8 kilograms and is 28.2 centimeters long. _____

   B. A child weighs 28.1 kilograms and is 133.4 centimeters tall. _____

   C. A child is 85.5 centimeters tall and weighs 25 kilograms. _____

16. Order: lomustine 100 mg/m^2
    Child's weight is 80 pounds; height is 40 inches tall.

   A. Calculate the BSA using the West nomogram. _____

   B. Calculate the BSA using the square root method and using the child's height and weight in inches and pounds. _____

   C. Using the calculated answer from B, determine the milligrams the child should receive per dose.
   _____

17. Drug X 50 mg/m^2 is ordered for a child who weighs 70 pounds and is 54 inches tall.

   A. What is the BSA? _____

   B. How many milligrams should the child receive? _____

18. Drug X 35 mg/m^2 is ordered for a child who weighs 43 pounds and is 52 inches tall.

   A. What is the BSA? _____

   B. What is the dosage? _____

19. Drug X 134 mg/m^2 is ordered for a child who is 100 pounds and is 54 inches tall.

   A. What is the BSA? _____

   B. What is the dosage? _____

20. Carmustine 225 mg/m^2 IV as a single dose every 4 weeks is ordered for a child who weighs 71 pounds and is 60 inches tall.

   A. What is the BSA? _____

   B. How many milligrams should the child receive? _____

21. Methotrexate 3.3 mg/m^2 IV daily every 4 weeks is ordered for an adolescent who is 104 pounds and is 64 inches tall.

   A. What is the BSA? _____

   B. How many milligrams should the adolescent receive? _____

22. Order: cyclophosphamide 350 mg/m^2
   Child's weight: 36.9 kg; height: 59 centimeters

   A. What is the child's BSA? _____

   B. How many milligrams should the child receive? _____

23. Order: imatinib 340 mg/m^2/day PO divided into two doses
   Child weighs 47.5 kilograms and is 160 centimeters tall.

   A. What is the BSA? _____

   B. How many milligrams should the child receive per dose? _____

SECTION 11C—CALCULATING DOSAGES: DRUGS THAT REQUIRE RECONSTITUTION

Use the basic formula, ratio and proportion/fractional equation, or dimensional analysis to calculate the following drug problems.

1. Order: oxacillin sodium 300 mg IM q6h
   Available:

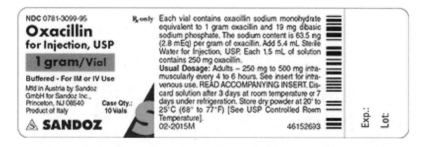

   A. The nurse must add _____ mL of sterile water to yield _____ mg/mL of drug solution.

   B. How many milliliters should be administered?
      a. 0.5 mL
      b. 1 mL
      c. 1.8 mL
      d. 2 mL

2. Order: nafcillin 500 mg IM q4h
   Available:

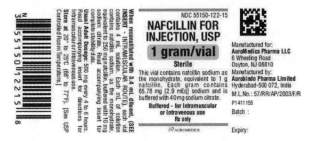

A. The nurse must add _____ mL of diluent to yield _____ mL of drug solution.

B. How many milliliters should be administered?
    a. 1 mL
    b. 2 mL
    c. 3 mL
    d. 4 mL

3. Order: cefotetan disodium 500 mg IM q12h
   Available: (NOTE: Mix 2 mL of diluent. Once reconstituted, each mL of solution contains cefotetan 400 mg.)

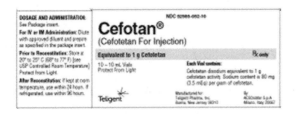

How many milliliters should be administered per dose?
a. 1 mL
b. 1.3 mL
c. 2 mL
d. 2.3 mL

4. Order: ampicillin sodium 350 mg IM q6h
   Available:

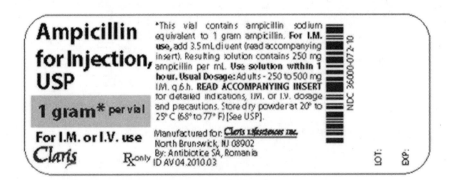

How many milliliters should be administered per dose?
a. 0.8 mL
b. 1 mL
c. 1.4 mL
d. 2 mL

5.   Order: tobramycin 3 mg/kg IM in three divided doses
     Patient's weight: 184 pounds
     Available:

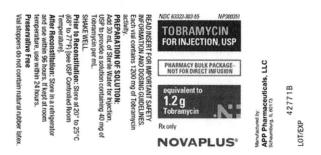

How many milliliters should be administered per dose?
a. 1.5 mL
b. 2.8 mL
c. 4.2 mL
d. 6.3 mL

SECTION 11D—CALCULATION METHODS: INSULIN DOSAGES

Select the best response.

1.   A tuberculin syringe (is/is not) used for insulin administration. *(Circle correct answer.)*

2.   Insulin syringes are calibrated in (units/mL). *(Circle correct answer.)*

3.   Circle the best insulin syringe to administer 23 units of regular insulin.

a.

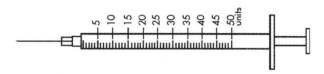

b.

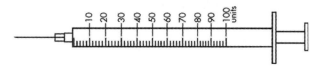

4.   Order: lente insulin 36 units subcut qam

Shade the appropriate amount to administer on the insulin syringe.

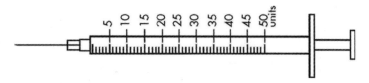

5. Order: regular insulin 8 units and isophane insulin 44 units subcut every am
   Available: (NOTE: These insulins can be mixed together in the same insulin syringe.)

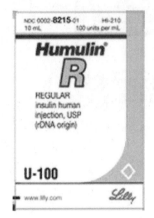 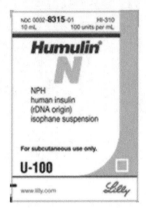

A. Using both syringes, indicate on the insulin syringes the amount of insulin to be withdrawn.

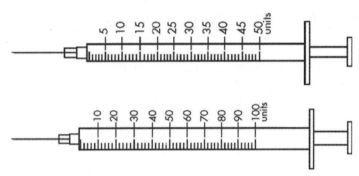

B. Which insulin should be drawn up first?
   a. Either one can be drawn first
   b. The isophane insulin
   c. The regular insulin
   d. Neither; they should not be given together

C. Indicate the combined dosages by shading the appropriate amount

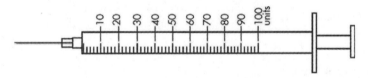

For problems 6–9, determine the size of insulin syringe and the units shaded.

6.

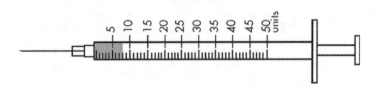

7.

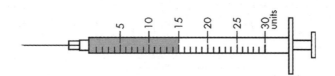

8.

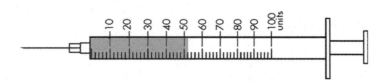

9.

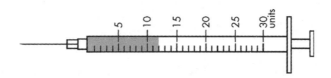

10.   A patient has an order for sliding scale insulin with regular insulin before meals and at bedtime according to the following sliding scale coverage:

Blood Sugar Results	Lispro Coverage Subcut
Less than 125	No coverage
>125–150	2 units
151–200	4 units
201–250	6 units
251–300	8 units
>300	Call physician

A.   Blood sugar before breakfast was 243. Shade the appropriate amount of insulin on the syringe.

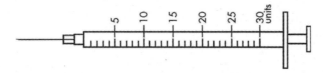

B.   Blood sugar before lunch was 218. Shade the appropriate amount of insulin on the syringe.

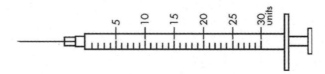

C.   Blood sugar before dinner was 450. What is the most appropriate action by the nurse?

Chapter **11** **Drug Calculations**

D. The nurse administered 15 units of insulin lispro for blood glucose of 450 before dinner. Now at bedtime, his blood glucose is 130. Shade the appropriate amount of insulin on the syringe to administer bedtime insulin.

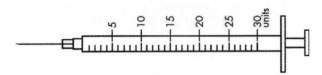

SECTION 11E—CALCULATION METHODS: INTRAVENOUS FLOW RATES

Select the best response.

1. The health care provider orders heparin infusion. The nurse should calculate the dosage for infusion in which of the following measurements?
    a. mL/h
    b. gtt/min
    c. units/h
    d. units/kg/h

2. The best method for calculating critical care drugs is:
    a. ratio and proportion method because it contains multiple steps.
    b. fractional equation method because conversion factors are not needed.
    c. basic formula method because it is the easiest.
    d. dimensional analysis because all the units of measurement and conversion factors are included in one equation.

3. When an electronic infusion device is used to deliver intravenous fluids or drugs, the nurse should calculate the dosage in which of the following units of measurement?
    a. gtt/min
    b. units/h
    c. gtt/mL
    d. mL/h

4. When infusing intravenous fluids by gravity, the nurse should calculate the dosage in which of the following units of measurement?
    a. gtt/min
    b. gtt/mL
    c. units/h
    d. mL/h

Match the common fluid abbreviation in Column I to the appropriate IV solution bags in Column II.

Column I

_____ 5. D_5 1/2NS

_____ 6. LR or RL

_____ 7. D_5W

_____ 8. D_5NS

Column II

a.

LOT   EXP

⊙   ⊙   2B2324
NDC 0338-0117-04
DIN 00061085

Lactated Ringer's Injection USP

1000 mL
EACH 100 mL CONTAINS   600 mg SODIUM CHLORIDE USP
310 mg SODIUM LACTATE   30 mg POTASSIUM CHLORIDE USP
20 mg CALCIUM CHLORIDE USP   pH 6.5 (6.0 TO 7.5)   mEq/L
SODIUM 130   POTASSIUM 4   CALCIUM 2.7   CHLORIDE 109
LACTATE 28   OSMOLARITY 273 mOsmol/L (CALC)   STERILE
NONPYROGENIC   SINGLE DOSE CONTAINER   NOT FOR USE IN THE
TREATMENT OF LACTIC ACIDOSIS   ADDITIVES MAY BE
INCOMPATIBLE   CONSULT WITH PHARMACIST IF AVAILABLE   WHEN
INTRODUCING ADDITIVES USE ASEPTIC TECHNIQUE   MIX
THOROUGHLY   DO NOT STORE   DOSAGE   INTRAVENOUSLY AS
DIRECTED BY A PHYSICIAN   SEE DIRECTIONS   CAUTIONS
SQUEEZE AND INSPECT INNER BAG WHICH MAINTAINS PRODUCT
STERILITY   DISCARD IF LEAKS ARE FOUND   MUST NOT BE USED IN
SERIES CONNECTIONS   DO NOT ADMINISTER SIMULTANEOUSLY
WITH BLOOD   DO NOT USE UNLESS SOLUTION IS CLEAR   FEDERAL
(USA) LAW PROHIBITS DISPENSING WITHOUT PRESCRIPTION
STORE UNIT IN MOISTURE BARRIER OVERWRAP AT ROOM
TEMPERATURE (25°C/77°F) UNTIL READY TO USE   AVOID
EXCESSIVE HEAT   SEE INSERT

Baxter
BAXTER HEALTHCARE CORPORATION
DEERFIELD IL 60015 USA
MADE IN USA
DISTRIBUTED IN CANADA BY
BAXTER CORPORATION
TORONTO ONTARIO CANADA

Viaflex® CONTAINER
PL 146® PLASTIC

FOR PRODUCT INFORMATION
CALL 1-800-933-0303

⊙   ⊙

1 2 3 4 5 6 7 8 9

b.

LOT   EXP

⊙   ⊙   2B0064
NDC 0338-0017-04

5% Dextrose Injection USP

1000 mL
EACH 100 mL CONTAINS   5 g DEXTROSE HYDROUS USP
pH 4.0 (3.2 TO 6.5)   OSMOLARITY 252 mOsmol/L (CALC)
STERILE   NONPYROGENIC   SINGLE DOSE CONTAINER   ADDITIVES
MAY BE INCOMPATIBLE   CONSULT WITH PHARMACIST IF AVAILABLE
WHEN INTRODUCING ADDITIVES USE ASEPTIC TECHNIQUE   MIX
THOROUGHLY   DO NOT STORE   DOSAGE   INTRAVENOUSLY AS
DIRECTED BY A PHYSICIAN   SEE DIRECTIONS   CAUTIONS   SQUEEZE
AND INSPECT INNER BAG WHICH MAINTAINS PRODUCT STERILITY
DISCARD IF LEAKS ARE FOUND   MUST NOT BE USED IN SERIES
CONNECTIONS   DO NOT ADMINISTER SIMULTANEOUSLY WITH BLOOD
DO NOT USE UNLESS SOLUTION IS CLEAR   FEDERAL (USA) LAW
PROHIBITS DISPENSING WITHOUT PRESCRIPTION   STORE UNIT IN
MOISTURE BARRIER OVERWRAP AT ROOM TEMPERATURE
(25°C/77°F) UNTIL READY TO USE   AVOID EXCESSIVE HEAT   SEE
INSERT

Baxter
BAXTER HEALTHCARE CORPORATION
DEERFIELD IL 60015 USA
MADE IN USA

FOR PRODUCT INFORMATION
CALL 1-800-933-0303

⊙   ⊙

1 2 3 4 5 6 7 8 9

c.

LOT   EXP

⊙   ⊙   2B1073
NDC 0338-0085-03

5% Dextrose and 0.45% Sodium Chloride Injection USP

500 mL
EACH 100 mL CONTAINS   5 g DEXTROSE HYDROUS USP   450 mg SODIUM
CHLORIDE USP   pH 4.0 (3.2 TO 6.5)   mEq/L   SODIUM 77   CHLORIDE 77
HYPERTONIC   OSMOLARITY   406 mOsmol/L (CALC)   STERILE
NONPYROGENIC   SINGLE DOSE CONTAINER   ADDITIVES MAY BE INCOMPATIBLE
CONSULT WITH PHARMACIST IF AVAILABLE   WHEN INTRODUCING ADDITIVES USE
ASEPTIC TECHNIQUE   MIX THOROUGHLY   DO NOT STORE   DOSAGE
INTRAVENOUSLY AS DIRECTED BY A PHYSICIAN   SEE DIRECTIONS   CAUTIONS
SQUEEZE AND INSPECT INNER BAG WHICH MAINTAINS PRODUCT STERILITY
DISCARD IF LEAKS ARE FOUND   MUST NOT BE USED IN SERIES CONNECTIONS
DO NOT USE UNLESS SOLUTION IS CLEAR   FEDERAL (USA) LAW PROHIBITS
DISPENSING WITHOUT PRESCRIPTION   STORE UNIT IN MOISTURE BARRIER
OVERWRAP AT ROOM TEMPERATURE (25°C/77°F) UNTIL READY TO USE
AVOID EXCESSIVE HEAT   SEE INSERT

Baxter
BAXTER HEALTHCARE CORPORATION
DEERFIELD IL 60015 USA
MADE IN USA

Viaflex® CONTAINER
PL 146® PLASTIC

FOR PRODUCT INFORMATION
CALL 1-800-933-0303

1 2 3 4

d.

LOT   EXP

⊙   ⊙   2B1064
NDC 0338-0089-04

5% Dextrose and 0.9% Sodium Chloride Injection USP

1000 mL
EACH 100 mL CONTAINS   5 g DEXTROSE HYDROUS USP
900 mg SODIUM CHLORIDE USP   pH 4.0 (3.2 TO 6.5)
mEq/L   SODIUM 154   CHLORIDE 154   HYPERTONIC
OSMOLARITY   560 mOsmol/L (CALC)   STERILE NONPYROGENIC
SINGLE DOSE CONTAINER   ADDITIVES MAY BE INCOMPATIBLE
CONSULT WITH PHARMACIST IF AVAILABLE   WHEN INTRODUCING
ADDITIVES USE ASEPTIC TECHNIQUE   MIX THOROUGHLY   DO NOT
STORE   DOSAGE   INTRAVENOUSLY AS DIRECTED BY A PHYSICIAN
SEE DIRECTIONS   CAUTIONS   SQUEEZE AND INSPECT INNER BAG
WHICH MAINTAINS PRODUCT STERILITY   DISCARD IF LEAKS ARE
FOUND   MUST NOT BE USED IN SERIES CONNECTIONS   DO NOT
USE UNLESS SOLUTION IS CLEAR   FEDERAL (USA) LAW PROHIBITS
DISPENSING WITHOUT PRESCRIPTION   STORE UNIT IN MOISTURE
BARRIER OVERWRAP AT ROOM TEMPERATURE (25°C/77°F) UNTIL
READY TO USE   AVOID EXCESSIVE HEAT   SEE INSERT

Baxter
BAXTER HEALTHCARE CORPORATION
DEERFIELD IL 60015 USA
MADE IN USA

Viaflex® CONTAINER
PL 146® PLASTIC

FOR PRODUCT INFORMATION
CALL 1-800-933-0303

⊙

1 2 3 4 5 6 7 8 9

59

Complete the following.

9. Macrodrip infusion sets deliver _____ gtt/mL; microdrip infusion sets deliver _____ gtt/mL.

10. KVO means _____. The preferred size of IV bag for KVO is (1000 mL/500 mL/250 mL). *(Circle correct answer.)*

11. The Buretrol is a (calibrated cylinder with tubing/small IV bag of solution with short tubing). *(Circle correct answer.)*

12. The pump infusion regulator that delivers mL/h is a (volumetric/nonvolumetric) IV regulator. *(Circle correct answer.)*

13. Patient-controlled analgesia is a method used to administer drugs intravenously. The purpose is to provide _____.

Calculating Intravenous Flow Rates: Milliliters per Hour, and Drops per Minute

Use the basic formula, ratio and proportion/fractional equation, or dimensional analysis methods to calculate the following drug problems.

14. Order: 1 liter or 1000 mL of D_5W to infuse over 6 hours
    Available: Macrodrip set: 10 gtt/mL
    The IV flow rate should be _____ gtt/min.

15. Order: 1000 mL of $D_5\frac{1}{2}NS$ with 1 ampule of multiple vitamins to infuse over 8 hours
    Available: Macrodrip set: 15 gtt/mL
    Calculate the IV flow rate in gtt/min. _____

16. Order: ceftriaxone 2 g in 100 mL of 0.9% NaCl (normal saline solution) over 30 minutes
    Available: Macrodrip set: 15 gtt/mL

    Calculate the IV flow rate in gtt/min. _____

17. Order: The following IV fluids to infuse over 24 hours are ordered. They include 1 L of D_5W, 1 L of $D_5\frac{1}{2}NS$, and 500 mL of 5% D/LR.
    Available:

    A. One liter is equal to _____ milliliters.

    B. Total number of milliliters of IV solutions to infuse in 24 hours is _____ milliliters.

    C. What is the flow rate? _____

18. A liter of IV fluid was started at 7:00 am and was to infuse for 8 hours. The IV set delivers 10 gtt/mL. At 12:00 pm, only 500 mL were infused.

    A. How much IV fluid is left?
        a. 100 mL
        b. 200 mL
        c. 300 mL
        d. 400 mL
        e. 500 mL

    B. Recalculate the flow rate for the remaining IV fluids in gtt/min. _____

19.   Order: cimetidine 200 mg IV q6h
      Set and solution: Buretrol with drop factor 60 gtt/mL; primary IV fluid of 500 mL of 0.9% NaCl
      Instruction: Dilute cimetidine 200 mg in 50 mL of normal saline and infuse in 15 minutes.

      A.   How much cimetidine will be infused per mL?
           a. 2 mg
           b. 3 mg
           c. 4 mg
           d. 5 mg

      B.   Calculate the flow rate in gtt/min.
           a. 50 gtt/min
           b. 100 gtt/min
           c. 150 gtt/min
           d. 200 gtt/min

20.   Order: cefazolin 1000 mg IV q8h
      Available:

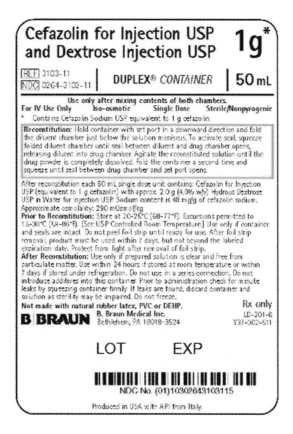

      IV tubing with drop factor, 15 gtt/mL
      Calculate IV flow rate in gtt/min to be infused over 1 hour.
      a. 6.5 gtt/min
      b. 7 gtt/min
      c. 12.5 gtt/min
      d. 13 gtt/min

Chapter **11** Drug Calculations

21. Order: nafcillin 1000 mg IV q4h
Available:

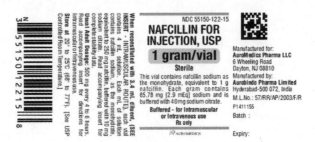

A. How many mL of diluent should be added? _____

B. What is the drug's concentration? _____

IV tubing available: Secondary set with drop factor 15 gtt/mL

Instruction: Dilute nafcillin 1000 mg in 100 mL of D_5W and infuse in 40 minutes.

C. Calculate the flow rate.
   a. 22 gtt/min
   b. 38 gtt/min
   c. 53 gtt/min
   d. 69 gtt/min

22. Order: fluconazole 400 mg IV daily
Available:

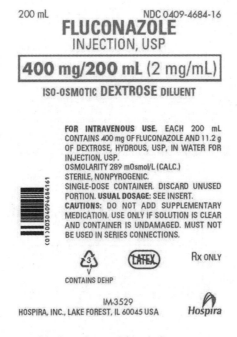

IV tubing available: Secondary set with drop factor 15 gtt/mL

Instruction: Infuse over 2 hours.

Calculate the flow rate _____

23. Order: imipenem; cilastatin 500 mg IV q8h
Available: imipenem; cilastatin 500 mg in 100-mL solution

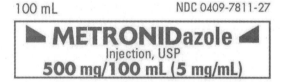

Instruction: Infuse over 30 minutes.

Calculate the gtt/min with an infusion set, 20 gtt/mL. _____

24. Order: sulfamethoxazole/trimethoprim 10 mcg/kg/d (trimethoprim component), IV divided in 3 doses. Patient weighs 135 pounds.
Available: sulfamethoxazole/trimethoprim 400 mg/80 mg per 5 mL

Instruction: Further dilute in 250 mL of D_5W and infuse over 2 hours.

A. What is the total dosage in micrograms for the day? _____

B. How many micrograms for each dose?_____

C. What is the flow rate?_____

D. The hospital is experiencing a power failure after 20 minutes of infusion. Recalculate the flow rate in gtt/min with IV tubing, 20 gtt/mL to be infused over 1 hour and 40 minutes.

25. Order: metronidazole 500 mg IV q6h
Available:

Instruction: Infuse in 30 minutes.

What is the flow rate?_____

Chapter **11** Drug Calculations

26. Order: amikacin sulfate 7.5 mg/kg q12h
    Adult weight: 64 kg
    Available:

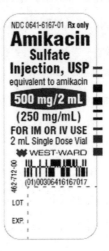

A. How many mL would equal amikacin 400 mg? _____

Instruction: Dilute amikacin 400 mg in 100 mL of D₅W and infuse in 30 min.

B. What is the flow rate?_____

27. Order: minocycline 100 mg IV q12h
    Available: Add 5 mL of sterile water.

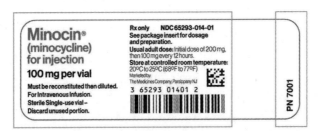

Instruction: Further dilute minocycline 100 mg in 500 mL of D₅W and infuse in 6 hours.

What is the flow rate? _____

28.   Order: cefepime hydrochloride 1 g IV q12h
       Available:

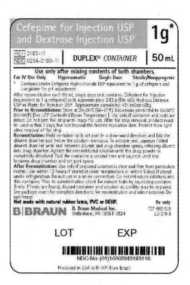

Instruction: Drop factor, 60 gtt/mL. Infuse over 30 minutes.

What is the flow rate?_____

29.   Order: ampicillin sodium/sulbactam sodium 1.5 g IV q6h
       Available: (NOTE: ADD-Vantage vials do not need further dilution.)

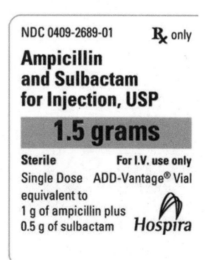

Set and solution: IV tubing with drop factor of 15 gtt/mL

Instruction: Infuse ampicillin sodium/sulbactam sodium 1.5 g solution in 100 mL of D₅W over 30 minutes.

What is the flow rate? _____

Calculating Intravenous Heparin and Critical Care Drug Infusions

Use the basic formula, ratio and proportion/fractional equation, or dimensional analysis to calculate the following drug problems.

30. Order: heparin 30,000 units/d continuous infusion
     Available:

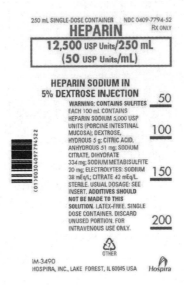

A. How many units/h is the patient receiving? _____
B. What is the flow rate? _____

31. Order: heparin bolus 80 units/kg, then maintenance infusion of 18 units/kg/h
     Patient's weight: 180 pounds
     Available:

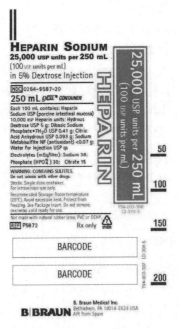

A. What is the patient's weight in kg? _____

B. How many units for the bolus? _____

C. Calculate the maintenance infusion flow rate. _____

32. A patient was prescribed heparin sodium 18 units/kg/h; titrate according to the weight-based heparin protocol. The patient's weight is 123 pounds. Heparin 25,000 units/250 mL (100 unit/mL) is available.

    A. Calculate the flow rate in mL/h _____

    B. aPTT is 40, and the protocol states to rebolus with 40 units/kg and increase the infusion rate by 2 units/kg/h.

    How many more units did the patient receive? _____ What is the new flow rate? _____

33. A patient was prescribed heparin sodium 18 units/kg/h; titrate according to the weight-based heparin protocol for a patient with pulmonary embolus. The patient's weight is 63 kilograms. Heparin 25,000 units/250 mL (100 units/mL) is available.

    A. Calculate the flow rate in mL/h _____

    B. aPTT is 45, and the protocol states to rebolus with 40 units/kg and increase infusion by 2 units/kg.

    How many more units did the patient receive? _____ What is the new flow rate? _____

34. A patient was prescribed heparin sodium 18 units/kg/h; titrate according to the weight-based heparin protocol. The patient's weight is 70 kilograms. Heparin 12,500/250 mL (50 unit/mL) is available.

    A. Calculate the flow rate in mL/h _____

    B. aPTT is >90, and the protocol states to hold the infusion for 1 hour and decrease rate by 3 units/kg/h.

    What is the new flow rate? _____

35. Order: diltiazem 0.25 mg/kg bolus over 2 minutes, then 15 minutes later, rebolus with 0.35 mg/kg IV, then start maintenance infusion at 10 mg/h.
Weight: 65 kg
Available:
For bolus:

For maintenance infusion:

    A. What is the total bolus in milligrams? _____

    B. What is the flow rate for the maintenance infusion? _____

Chapter **11** **Drug Calculations**

36. Order: dobutamine 2 mcg/kg/min as a continuous infusion. Titrate according to patient's hemodynamic response.
Weight: 63 kg
Available:

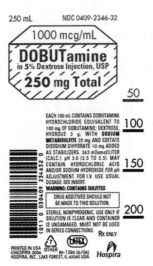

250 mL NDC 0409-2346-32

1000 mcg/mL

DOBUTamine
in 5% Dextrose Injection, USP

250 mg Total

50
100
150
200

EACH 100 mL CONTAINS DOBUTAMINE HYDROCHLORIDE EQUIVALENT TO 100 mg OF DOBUTAMINE; DEXTROSE, HYDROUS 5 g; WITH **SODIUM METABISULFITE** 25 mg AND EDETATE DISODIUM DIHYDRATE 10 mg ADDED AS STABILIZERS. 263 mOsmol/LITER (CALC.). pH 3.0 (2.5 TO 5.5). MAY CONTAIN HYDROCHLORIC ACID AND/OR SODIUM HYDROXIDE FOR pH ADJUSTMENT. FOR I.V. USE. USUAL DOSAGE: SEE INSERT.
WARNING: CONTAINS SULFITES
DRUG ADDITIVES SHOULD NOT BE MADE TO THIS SOLUTION.
STERILE, NONPYROGENIC. USE ONLY IF SOLUTION IS CLEAR AND CONTAINER IS UNDAMAGED. MUST NOT BE USED IN SERIES CONNECTIONS. Rx ONLY

PRINTED IN USA OTHER M-1286 (6/06)
©HOSPIRA 2006
HOSPIRA, INC., LAKE FOREST, IL 60045 USA *Hospira*

What is the flow rate? _____

37. Order: dobutamine 5 mcg/kg/min as a continuous infusion. Titrate according to patient's hemodynamic response.
Weight: 78 kg
Available:

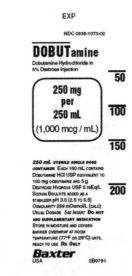

LOT   EXP

NDC 0338-1073-02

DOBUTamine
Dobutamine Hydrochloride in 5% Dextrose Injection

50

250 mg
per
250 mL
(1,000 mcg / mL)

100

150

200

250 mL *STERILE SINGLE DOSE*
CONTAINER EACH 100 mL CONTAINS
DOBUTAMINE HCl USP EQUIVALENT TO
100 mg DOBUTAMINE AND 5 g
DEXTROSE HYDROUS USP 5 mEq/L
SODIUM BISULFITE ADDED AS A
STABILIZER pH 3.5 (2.5 TO 5.5)
OSMOLARITY 259 mOsmol/L (CALC)
USUAL DOSAGE *SEE INSERT* DO NOT
ADD SUPPLEMENTARY MEDICATION
STORE IN MOISTURE AND OXYGEN
BARRIER OVERWRAP AT ROOM
TEMPERATURE (77°F OR 25°C) UNTIL
READY TO USE Rx ONLY

Baxter
USA   2B0791

A. What is the flow rate? _____

B. Nurse is to increase the dobutamine infusion by 2 mcg/kg/min. What is the new flow rate? _____

38.   Order: amiodarone 0.5 mg/min
        Available:

Amiodarone 900 mg
HCl

Added to 5% Dextrose
500 mL* Bag **(1.8 mg/mL*)**

*Volume and Concentration Exclude Manufacturer Overfill.
Store at Room Temperature. Protect from Light.
Contains Preservatives. Single-Dose Bag.
Recommend In-Line Filter During Administration.
Injection Solution for IV Use.
Each mL Contains: Amiodarone HCl 1.8 mg; Polysorbate 80, 3.6 mg;
Benzyl Alcohol 0.73 mg; Dextrose 50 mg.

NDC: 52533-101-59

HIGH ALERT   **Rx Only**
(01) 0 0352533 10159 5
Hospital/Office Use Only
Outsourced Compounded Drug. Not for Resale   00003

CANTRELL DRUG COMPANY   LOT: xxxxx
7321 Cantrell Road Little Rock, AR 72207   BUD:
(877) 666-5222 www.cantrelldrug.com   CMPD Date: 03/13

What is the flow rate? _____

39.   Patient is receiving nitroglycerin 0.25 mg/min for unstable angina.
        Available:

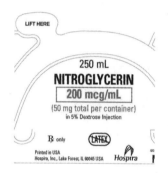

LIFT HERE

250 mL
NITROGLYCERIN
200 mcg/mL
(50 mg total per container)
in 5% Dextrose Injection

℞ only   LATEX

Printed in USA
Hospira, Inc., Lake Forest, IL 60045 USA   Hospira

What is the flow rate? _____

40.   Patient is receiving nitroglycerin 55 mcg/min.
        Available:

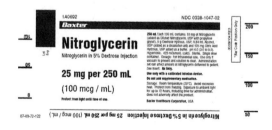

1A0692   NDC 0338-1047-02
Baxter
Nitroglycerin
Nitroglycerin in 5% Dextrose Injection

25 mg per 250 mL
(100 mcg / mL)
Protect from light until time of use.

250 mL Each 100 mL contains: 10 mg of Nitroglycerin
(added as Diluted Nitroglycerin, USP with propylene
glycol), 5 g Dextrose Hydrous, USP, 0.84 mL Alcohol,
USP (added as a dissolution aid) and 505 mg Citric Acid
Hydrous, USP added as a buffer. pH 4.0 (3.0 to 6.0).
Hyperosmolar, 425 mOsmol/L (calc.). Sterile. Single dose
container. Dosage: For intravenous use. Use only if
vacuum is present and solution is clear. Administration
set can affect amount of nitroglycerin delivered to patient.
See insert. **Rx Only.**
Use only with a calibrated infusion device.
Do not add supplementary medication.
Storage: Room temperature (25°C). Avoid excessive
heat. Protect from freezing. Exposure to ambient light
for up to 72 hours, including time for administration,
does not adversely affect the product.
Baxter Healthcare Corporation, USA

07-09-72-122   Nitroglycerin in 5% Dextrose Injection 25 mg per 250 mL (100 mcg / mL)

What is the flow rate? _____

41.   Order: dobutamine 5 mcg/kg/min
        Patient's weight: 152 lb
        Available: dobutamine 500 mg in 250 mL D₅W

        What is the flow rate? _____

42. Order: dobutamine 10 mcg/kg/min

Patient's weight: 95 kg

Available: dobutamine 1000 mg in 250 mL D$_5$W

What is the flow rate? _____

43. Order: dopamine 5 mcg/kg/min

Patient weights 130 lb

Available: dopamine 800 mg in 500 mL of D$_5$W

What is the flow rate? _____

44. Order: dopamine 300 mcg/min

Available: dopamine 400 mg in 250 mL of D$_5$W

What is the flow rate? _____

45. Order: heparin at 800 units/h

Available: heparin 25,000 units in 250 mL of D$_5$W

What is the flow rate? _____

46. Order: lidocaine 2 g in 250 mL of D$_5$W at 30 mL/h

A.   How many mg/min is the patient receiving? _____

B.   What is the flow rate? _____

47. Order: nitroprusside 100 mg/250 mL D$_5$W at 25 mL/hour for hypertension

The patient weighs 143 lb.

A.   How many mcg/kg/min of nitroprusside is the patient receiving? _____

B.   What is the flow rate? _____

12 Fluid Volume and Electrolytes

STUDY QUESTIONS

Match the electrolytes in Column I with its normal value in Column II.

Column I

_____ 1. Magnesium

_____ 2. Calcium

_____ 3. Sodium

_____ 4. Potassium

_____ 5. Chloride

_____ 6. Phosphorus

Column II

a. 96–106 mEq/L
b. 135–145 mEq/L
c. 2.4–4.4 mEq/L
d. 1.5–2.5 mEq/L
e. 3.5–5 mEq/L
f. 8.6–10.2 mg/dL

Match the description in Column I with its term in Column II.

Column I

_____ 7. Similar to plasma concentration

_____ 8. Based on milliosmoles per kilogram of water

_____ 9. Fluids contain fewer particles and more water

_____ 10. Fluids have a higher solute/particle concentration

Column II

a. Osmolality
b. Isoosmolar
c. Hypoosmolar
d. Hyperosmolar

NCLEX REVIEW QUESTIONS

11. The nurse has taught the patient how to take his oral potassium supplement. Which statement by the patient indicates that he requires more education on taking this drug?
    a. "I can take this with a few sips of water."
    b. "It may upset my stomach."
    c. "I should drink at least six ounces of water or juice when I take it."
    d. "I must not chew up the tablet."

12. 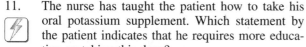 The patient has been diagnosed with hypokalemia and will be admitted to the hospital for IV potassium replacement. What is the nurse's best action when preparing to give this drug?
    a. Prepare the syringe with the ordered amount of drug to give IV push.
    b. Push the potassium into the IV bag and keep it still before administration.
    c. Push the potassium chloride into the IV bag and shake vigorously.
    d. Obtain an IV pump and pump tubing since this IV drug must be controlled.

13. 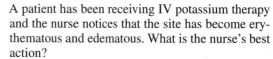 A patient has been receiving IV potassium therapy and the nurse notices that the site has become erythematous and edematous. What is the nurse's best action?
    a. Flush the IV site with normal saline and increase the rate.
    b. Flush the IV site with heparin.
    c. Stop the IV and check for blood return.
    d. Discontinue the IV and restart in another site.

14. 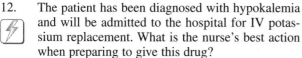 A patient has been receiving IV potassium supplements. The nurse notices that the patient's heart rate is now 116 beats/minute. What other symptom(s) might the nurse expect to see if the patient is becoming hyperkalemic? *(Select all that apply.)*
    a. Abdominal distention
    b. Nausea
    c. Numbness in extremities
    d. Polyuria
    e. Confusion

15. The patient presents to the hospital and is found to be hyperkalemic. What will the nurse anticipate administering?
    a. 10 mEq/L magnesium mixed in 1000 mL of normal saline
    b. 0.9% saline bolus of 500 mL
    c. A fluid challenge of 250 mL of high-molecular-weight dextran
    d. Sodium bicarbonate

16. The patient has been started on a potassium supplement. What should be included in the teaching plan for this patient? *(Select all that apply.)*
    a. List the signs and symptoms of both hypokalemia and hyperkalemia.
    b. Regular testing of serum potassium levels is required.
    c. The patient should increase his intake of potassium-rich foods.
    d. The drug must be taken on a full stomach or with a glass of water.
    e. The patient should sit up for 30 minutes after taking the drug.

17. What is the normal range for serum osmolality?
    a. 175–195 mOsm/kg
    b. 275–295 mOsm/kg
    c. 330–350 mOsm/kg
    d. 475–495 mOsm/kg

18. What is the term used to describe the body fluid when the serum osmolality is 285 mOsm/kg?
    a. Hypoosmolar
    b. Hyperosmolar
    c. Isoosmolar
    d. Neoosmolar

19. A patient with severe head trauma is receiving 3% saline. It has an osmolality of 900 mOsm/kg. This is considered to be what type of solution?
    a. Hypotonic
    b. Hypertonic
    c. Isotonic
    d. Neotonic

20. How is the majority of potassium excreted?
    a. Feces
    b. Kidneys
    c. Liver
    d. Lungs

21. The patient has pancreatitis. The nurse knows he is at risk for which electrolyte abnormality?
    a. Hypocalcemia
    b. Hypernatremia
    c. Hypomagnesemia
    d. Hyperkalemia

22. The nurse is teaching the patient about calcium absorption and includes the health teaching that vitamin D is needed for calcium absorption. Where in the body does vitamin D help in calcium absorption?
    a. Colon
    b. GI tract
    c. Kidneys
    d. Liver

23. Calcium is distributed intercellularly and intracellularly in what proportions?
    a. 25%:75%
    b. 50%:50%
    c. 75%:25%
    d. 90%:10%

24. A patient is prescribed 2 L of IV fluids: 1000 mL of D_5W followed by 1000 mL of $D_5\frac{1}{2}$ NS. What are these fluids classified as?
    a. Colloids
    b. Crystalloids
    c. Lipids
    d. Parenteral nutrition

25. The patient is in the hospital overnight after having surgery and the nurse has received an order to start an IV of $D_5\frac{1}{2}$ NS. What type of fluid is $D_5\frac{1}{2}$ NS?
    a. Hypotonic
    b. Hypertonic
    c. Isotonic
    d. Normotonic

26. A patient is receiving high-molecular-weight dextran after an explosion has burned over 50% of his body. What is the purpose of this fluid?
    a. Temporarily restore circulating volume
    b. Serve as a line to infuse blood into
    c. Piggyback fluid for antibiotics
    d. Whole blood substitute

27. Which body fluid has a similar composition to lactated Ringer's IV solution?
    a. Plasma
    b. Skin
    c. Tears
    d. White blood cells

28. The patient is taking potassium chloride. She is also taking hydrochlorothiazide 50 mg daily to control her hypertension. The patient's serum potassium level is 2.4 mEq/L. What clinical manifestations would the nurse expect to see in this patient? *(Select all that apply.)*
    a. Bradycardia
    b. Headache
    c. Muscle weakness
    d. Nausea

29. Magnesium deficiencies are frequently associated with which other electrolyte imbalance?
    a. Hypocalcemia
    b. Hyperkalemia
    c. Hyponatremia
    d. Hyperphosphatemia

30. The patient has a serum potassium level of 3.2 mEq/L and has been prescribed an extended-release potassium supplement. She asks the nurse why she has to take the supplement. What is the nurse's best response?
    a. "A low potassium level can be dangerous, and your level of 3.2 mEq/L is low and should be corrected."
    b. "You will only be on the drug for a few days, so don't worry."
    c. "You obviously aren't taking enough in your diet, so you have to take this."
    d. "Have you been constipated lately? Constipation will cause a low potassium level."

31. The patient has the following lab results: Na^+ 150 mEq/L, K^+ 4.2 mEq/L, Cl^- 100 mEq/L, Ca 9.8 mEq/L, Mg^{2+} 1.8 mg/dL, PO_4^- 3.1 mEq/L. What electrolyte abnormality is present?
    a. Hypocalcemia
    b. Hyperkalemia
    c. Hypernatremia
    d. Hypomagnesemia

32. The patient has a serum potassium level of 6.1 mEq/L. What clinical manifestation(s) should the nurse expect to assess in this patient? *(Select all that apply.)*
    a. Abdominal cramps
    b. Muscle weakness
    c. Oliguria
    d. Paresthesias of the face
    e. Tachycardia and later bradycardia

33. Which drugs are used to treat hyperkalemia? *(Select all that apply.)*
    a. Digoxin and furosemide
    b. Glucagon and magnesium
    c. Glucose and insulin
    d. Sodium polystyrene sulfonate and sorbitol
    e. Sodium bicarbonate and calcium gluconate

34. The patient has had diarrhea for several days and has a serum calcium level of 7.2 mg/dL. What clinical manifestations will the nurse expect to see in this patient? *(Select all that apply.)*
    a. Hyperactive deep tendon reflexes
    b. Irritability
    c. Numbness of the fingers
    d. Pathologic fractures
    e. Tetany

CASE STUDY

Read the scenario and answer the following questions on a separate sheet of paper.

D.M., 28 years old, has been stabbed multiple times in the chest and abdomen. His vital signs on arrival are blood pressure 84/62 mm Hg, heart rate 118 beats/minute, respiratory rate 30 breaths/minute, pulse oximetry 94% on room air, and temperature 35.2° C.

1. What is the priority assessment for this patient?

2. What types of fluids would the nurse anticipate to be ordered?

3. Explain the advantage of using whole blood versus packed red blood cells.

73

13 Vitamin and Mineral Replacement

STUDY QUESTIONS

Match the letter of the fat- or water-soluble vitamins in Column II with the appropriate word or phrase in Column I.

Column I

_____ 1. Vitamin A

_____ 2. Vitamin B complex

_____ 3. Vitamin C

_____ 4. Vitamin D

_____ 5. Vitamin E

_____ 6. Vitamin K

_____ 7. Toxic in excessive amounts

_____ 8. Metabolized slowly

_____ 9. Minimal protein binding

_____ 10. Readily excreted in urine

_____ 11. Slowly excreted in urine

Column II

a. Fat-soluble vitamins

b. Water-soluble vitamins

Match the letter of the common food sources in Column II with the appropriate vitamin in Column I.

Column I

_____ 12. Vitamin A

_____ 13. Vitamin B_{12}

_____ 14. Vitamin C

_____ 15. Vitamin D

_____ 16. Vitamin E

Column II

a. Salmon, egg yolk, milk

b. Wheat germ, egg yolk, avocado

c. Fish, liver, egg yolk

d. Green and yellow vegetables

e. Tomatoes, pepper, citrus fruits

Label the *ChooseMyPlate* diagram with the appropriate food groups.

17.

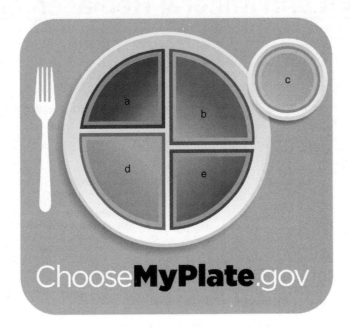

a. _____

b. _____

c. _____

d. _____

e. _____

NCLEX REVIEW QUESTIONS

Select the best response.

18. Regulation of calcium and phosphorous metabolism and calcium absorption from the intestine is a major role of which of the following vitamins?
    a. A
    b. B_{12}
    c. C
    d. D

19. The patient has just given birth, and the nurse is preparing to administer vitamin K to the newborn. The patient asks, "Why do you have to give that to my baby?" What is the nurse's best response?
    a. "It will help the baby's digestive tract work better."
    b. "Vitamin K helps a baby maintain its temperature."
    c. "Newborns are vitamin K–deficient at birth."
    d. "This will help prevent infections for the first month."

20. Protection of red blood cells from hemolysis is a role of which vitamin?
    a. A
    b. D
    c. E
    d. K

21. The patient presents for her annual well-woman exam. She states that she does not take any drugs but she knows she is supposed to take "some supplement in case I get pregnant." What is the nurse's best response?
    a. "Folic acid supplements are recommended in women who may become pregnant to prevent neural tube defects."
    b. "Vitamin A 8000 units should be taken to promote bone growth."
    c. "Megadoses of iron are important for blood formation."
    d. "Vitamin C 1600 mg should be taken to prevent colds, which are more common in pregnancy."

22. The patient has been involved in a motorcycle collision and has lost 1500 mL of blood from a pelvic fracture. Which mineral is essential for regeneration of hemoglobin?
    a. Chromium
    b. Copper
    c. Iron
    d. Selenium

23. The patient has a history of heavy alcohol abuse. He presents to the emergency department confused, combative, and complaining of double vision. The patient's family states he has become very forgetful recently. The nurse will anticipate that the provider will order which substance for this patient?
    a. Vitamin C
    b. Vitamin B_1
    c. Dextrose
    d. Vitamin B_6

24. Which vitamin or mineral is responsible for collagen synthesis?
    a. Vitamin C
    b. Vitamin D
    c. Iron
    d. Zinc

25. The patient takes an antacid for reflux and an iron supplement for anemia. What information will the nurse be sure to include in patient education regarding these drugs?
    a. "The drugs have a synergistic effect."
    b. "Iron and antacids must be taken on alternate days."
    c. "Antacids will decrease iron absorption."
    d. "Iron will decrease the effectiveness of the antacids."

26. A patient is advised to drink a liquid iron preparation through a straw because it may cause which effect?
    a. Bleeding gums
    b. Esophageal varices
    c. Corroded tooth enamel
    d. Tooth discoloration

27. Which patient might be most at risk for vitamin A deficiency?
    a. A 36-year-old pregnant patient
    b. An 18-year-old patient with celiac disease
    c. A 74-year-old patient with a urinary tract infection
    d. A 33-year-old patient with sickle cell anemia

28. Vitamin A is stored in the liver, kidneys, and fat. How is it excreted?
    a. Rapidly through the bile and feces
    b. Slowly through the urine and feces
    c. Rapidly through the bile only
    d. Slowly through the feces only

29. A 24-year-old patient has been prescribed large doses of vitamin A as treatment for acne. What will the nurse advise this patient? *(Select all that apply.)*
    a. Contact the health care provider concerning drug dosing.
    b. Report peeling skin, anorexia, or nausea and vomiting to the health care provider.
    c. Do not exceed the recommended dosage without consulting the health care provider.
    d. Avoid alcohol consumption.
    e. Megadoses of vitamin A are necessary for several months to alleviate acne.

30. The patient has a history of tuberculosis and is on isoniazid therapy. The patient presents to the clinic with complaints of numbness and weakness in his hands and feet. He has no other significant medical history. Which vitamin supplement might be considered for his condition?
    a. Niacin
    b. Pyridoxine
    c. Riboflavin
    d. Thiamine

31. The patient has sustained burns to 40% of his body and is receiving long-term parenteral nutrition. This patient is at risk for which mineral deficiency?
    a. Copper
    b. Iron
    c. Selenium
    d. Zinc

32. Chromium is thought to be helpful in control of which condition?
    a. Alzheimer disease
    b. Common cold
    c. Type 2 diabetes
    d. Raynaud phenomenon

33. Which food is high in copper?
    a. Broccoli
    b. Grapefruit
    c. Lamb
    d. Shellfish

34. The patient presents to the emergency department with an overdose of the oral anticoagulant warfarin. The nurse will anticipate administration of which vitamin for this patient?
   a. B_2
   b. C
   c. E
   d. K

CASE STUDY

Read the scenario and answer the following questions on a separate sheet of paper.

A patient with a history of atrial fibrillation and on the anticoagulant warfarin is seen in the clinic for routine blood work to monitor the INR. While obtaining the drug history, it was discovered that the patient has been taking various vitamins, including vitamins E, C, and A. The patient also has been on a "health conscious" diet, consuming large amounts of fresh fruits and vegetables and fresh fish.

1. Describe the mechanisms of action for vitamins A, C, and E and the potential complications of hypervitaminosis.

2. Discuss the drug–drug and drug–food interactions that can occur with warfarin.

3. What education should the nurse provide?

14 Nutritional Support

Complete the following.

1. Adequate nutritional support is needed for the body's _____ _____.

2. A critically ill person requires _____ more than the normal energy requirement.

3. In addition to nutritional support, _____ and _____ balance must be considered.

4. A _____ _____ _____ should be used when considering enteral nutrition.

5. The gastrostomy tube, also known as the _____ tube, is placed _____, _____, or _____.

Answer the following questions as true or false.

_____ 6. Early enteral nutrition restores intestinal motility and maintains GI function.

_____ 7. Nutritional support is considered if the patient has had little or no nutrition for more than 5 days.

_____ 8. Parenteral and enteral nutrition are synonymous and are delivered through the same route.

_____ 9. Nasoduodenal, nasojejunal, and jejunostomy enteral nutrition deliver food below the pyloric sphincter.

Label the following.

10. Label the routes for enteral feedings.

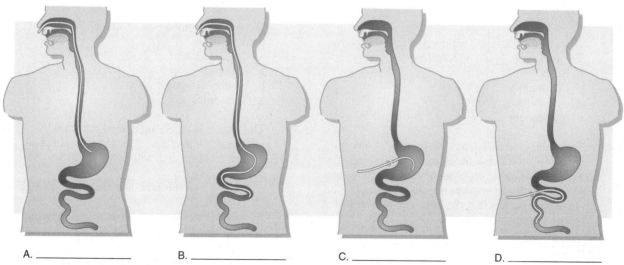

A. _____   B. _____   C. _____   D. _____

Match the terms in Column I with the descriptions in Column II.

Column I

_____ 11. Bolus

_____ 12. Intermittent

_____ 13. Continuous

_____ 14. Cyclic

Column II

a. Feeding given every 3–6 hours for 30–60 minutes by gravity infusion
b. Feeding given continuously into the small intestine
c. Feeding infused over 8–16 hours per day
d. 250–400 mL given at one time; used for ambulatory patients

NCLEX REVIEW QUESTIONS

Select the best response.

15. The older adult patient has a history of hypertension, arthritis, and diabetes. Which formula does the nurse anticipate will be ordered?
    a. Glucerna
    b. Ensure
    c. Criticare HN
    d. Peptamen

16. The patient with a functional GI system is at risk for aspiration because of difficulty swallowing. Which supplemental nutrition does the nurse anticipate will be ordered?
    a. Enteral via nasogastric tube
    b. Parenteral via peripheral IV
    c. Parenteral via central IV
    d. Enteral via jejunostomy tube

17. Ensure and Isocal are examples of which type of solution?
    a. Blenderized solutions
    b. Elemental or monomeric solutions
    c. Polymeric
    d. Modular

18. What type of enteral feeding is administered over 30–60 minutes by pump infusion?
    a. Bolus
    b. Continuous
    c. Gravity
    d. Intermittent

19. The patient is a full-time college student who sustained full-thickness burns to her face 2 months ago. She is now undergoing skin grafting and wound repair and requires nutritional support. The nurse understands that the best way to administer nutrition to this patient is
    a. continuous.
    b. cyclic.
    c. gravity.
    d. TPN.

20. The patient has ulcerative colitis and is in the midst of a flare-up. He has been prescribed TPN. Which site will the nurse select to administer TPN?
    a. Accessory vein
    b. Brachiocephalic vein
    c. Radial vein
    d. Subclavian vein

21. What is the average percentage of carbohydrates provided by TPN?
    a. <10%
    b. 10–20%
    c. 25–50%
    d. 60–70%

22. The patient has sustained a severe head injury and is on continuous tube feedings. These feedings are commonly infused
    a. over 30–60 minutes.
    b. over 24 hours.
    c. over 15 minutes.
    d. over 8–16 hours.

23. What is a common side effect associated with enteral nutrition?
    a. Constipation
    b. Diarrhea
    c. Urinary retention
    d. Yeast infection

24. The patient is receiving enteral nutrition by means of continual feeding. The nurse is checking for gastric residual and withdraws 170 mL. What is the best action by the nurse?
    a. Discontinue enteral nutrition and change to TPN.
    b. Immediately notify the health care provider.
    c. Stop the feeding for 30–60 minutes and recheck.
    d. Switch to a formula with more fiber.

25. What are the best reasons enteral feedings should be used before TPN? *(Select all that apply.)*
   a. Less costly
   b. Less risk of aspiration
   c. Lower risk of infection
   d. Maintenance of GI integrity
   e. Promotes better wound healing

26. Which complication(s) is/are associated with the use of TPN? *(Select all that apply.)*
   a. Air embolism
   b. Aspiration
   c. Hyperglycemia
   d. Pneumothorax

CASE STUDY

Read the scenario and answer the following questions on a separate sheet of paper.

M.B., 35 years old, sustained severe trauma from a rollover motor vehicle collision. He has been on TPN for several weeks and is being transitioned to enteral feeding through a nasogastric tube before a gastrostomy tube is placed.

1. What steps must be performed to transition a patient from TPN to enteral nutrition?

2. What precautions will the nurse take to prevent aspiration?

15 Adrenergic Agonists and Antagonists

Match the description in Column I with the letter of the reference in Column II.

Column I

_____ 1.   Alpha blocker

_____ 2.   Beta blocker

_____ 3.   Selectivity

_____ 4.   Sympathomimetic

_____ 5.   Sympatholytic

Column II

a.   Blocks action of sympathetic nervous system
b.   Has a greater affinity for certain receptors
c.   Causes vasodilation
d.   Causes decreased heart rate
e.   Similar in action to stimulation of the sympathetic nervous system

Complete the following.

6.   Adrenergic receptors are located on the _____ cells of smooth muscles.

7.   Bladder relaxation and urinary sphincter constriction resulting in urinary retention may occur with high doses of _____ agonists.

8.   Sympathomimetics (do/do not) pass into the breast milk. *(Circle correct answer.)*

9.   Adrenergic blockers are also called _____.

10.   The antidote for IV infiltration of alpha- and beta-adrenergic drugs such as norepinephrine and dopamine is _____.

11.   A beta-adrenergic blocker that can be given for migraine or hypertension is _____.

12.   Mood changes such as depression and suicidal tendencies are possible when taking which type of adrenergic blocker? _____

13.   Carvedilol, penbutolol, and pindolol are examples of selective/nonselective beta blockers. *(Circle correct answer.)*

14.   Nonselective beta blockers, such as propranolol, are contraindicated in patients with _____ and _____.

15.   What is most likely to occur if a patient is taking an adrenergic agonist with an adrenergic blocker? _____

Match the letter of the receptor in Column II with the associated adrenergic response in Column I. (Answers may be used more than once, and response may affect more than one receptor type.)

Column I

_____ 16. Increases gastrointestinal relaxation

_____ 17. Increases force of heart contraction

_____ 18. Dilates pupils

_____ 19. Decreases salivary secretions

_____ 20. Inhibits release of norepinephrine

_____ 21. Dilates bronchioles

_____ 22. Increases heart rate

_____ 23. Promotes uterine relaxation

_____ 24. Dilates blood vessels

Column II

a. Alpha$_1$
b. Alpha$_2$
c. Beta$_1$
d. Beta$_2$

NCLEX REVIEW QUESTIONS

Select the best response.

25. A patient with asthma asks the nurse how his albuterol inhaler will work to help him breathe better. What is the best response for the nurse to explain the action of the drug?
    a. "Albuterol will increase your heart rate so you will feel like you are able to breathe better."
    b. "Albuterol causes bronchodilation in the lungs, improving function."
    c. "Albuterol will cause an increase in urinary output to remove extra fluid from the lungs."
    d. "Albuterol causes bronchial smooth muscle contraction that forces air into the lungs."

26. A patient presents to the clinic with a swollen face and tongue, difficulty breathing, and audible wheezes after eating a peanut butter sandwich for lunch. What is the first action the nurse should take?
    a. Ensure a patent airway.
    b. Obtain an electrocardiogram (ECG).
    c. Administer 1 mg of 1:1000 epinephrine subcut.
    d. Start an IV of normal saline.

27. A patient calls the home health agency to tell the nurse she is having a reaction to her albuterol inhaler. She tells the nurse she is shaking and trembling. What is the first question the nurse should ask the patient?
    a. "Are you having any other symptoms?"
    b. "How long ago did this start?"
    c. "When was the last time you used your inhaler?"
    d. "How many puffs on the inhaler did you take?"

28. Which drug(s) is/are classified as beta blockers? (*Select all that apply.*)
    a. Albuterol
    b. Atenolol
    c. Propranolol
    d. Amphetamine
    e. Acebutolol

29. The nurse discovers an IV has infiltrated on a patient receiving IV dopamine. The nurse prepares to administer _____ as an antidote.
    a. dobutamine
    b. epinephrine
    c. phentolamine
    d. reserpine

30. When completing the patient health history, the nurse finds a history of narrow-angle glaucoma. When performing the drug reconciliation, which drug would concern the nurse? (*Select all that apply.*)
    a. Pseudoephedrine
    b. Midodrine
    c. Albuterol
    d. Carvedilol

31. Some over-the-counter (OTC) medications for cold symptoms contain substances that have sympathetic properties. These drugs are contraindicated in patients with which disease process?
    a. Allergic rhinitis
    b. Hypertension
    c. Orthostatic hypotension
    d. Chronic bronchitis

32. Which adrenergic drug used in emergency settings does not decrease renal function?
    a. Norepinephrine
    b. Dopamine
    c. Phenylephrine
    d. Dobutamine

33. Where are beta$_1$ receptors located? *(Select all that apply.)*
    a. Gastrointestinal tract
    b. Lungs
    c. Kidneys
    d. Brain
    e. Heart

34. A patient tells the nurse during the admitting history that he utilizes alternative and complementary therapies to help manage his medical conditions. Which drug would raise a concern in a patient taking St. John's wort?
    a. Reserpine
    b. Albuterol
    c. Propranolol
    d. Pseudoephedrine

35. The nurse has been floated to the cardiac telemetry unit and is preparing to give a new drug to the patient. The health care provider's order is for timolol 100 mg b.i.d. Which is the nurse's best action?
    a. Give the patient the drug after proper identification.
    b. Hold the drug, and contact the health care provider regarding the dosage.
    c. Give the drug now, and request a new order during patient rounds.
    d. Assess the patient's vital signs, and give the drug.

36. What is a catecholamine?
    a. A substance that can produce a sympathomimetic response
    b. Another name for a beta blocker
    c. A type of decongestant
    d. A receptor site in the lungs

CASE STUDY

Read the scenario, and answer the following questions on a separate sheet of paper.

R.G. is a 34-year-old patient who sustained a bee sting and had an allergic reaction. He has been prescribed an epinephrine auto-injector.

1. What are the mechanisms of action and indications for the epinephrine auto-injector?

2. How should the drug be stored?

3. Describe how the patient should administer the drug.

16 Cholinergic Agonists and Antagonists

Match the term in Column I with the definition in Column II.

Column I

_____ 1.   Acetylcholine

_____ 2.   Anticholinergic

_____ 3.   Anticholinesterase

_____ 4.   Cholinergic agonists

_____ 5.   Cholinesterase

_____ 6.   Muscarinic receptor

_____ 7.   Nicotinic receptor

_____ 8.   Parasympathomimetic

Column II

a.   Stimulates smooth muscle and slows heart rate
b.   Impacts skeletal muscles
c.   Stimulates muscarinic and nicotinic receptors
d.   Types of drugs that stimulate the parasympathetic system
e.   Blocks the action of acetylcholine
f.   Mimics cholinergic actions
g.   Blocks the breakdown of acetylcholine
h.   Causes the breakdown of acetylcholine

Labeling

9.   Identify the parts of the parasympathetic nervous system and its cholinergic effects to the different organs.

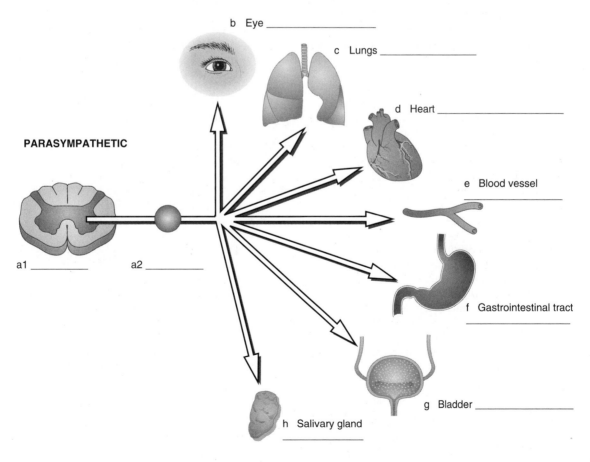

PARASYMPATHETIC

a1 _____   a2 _____

b Eye _____

c Lungs _____

d Heart _____

e Blood vessel _____

f Gastrointestinal tract
_____

g Bladder _____

h Salivary gland
_____

Select the best response.

10. The patient has ingested an organophosphate poison in a suicide attempt. What drug does the nurse anticipate the health care provider will order to treat this patient?
    a. Bethanechol
    b. Edrophonium chloride
    c. Metoclopramide
    d. Pralidoxime chloride

11. The pediatric patient has urinary retention. Which cholinergic drug does the nurse anticipate will be prescribed to increase urination?
    a. Bethanechol
    b. Edrophonium chloride
    c. Metoclopramide
    d. Neostigmine bromide

12. The patient is scheduled for a comprehensive eye examination. Anticholinergic eyedrops are used for which purpose?
    a. Constrict the pupils
    b. Dilate the pupils
    c. Decrease the intraocular pressure
    d. Detect astigmatism

13. The 80-year-old patient has narrow-angle glaucoma and is prescribed an anticholinergic drug. What is the nurse's priority action?
    a. Administer the medication as ordered after verifying the patient's identity.
    b. Give only one-half of the prescribed dose.
    c. Hold the dose, and contact the health care provider.
    d. Wait until after the patient has taken glaucoma medication and then give the drug.

14. Which type of medication is bethanechol?
    a. Anticholinergic
    b. Cholinergic agonist
    c. Cholinesterase inhibitor
    d. Sympatholytic

15. How does bethanechol work in the body?
    a. Inhibits muscarinic receptors
    b. Inhibits nicotinic receptors
    c. Stimulates muscarinic receptors
    d. Stimulates nicotinic receptors

16. The patient has been prescribed bethanechol and asks the nurse how it works. What is the nurse's best response?
    a. "This drug decreases bladder tone."
    b. "This drug inhibits bladder contraction."
    c. "This drug promotes contraction of the bladder."
    d. "This drug stimulates urine production."

17. How does the body respond to large doses of cholinergic drugs? *(Select all that apply.)*
    a. Decreased blood pressure
    b. Decreased salivation
    c. Increased bronchial secretions
    d. Mydriasis
    e. Urinary retention

18. The patient has been prescribed bethanechol and is experiencing decreased urinary output. What is the nurse's priority action?
    a. Catheterize the patient to drain the bladder and measure output.
    b. Encourage the patient to increase fluid intake to increase urinary output.
    c. Encourage the patient to relax when urinating.
    d. Notify the health care provider with current intake and output values.

19. The patient has been taking bethanechol and is experiencing flushing, sweating, nausea, and abdominal cramps. What is the nurse's best action?
    a. Document the patient's manifestations.
    b. Give the patient a laxative.
    c. Increase the patient's fluid intake.
    d. Prepare to administer atropine.

20. Which medication treats myasthenia gravis by increasing muscle strength?
    a. Bethanechol
    b. Edrophonium chloride
    c. Neostigmine bromide
    d. Pilocarpine

21. The nurse is taking care of five patients in the emergency department. Which patient(s) would be candidate(s) to receive atropine? *(Select all that apply.)*
    a. A 25-year-old having surgery for appendicitis
    b. A 42-year-old with a heart rate of 38 beats/minute and dizziness
    c. A 50-year-old with paralytic ileus
    d. A 61-year-old with urinary retention
    e. A 68-year-old with gastric ulcers

22. The nurse would question an order for atropine for which patient?
    a. A 35-year-old with a peptic ulcer
    b. A 50-year-old with parkinsonism
    c. A 55-year-old with cirrhosis
    d. A 60-year-old with narrow-angle glaucoma

23. The patient is admitted for evaluation of peptic ulcers. She is taking propantheline three times per day. The nurse is teaching this patient about nutrition while taking this drug. The priority nutrition teaching point is that the patient should eat foods that are high in which component?
    a. Calcium
    b. Fat
    c. Fiber
    d. Protein

24. What teaching point(s) will the nurse include for a 30-year-old patient who is taking hyoscyamine for irritable bowel syndrome? *(Select all that apply.)*
    a. Ensure adequate fluid intake.
    b. Do not drive until you are aware of how this drug will affect your vision.
    c. Sucking on hard candy may help with dry mouth.
    d. Increased sweating is a common side effect.
    e. Report a rapid heart rate to your health care provider.

25. Anticholinergic drugs are contraindicated in patients with which other disease processes? *(Select all that apply.)*
    a. Coronary artery disease
    b. Diabetes mellitus
    c. Gastrointestinal obstruction
    d. Supraventricular tachycardia

26. A specific group of anticholinergics may be prescribed in the early treatment of which neuromuscular disorder?
    a. Multiple sclerosis
    b. Muscular dystrophy
    c. Myasthenia gravis
    d. Parkinsonism

27. The older adult patient is taking benztropine for symptoms associated with parkinsonism. The nurse will instruct the patient to report which clinical manifestation(s) to the health care provider? *(Select all that apply.)*
    a. Diarrhea
    b. Dizziness
    c. Hallucinations
    d. Hyperthermia
    e. Palpitations

CASE STUDY

Read the scenario, and answer the following questions on a separate sheet of paper.

H.H., 65 years old, has just received a prescription for tolterodine tartrate for treatment of urinary incontinence.

1. What is the mechanism of action of this drug?

2. What are some of the major side effects?

3. What are some contraindications?

4. Discuss key teaching points for the nurse to provide when educating the patient.

Chapter **16** Cholinergic Agonists and Antagonists

17 Stimulants

STUDY QUESTIONS

Complete the following.

1. The central nervous system involves the _____ and _____ _____.

2. Attention-deficit/hyperactivity disorder can be caused by a _____ of neurotransmitters.

3. Amphetamines stimulate the release of neurotransmitters _____ and _____, and can lead to cardiovascular problems.

4. Anorexiants have a/an _____ effect on the brain to _____ _____.

5. Central nervous system stimulants, also referred to as _____, stimulate respiration.

NCLEX REVIEW QUESTIONS

Select the best response.

6. Which medical condition(s) is/are central nervous system (CNS) stimulants approved to treat? *(Select all that apply.)*
   a. Attention-deficit/hyperactivity disorder (ADHD)
   b. Anorexia
   c. Narcolepsy
   d. Obesity
   e. Posttraumatic stress disorder

7. A new nurse is admitting a patient who has received doxapram. The nurse recognizes that this is which type of drug?
   a. Inhaled respiratory stimulant
   b. Narcotic antagonist
   c. Postanesthetic respiratory stimulant
   d. Long-acting narcotic

8. The patient has been prescribed methylphenidate for the treatment of narcolepsy. What priority teaching consideration(s) should be included for this patient? *(Select all that apply.)*
   a. Avoid operating hazardous equipment.
   b. Caffeine should be avoided.
   c. Nervousness and tremors may occur.
   d. Take the medication before meals.
   e. Report any weight gain.

9. Which drug group acts on the brainstem and medulla to stimulate respiration?
   a. Amphetamine
   b. Analeptic
   c. Anorexiant
   d. Triptan

10. The patient is being treated with methylphenidate for attention-deficit/hyperactivity disorder (ADHD). What common side/adverse effect(s) should the patient and family be informed might occur? *(Select all that apply.)*
    a. Euphoria
    b. Headache
    c. Hypertension
    d. Irritability
    e. Orthostatic hypotension
    f. Vomiting

11. To maintain the half-life of immediate-release methylphenidate, how often should this drug be taken?
    a. Daily
    b. 2 to 3 times a day
    c. 4 times a day
    d. Every other day

12. The patient has been prescribed phentermine hydrochloride for obesity. The patient also has Parkinson"s disease and takes selegiline. What should the nurse do before the patient starts the new drug?
   a. Contact the patient's primary health care provider to verify the prescription.
   b. Have baseline lab work drawn to assess liver function.
   c. Tell the patient to immediately stop taking the selegiline.
   d. Tell the patient to increase fluid intake with the next meal.

13. The patient has a history of migraines, depression, and hypertension and has been started on phentermine-topiramate. For which condition is phentermine-topiramate used?
   a. Attention-deficit/hyperactivity disorder (ADHD)
   b. Asthma
   c. Narcolepsy
   d. Short-term weight management

14. The pediatric patient has been started on methylphenidate for attention-deficit/hyperactivity disorder (ADHD). What information should the nurse include in the health teaching?
   a. Constipation is a common side effect.
   b. Counseling should be combined with drug.
   c. This drug will only be used for a few weeks.
   d. Weight gain is to be expected.

15. Which statement(s) is/are true of methylphenidate? *(Select all that apply.)*
   a. If taken with monoamine oxidase inhibitors (MAOIs), it may increase a hypertensive crisis.
   b. The effects of anticoagulants may increase.
   c. Hyperglycemia may occur.
   d. Insulin will be more effective.
   e. There may be increased effects if taken with caffeinated beverages.

16. The 18-year-old patient is brought to the emergency department by her roommates. Her blood pressure is 220/136 mm Hg, heart rate 142 beats/minute, and respiratory rate 20 breaths/minute. She is responsive only to deep pain. Her roommates say she has been trying to lose weight and has been taking "these pills she gets over the Internet." What will the nurse consider as the most likely cause for this patient's symptoms?
   a. Cardiac arrest
   b. Food poisoning
   c. Hemorrhagic stroke
   d. Pregnancy-induced hypertension

17. Central nervous system (CNS) stimulants are absolutely contraindicated for patients with a history of which condition(s)? *(Select all that apply.)*
   a. Coronary artery disease
   b. Diabetes
   c. Hypothyroidism
   d. Hypertension
   e. Glaucoma

18. The patient is born at 28 weeks' gestation and is scheduled to receive caffeine citrate 20 mg IV shortly after birth. The patient's mother asks, "Why are you giving my baby stuff that is in coffee?" What is the nurse's best response?
   a. "Caffeine can help your baby breathe better."
   b. "It will help your baby gain weight faster."
   c. "The baby's temperature will be warmer with caffeine."
   d. "This isn't the same substance that is in coffee."

CASE STUDY

Read the scenario, and answer the following question on a separate sheet of paper.

A new nurse at a school where there are more than 75 students who take methylphenidate for attention-deficit/hyperactivity disorder (ADHD). The majority of the students come in between 11:30 AM and 12:30 PM for their drug.

1. What is the pharmacokinetics and pharmacodynamics for methylphenidate?

2. What are the nursing implications for giving these drugs at school regarding timing, monitoring, and health teaching for the students, families, and teachers?

18 Depressants

STUDY QUESTIONS

Identify the induction time for the following anesthetics—slow or rapid:

1. Halothane _____

2. Enflurane _____

3. Methoxyflurane _____

4. Midazolam _____

5. Propofol _____

6. Nitrous oxide _____

Complete the following.

7. The broad classification of CNS depressants includes the following seven groups: _____, _____, _____, _____, _____, _____, and _____.

8. The two phases of sleep are _____ and _____.

9. The mildest form of CNS depression is _____.

10. Anesthesia (may/may not) be achieved with high doses of sedative-hypnotics. *(Circle correct answer.)*

11. Procaine hydrochloride is used in local anesthesia as a short/moderate/long-acting anesthetic *(Circle correct answer.)*

12. General anesthesia depresses the _____ system, alleviates _____, and causes a loss of _____.

13. Surgery is performed during the _____ stage of anesthesia. The other three stages are _____, _____, and _____.

14. Bupivacaine and tetracaine are drugs commonly used for _____ anesthesia.

15. A major potential adverse effect of spinal anesthesia is _____.

16. A type of spinal anesthesia used for patients in labor is a(n) _____.

17. Muscle relaxants (are/are not) part of balanced anesthesia. *(Circle correct answer.)*

18. Drugs used to induce sleep in those who have difficulty getting to sleep are _____-acting barbiturates.

19. One example of a nonbenzodiazepine drug for the treatment of insomnia is _____. (*Answers may vary.*).

20. The drug of choice for the management of benzodiazepine overdose is _____.

21. Local anesthetics are divided into two groups: _____ and _____.

Match the letter of the description in Column II with the common side effect of sedative-hypnotics in Column I.

Column I

_____ 22. Hangover

_____ 23. REM rebound

_____ 24. Dependence

_____ 25. Tolerance

_____ 26. Respiratory depression

_____ 27. Hypersensitivity

Column II

a. Need to increase dosage to get desired effect
b. Suppression of respiratory center in the medulla
c. Skin rashes
d. Residual drowsiness
e. Results in withdrawal symptoms
f. Vivid dreams and nightmares

NCLEX REVIEW QUESTIONS

Select the best response.

28. What is the most commonly prescribed drug to assist patients with sleep disorders?
    a. Analeptic
    b. Anesthetic
    c. Sedative-hypnotic
    d. Triptan

29. The patient has been diagnosed with a seizure disorder. The nurse knows that which drugs may be prescribed to control seizures?
    a. Intermediate-acting barbiturates
    b. Long-acting barbiturates
    c. Short-acting barbiturates
    d. Ultra–short-acting barbiturates

30. A patient returns to the unit after having surgery with spinal anesthesia. What does the nurse know is/are the best action(s) to take to decrease the possibility of spinal headache? (Select all that apply.)
    a. Administer morphine 1 to 2 mg IV.
    b. Ambulate the patient as soon as she regains sensation.
    c. Encourage the patient to stay flat in bed.
    d. Increase fluid intake.
    e. Position the patient in high-Fowler's position.

31. The 61-year-old patient will be receiving spinal anesthesia for surgery. She states, "Why do I have to sit a certain way? Why can't I just be comfortable?" What is the nurse's best response?
    a. "It is easier for the anesthesiologist if you sit this way."
    b. "Because of your age, you have to sit straight up."
    c. "The anesthesia is injected in a specific area so it distributes evenly."
    d. "You can sit however you like."

32. The patient is postoperative day 3 from major orthopedic surgery and is unable to sleep. If nonpharmacologic measures have not been effective, what drug does the nurse anticipate may be ordered?
    a. Flumazenil
    b. Phenobarbital
    c. Triazolam
    d. Zolpidem

33. Which type(s) of anesthesia is/are administered using lidocaine? (*Select all that apply.*)
    a. General
    b. Inhaled
    c. Intravenous
    d. Local
    e. Spinal

34. The patient works 12-hour night shifts one week and 12-hour day shifts the next week. He tells the nurse he has been taking "some kind of sleeping pill from the drugstore." What does the nurse suspect is the most likely main ingredient in the over-the-counter sleep drug?
   a. Antihistamines
   b. Barbiturates
   c. Benzodiazepines
   d. Melatonin

35. The 71-year-old patient presents to the health care provider with complaints of inability to go to sleep and inability to stay asleep. What question(s) will the nurse ask to further evaluate her complaint? *(Select all that apply.)*
   a. "Do you have a bedtime routine?"
   b. "How many caffeinated beverages do you drink per day?"
   c. "Do you take naps?"
   d. "Do you sleep with the windows open?"
   e. "Are you taking diuretics?"

36. What is/are the possible complication(s) of spinal anesthesia? *(Select all that apply.)*
   a. Drowsiness
   b. Dysrhythmias
   c. Dizziness
   d. Headache
   e. Hypertension
   f. Respiratory distress

CASE STUDY

Read the scenario, and answer the following questions on a separate sheet of paper.

F.B., 42 years old, is scheduled for a laparoscopic cholecystectomy next week. She has had a bad experience with anesthesia before and is very anxious.

1. What drugs might be prescribed before her surgery for anxiety?

2. Explain the principles of balanced anesthesia.

19 Antiseizure Drugs

Match the seizure type in Column I with its definition in Column II.

1. Absence seizure
2. Partial seizure
3. Generalized seizure
4. Myoclonic seizure
5. Simple seizure

a. Involves one hemisphere of the brain with no loss of consciousness
b. Can be focal or massive with jerky movements lasting 10 seconds or less
c. No loss of consciousness and can have a motor, sensory, autonomic, or psychic form
d. Loss of consciousness usually lasts less than 10 seconds; also called petit mal seizures
e. A seizure that involves both hemispheres of the brain with loss of consciousness

Complete the following.

6. To diagnose epilepsy, results of a(n) _____ are useful.

7. Seventy-five percent of all epilepsy is considered to be primary or _____.

8. The International Classification of Seizures describes the two categories of seizures as _____ and

   _____.

9. Anticonvulsant drugs suppress abnormal electrical impulses, thus _____ the seizure, but they (do/do not) eliminate the cause. *(Circle correct answer.)*

10. Anticonvulsants (are/are not) used for all types of seizures. *(Circle correct answer.)*

11. The first anticonvulsant used to treat seizures was _____, discovered in 1938, and today is the most commonly used drug for seizures.

12. It is strongly recommended that the patient check with the health care provider before taking _____ preparations.

13. Administration of phenytoin via the (oral/intramuscular/intravenous) route is not recommended because of its erratic absorption rate. *(Circle correct answer.)*

NCLEX REVIEW QUESTIONS

Select the best response.

14. The patient with a history of bipolar disorder recently experienced tonic-clonic seizures. Which drug would the nurse expect to be prescribed for this patient? *(Select all that apply.)*
    a. Carbamazepine
    b. Diazepam
    c. Ethosuximide
    d. Acetazolamide

15. The patient has a seizure disorder and has just discovered that she is pregnant. At her first prenatal visit, she tells the nurse, "I quit taking all of my drugs because I don't want anything to be wrong with my baby." What is the nurse's best response?
    a. "You can't do that. You have to take your medications."
    b. "What drugs have been prescribed for you?"
    c. "How long have you had seizures?"
    d. "When was your last seizure?"

16. Which anticonvulsant(s) is/are appropriate for status epilepticus? *(Select all that apply.)*
    a. Fosphenytoin
    b. Carbamazepine
    c. Phenobarbital
    d. Diazepam
    e. Topiramate

17. The patient has just been diagnosed with epilepsy and will be starting phenytoin. The patient's spouse asks how this drug works in the body. What is the nurse's best response?
    a. "It inhibits the enzyme that destroys one of the neurotransmitters."
    b. "It helps stop the entry of sodium into the cell."
    c. "It has not been determined exactly how it prevents seizures."
    d. "It increases the amount of calcium that enters the cell."

18. The patient has just been diagnosed with a seizure disorder and has been started on valproic acid. What statement(s) by the patient indicate(s) to the nurse the patient needs more instruction regarding his drug? *(Select all that apply.)*
    a. "I just have to remember to take it once a day."
    b. "I do not have to worry about labs."
    c. "I need to take it at the same times every day."
    d. "This drug will cure my seizures."

19. The nurse has received an order to administer an initial dose of IV phenytoin to a patient with new-onset seizures. What will the nurse check before administering the first dose? *(Select all that apply.)*
    a. Hourly urine output
    b. Blood glucose levels
    c. Cardiac rhythm
    d. Blood pressure measurements

20. The nurse is working on a neurosurgery unit. The patient calls the desk to complain that his arm is really burning and feels hot. The patient is receiving IV phenytoin for his grand mal seizures. What is the nurse's best action?
    a. Call the health care provider immediately to change the drug to oral.
    b. Continue the infusion and reassure the patient.
    c. Flush the line with 10 mL of normal saline and continue the infusion.
    d. Discontinue the IV and restart the IV infusion at a different site.

21. A 38-year-old male patient has been started on an anticonvulsant for a seizure disorder of unknown cause and asks how long he will need to take the drug. What is the nurse's best response?
    a. "You will need to take an anticonvulsant of some type for your lifetime."
    b. "This drug should be taken until you haven't had a seizure for a month."
    c. "Seizures are unpredictable and so is the duration of the treatment."
    d. "You will only need to take it for a short period of time because anticonvulsants will cure the seizure disorder."

22. Phenytoin levels must be monitored carefully because there is a narrow therapeutic range. Which result is within the therapeutic range?
    a. 8 mcg/mL
    b. 18 mcg/mL
    c. 28 mcg/mL
    d. 38 mcg/mL

23. A nurse working triage in the emergency department witnesses a patient having a seizure. What information will be included in the nurse's documentation? *(Select all that apply.)*
    a. Types of movements
    b. Duration of movements
    c. Ability to stop movements
    d. Progression of movements
    e. Preceding events

24. The nurse is preparing discharge teaching for a patient who has been started on phenytoin for a seizure disorder. What information about side effects of this drug should the nurse provide to the patient and his family?
    a. "There may be a green discoloration of the patient's urine."
    b. "It is best to use a hard-bristle toothbrush for dental care."
    c. "Nosebleeds and sore throats should be reported to the health care provider."
    d. "The patient should get up slowly to prevent fainting."

25. What would the nurse expect to see if the patient is experiencing a common side effect of phenytoin?
    a. Gingival hyperplasia
    b. Excessive thirst
    c. Weight gain
    d. Muscle tremors

26. A patient presents to the emergency department in status epilepticus. Which drug would the nurse anticipate to be ordered first?
   a. Diazepam
   b. Midazolam
   c. Propofol
   d. Phenobarbital

27. Which statement(s) is/are true about seizures and anticonvulsant use in pregnancy? *(Select all that apply.)*
   a. Seizures may increase up to 25% in epileptic women.
   b. Many anticonvulsants have teratogenic properties.
   c. Anticonvulsant use increases loss of folic acid.
   d. Anticonvulsants increase the effects of vitamin K.
   e. Valproic acid causes malformation in 40% to 80% of fetuses.

28. Which anticonvulsant may also be used as prophylaxis for migraine headaches?
   a. Diazepam
   b. Phenytoin
   c. Valproic acid
   d. Clorazepate

CASE STUDY

Read the scenario, and answer the following question on a separate sheet of paper.

A 30-year-old elementary school teacher has missed several appointments with her primary care provider. She has a history of tonic-clonic seizure activity. She states, "I just can't take the carbamazepine. I can't function with it." Her provider prescribes oxcarbazepine.

1. What will the nurse discuss with the patient regarding oxcarbazepine?

2. What information should the nurse provide about antiseizure drugs and pregnancy?

20 Drugs for Parkinsonism and Alzheimer Disease

Match the description in Column I with the letter of the reference in Column II.

Column I

_____ 1. Acetylcholinesterase inhibitor

_____ 2. Dopamine agonist

_____ 3. Dystonic movement

_____ 4. Bradykinesia

_____ 5. Pseudo parkinsonism

Column II

a. Stimulates dopamine receptors
b. Adverse reaction to drugs, exposure to poisons, or disorders
c. Allows more acetylcholine in the neuron receptors
d. Involuntary abnormal movements
e. Slowed movements

Complete the following.

6. The two neurotransmitters within the neurons of the striatum of the brain that have opposing effects are

   _____ and _____.

7. Which of the neurotransmitters is deficient in parkinsonism? _____

8. A drug used in a combination therapy to treat parkinsonism by replacing the neurotransmitter is _____.

9. The substance that inhibits the enzyme dopa decarboxylase and allows more levodopa to reach the brain is

   _____.

10. An example of an acetylcholinesterase inhibitor is _____.

11. Acetylcholinesterase inhibitors _____ transmission at the cholinergic synapses.

12. The drug _____ prolongs action of levodopa and can decrease "on-off" fluctuations in patients with parkinsonism.

13. The drugs that are a combination of dopaminergic and a COMT inhibitor that provides the greatest dosing flexibility include _____, _____, and _____.

14. An example of a Food and Drug Administration (FDA)–approved anticholinergic drug used for parkinsonism is

   _____.

Select the best response.

15. The nurse is administering a carbidopa-levodopa tablet to an older adult patient with parkinsonism. Which order(s) would the nurse question before administering the medication? *(Select all that apply.)*
    a. Carbidopa 5 mg/levodopa 50 mg tid
    b. Carbidopa 10 mg/levodopa 100 mg tid
    c. Carbidopa 15 mg/levodopa 150 mg tid
    d. Carbidopa 20 mg/levodopa 200 mg tid
    e. Carbidopa 25 mg/levodopa 250 mg tid

16. A patient taking carbidopa-levodopa tablets for parkinsonism is complaining of dizziness, diarrhea, anxiety, and nasal stuffiness. Which of these complaints does the nurse recognize as a possible side effect of carbidopa-levodopa?
    a. Dizziness
    b. Diarrhea
    c. Anxiety
    d. Nasal stuffiness

17. The nurse is teaching a patient with parkinsonism about extended-release carbidopa-levodopa. Which statement(s) by the patient indicate(s) the need for further teaching? *(Select all that apply.)*
    a. "This drug may make my movements smoother."
    b. "My skin may turn yellow if I miss too many doses."
    c. "If I have trouble swallowing, I can crush my drug and mix it with applesauce."
    d. "I must take this medicine on an empty stomach."
    e. "I need to check my blood sugar regularly while taking this drug."

18. The nurse is helping a family prepare for a grocery shopping trip for a patient who has been prescribed selegiline. Which food(s) should be avoided? *(Select all that apply.)*
    a. Aged cheeses
    b. Chocolate
    c. Peanut butter
    d. Wheat bread
    e. Yogurt

19. A patient with Alzheimer's disease is taking rivastigmine and has also been started on a drug for depression. Which order will the nurse question before administering the new drug?
    a. Atypical antidepressant
    b. Monoamine oxidase inhibitor (MAOI) antidepressant
    c. Selective serotonin reuptake inhibitor (SSRI) antidepressant
    d. Tricyclic antidepressant

20. A patient with parkinsonism currently takes carbidopa-levodopa, and the patient's health care provider adds the drug entacapone to the patient's drug regimen. What would the nurse expect to occur with the carbidopa-levodopa dosing?
    a. There should be no change in the drug dosage.
    b. Both carbidopa and levodopa dosages should be decreased.
    c. Only the levodopa dosage should decrease.
    d. Only the carbidopa dosage should decrease.

21. Anticholinergics are contraindicated for which patient(s)? *(Select all that apply.)*
    a. A 45-year-old with glaucoma
    b. A 60-year-old with shingles
    c. A 65-year-old with urinary frequency
    d. A 71-year-old with diabetes
    e. A 77-year-old with angina

22. A patient with a history of parkinsonism is brought into the emergency department after the family reports the patient is talking to "rabbits coming out of the walls" at home. Which drug does the nurse suspect may have caused this symptom? *(Select all that apply.)*
    a. Bromocriptine mesylate
    b. Selegiline hydrochloride
    c. Pramipexole dihydrochloride
    d. Tolcapone

23. A patient's wandering and hostility levels have increased per family reports. What should concern the nurse in this patient who is taking memantine 10 mg/day?
    a. The patient is taking too high a daily dose to maintain mental status.
    b. The patient has taken an overdose of the drug.
    c. The patient is not taking enough of the drug.
    d. The patient needs to take a combination of memantine and amantadine.

24. What statement by the patient indicates an understanding of how to relieve some of the side effects associated with the use of benztropine mesylate?
   a. "I can suck on hard candy or chew sugarless gum to prevent dry mouth."
   b. "I need to take my drug every 6 hours so I don't get constipated."
   c. "I should decrease the doses of all of my other drugs so I don't get dizzy."
   d. "I should urinate after meals so I do not retain urine."

CASE STUDY

Read the scenario, and answer the following questions on a separate sheet of paper.

J.T. is a 75-year-old woman who has been diagnosed with Alzheimer's disease. She will be living with her daughter and granddaughter. J.T.'s health care provider has prescribed rivastigmine 3 mg bid.

1. Explain the progressive decline of Alzheimer's disease.

2. How does rivastigmine work?

3. What are some of the safety measures the daughter and granddaughter can utilize to help the patient stay safe in her new home?

21 Drugs for Neuromuscular Disorders and Muscle Spasms

STUDY QUESTIONS

Match the definition in Column II to the classifications of multiple sclerosis in Column I.

Column I

_____ 1. Relapsing remitting MS

_____ 2. Primary progressive MS

_____ 3. Secondary progressive MS

_____ 4. Progressive relapsing MS

Column II

a. May have relapses, remissions, and plateaus
b. Relapse with full recovery and residual deficit
c. Clear acute relapses with or without full recovery
d. Will have slowly worsening symptoms with no relapses or remissions

Complete the following.

5. Muscle spasms can result from _____ injuries and spasticity from chronic _____ _____.

6. Muscle relaxants suppress the _____ reflex and are prescribed for muscle spasms that do not respond

to _____ drugs or other forms of therapy.

7. Baclofen, dantrolene, and tizanidine are some drugs to _____ pain and _____ mobility for hyperexcitable, spastic muscles.

SHORT ANSWER QUESTIONS

Identify the affected neuromuscular site(s) for each of the autoimmune neuromuscular disorders and the drugs to treat the disorders.

8. Myasthenia gravis

9. Multiple sclerosis

Select the best response.

10. The patient is receiving treatment for myasthenia gravis with pyridostigmine. The nurse is assessing the patient. What clinical manifestations would be noted if the drug is working?
    a. Increased salivation
    b. Maintenance of muscle strength
    c. Miosis
    d. Tachycardia

11. The patient is receiving treatment for myasthenia gravis with an acetylcholinesterase inhibitor. The nurse observes that the patient is drooling, her eyes are tearing, and she is diaphoretic. What will concern the nurse about the patient exhibiting these clinical manifestations?
    a. She is having an anaphylactic reaction.
    b. She is having a cholinergic crisis.
    c. She is in the early stages of myasthenic crisis.
    d. She is having a vascular spasm.

12. What emergency medication will be administered to a patient exhibiting the signs of cholinergic crisis?
    a. Atropine
    b. Diazepam
    c. Edrophonium
    d. Pyridostigmine

13. The patient presents to her health care provider with complaints of double vision, headache, and muscle weakness. She states that these symptoms come and go every few weeks, but her "spells" seem to be getting closer together. If her health care provider is considering a diagnosis of multiple sclerosis, what test is likely to be ordered?
    a. Angiography
    b. Computerized tomography (CT) scan
    c. Magnetic resonance imaging (MRI)
    d. Myelogram

14. The patient has been receiving pyridostigmine. Which drug when ordered by the health care provider should the nurse question before administering to the patient?
    a. Histamine$_2$ blocker
    b. Propranolol
    c. Cephalosporin
    d. Tetracycline

15. The patient has had multiple sclerosis for several years, during which time he has had many remissions and exacerbations. He has been prescribed azathioprine and interferon-β. The patient inquires, "How will this help me feel better?" What is the nurse's best response?
    a. "These drugs will help form new neurons and axons."
    b. "They will improve muscle strength."
    c. "They will reduce spasticity and improve muscular movement."
    d. "They will stop the progression of the disease."

16. The patient has multiple sclerosis and is experiencing muscle spasms. How will centrally acting muscle relaxants improve his status?
    a. They affect mu receptors to decrease pain.
    b. They decrease pain and increase range of motion.
    c. They decrease inflammation of the peripheral nerves.
    d. They speed conduction to improve flexibility.

17. The patient has been involved in a motor vehicle collision and has been prescribed methocarbamol for muscle spasms in her neck and back. What side effect(s) should the nurse discuss with the patient before discharge? *(Select all that apply.)*
    a. Brown urine
    b. Diarrhea
    c. Drowsiness
    d. Increased appetite

18. The nurse is administering medications to her patients on a medical-surgical floor. Which drug order should the nurse question before administration?
    a. Dantrolene sodium for a 50-year-old with muscle spasms
    b. Diazepam for a 60-year-old who also has glaucoma
    c. Edrophonium for a 30-year-old who is undergoing diagnostic testing for myasthenia gravis
    d. Chlorzoxazone for a 33-year-old with muscle trauma

Chapter **21** **Drugs for Neuromuscular Disorders and Muscle Spasms**

Read the scenario and answer the following questions on a separate sheet of paper.

G.D., 24 years old, was involved in a high-speed rollover motor vehicle accident and has a spinal cord injury. He has muscle spasms and some spasticity in his lower extremities bilaterally. He has intermittently been prescribed carisoprodol and will be started on baclofen.

1. Why do muscle spasms occur in patients with spinal cord injuries?

2. What is the mechanism of carisoprodol? How does baclofen work?

3. What are the side effects of each drug?

22 Antipsychotics and Anxiolytics

STUDY QUESTIONS

Match the term in Column I to the corresponding statement in Column II.

Column I

_____ 1. Acute dystonia

_____ 2. Akathisia

_____ 3. Anxiolytics

_____ 4. Neuroleptic

_____ 5. Psychosis

_____ 6. Schizophrenia

_____ 7. Tardive dyskinesia

_____ 8. Extrapyramidal symptoms

Column II

a. Losing contact with reality

b. Protrusion and rolling of the tongue, sucking and smacking movements of the lips, chewing motion

c. Muscle tremors, rigidity, shuffling gait

d. Restlessness, inability to sit still, foot-tapping

e. Spasms of tongue, face, neck, and back

f. Used to treat anxiety and insomnia

g. Drug that modifies psychotic behavior

h. Chronic psychotic disorder

Complete the following.

9. Antipsychotic drugs were developed to improve the _____ _____ and _____ of patients with psychotic symptoms resulting from an imbalance of _____, a neurotransmitter.

10. Typical antipsychotics are subdivided into phenothiazines and nonphenothiazines. Nonphenothiazines are divided into four classes: _____, _____, _____, and _____.

11. The most common side effect of all antipsychotics is _____.

12. Antipsychotics may lead to dermatologic side effects that include _____ and _____.

13. Phenothiazines (increase/decrease) the seizure threshold; adjustment of anticonvulsants may be required. *(Circle correct answer.)*

14. Anxiolytics (are/are not) usually given for secondary anxiety. *(Circle correct answer.)*

15. Long-term use of anxiolytics is not recommended because _____ may develop within a short time.

16. The action of anxiolytics resembles that of _____, not antipsychotics.

Match the following drugs in Column I with their drug classification in Column II. Drug classifications in Column II may be used more than once.

Column I

_____ 17. Clozapine

_____ 18. Chlorpromazine

_____ 19. Fluphenazine

_____ 20. Molindone hydrochloride

_____ 21. Haloperidol

_____ 22. Risperidone

Column II

a. Phenothiazine
b. Nonphenothiazine
c. Atypical antipsychotic

NCLEX REVIEW QUESTIONS

Select the best response.

23. Neuroleptic drugs are useful in the management of which type of illness?
    a. Anxiety disorders
    b. Depressive disorders
    c. Psychotic disorders
    d. Psychosomatic disorders

24. The patient has been started on an antipsychotic drug for treatment of her schizophrenia. She asks the nurse when she will start to feel better. What is the nurse's best response?
    a. "It may take up to one week to start to feel the effects."
    b. "Responses vary, but it may be about 6 weeks."
    c. "You will only feel better when you start psychotherapy, too."
    d. "You should start to feel better within 30-60 minutes."

25. The patient has been started on chlorpromazine hydrochloride for treatment of intractable hiccups. What information will the nurse include in patient education about this class of drug?
    a. "A therapeutic response to this drug will be immediate."
    b. "Change positions slowly from sitting to standing to prevent orthostatic hypotension."
    c. "It is all right to have alcohol when taking this drug."
    d. "This drug may be stopped abruptly as soon as your pain stops."

26. Typical antipsychotics may cause extrapyramidal symptoms (EPS) or pseudoparkinsonism. Which symptom is considered an extrapyramidal symptom?
    a. Downward eye movement
    b. Intentional tremors
    c. Loss of hearing
    d. Shuffling gait

27. What drug would the nurse expect to give to decrease EPS?
    a. Benztropine
    b. Bethanechol
    c. Buspirone hydrochloride
    d. Doxepin

28. Phenothiazines are grouped into three categories based on their side effects. In which group is fluphenazine?
    a. Aliphatic
    b. Piperazine
    c. Piperidine
    d. Thioxanthene

29. The patient has been prescribed fluphenazine for treatment of schizophrenia. What information should the nurse include in the patient teaching for this drug? *(Select all that apply.)*
    a. "Blood pressure changes are not an indication of an adverse reaction."
    b. "It is all right to take all herbal drugs when taking fluphenazine."
    c. "Notify your health care provider if you have dizziness, headache, or nausea."
    d. "This medication must be taken every day."
    e. "You should not drink alcohol when taking this drug."

30. The 72-year-old patient diagnosed with schizophrenia was prescribed fluphenazine 20 mg/day. In reviewing his drugs before discharge from the hospital, the nurse notes the dose. What should concern the nurse about the amount of the drug prescribed?
    a. Nothing. The patient is an adult and this is in the normal adult range.
    b. The patient's dose should be 10% less than the adult dose.
    c. The patient's dose should be 25% to 50% less than the usual adult dose.
    d. This drug is contraindicated in patients more than 70 years old.

31. A patient presents to the emergency department with an overdose of chlorpromazine hydrochloride. What is the priority action by the nurse?
   a. Administer activated charcoal.
   b. Administer anticholinergic drugs.
   c. Establish an IV.
   d. Maintain the airway.

32. The 58-year-old patient presents to the emergency department. He is highly agitated and combative and is presenting a danger to self and others. The health care provider has ordered haloperidol 5 mg IM. What should the nurse know about this medication when giving it as an antipsychotic?
   a. It has a sedative effect on agitated, combative patients.
   b. It is the drug of choice for older patients with liver disease.
   c. It will not cause EPS.
   d. It can safely be used in patients with narrow-angle glaucoma.

33. Which of the following is a drug class of atypical antipsychotics?
   a. Butyrophenones
   b. Phenothiazines
   c. Serotonin/dopamine antagonists
   d. Thioxanthenes

34. The atypical antipsychotics have a weak affinity for the D_2 receptors. Consequently, what happens to the occurrence of EPS when taking these drugs?
   a. An absence of EPS
   b. An increase in EPS
   c. Fewer EPS
   d. No effect on EPS

35. Atypical antipsychotics have a stronger affinity for which type of receptors that block serotonin receptors?
   a. D_1
   b. D_2
   c. D_3
   d. D_4

36. A 34-year-old patient with bipolar disorder has just been prescribed risperidone. What side effects should the nurse include in the health teaching about this drug?
   a. Hepatotoxicity
   b. Hyperglycemia
   c. Hearing loss
   d. Urinary frequency

37. The drug alprazolam belongs to which anxiolytic drug group?
   a. Antihistamines
   b. Benzodiazepines
   c. Buspirinones
   d. Phenothiazines

38. In which patient(s) is/are fluphenazine contraindicated? *(Select all that apply.)*
   a. 32-year-old with narrow-angle glaucoma
   b. 35-year-old in a coma
   c. 47-year-old with subcortical brain damage
   d. 53-year-old with continued blood dyscrasias despite lowering dose
   e. 62-year-old with neuromuscular pain

39. Lorazepam is an anxiolytic drug; however, it may be prescribed for other purposes. For which other condition(s) might it be prescribed? *(Select all that apply.)*
   a. Alcohol withdrawal
   b. Anxiety associated with depression
   c. Muscle spasms
   d. Preoperative induction
   e. Status epilepticus

CASE STUDY

Read the scenario, and answer the following questions on a separate sheet of paper.

H.K., 20 years old, is brought to the emergency department. Her friends say she had been trying to "cram for finals." They have been unable to awaken her in 18 hours. An empty bottle of clonazepam and a bottle of vodka are found at the bedside. Vital signs are temperature 37.2° C, heart rate 64 beats/minute, respiratory rate 8 breaths/minute, blood pressure 82/40 mm Hg, O_2 saturation 78%. She is only responsive to deep pain.

1. What class of drug is clonazepam?

2. What is its mechanism of action?

3. What are the side effects associated with this category of drug?

4. With the above history, what is concerning to the nurse, and what are the priority actions?

111

Chapter **22** **Antipsychotics and Anxiolytics**

Antidepressants and Mood Stabilizers

STUDY QUESTIONS

Answer the following questions as true or false.

1. _____ Herbal supplements, such as St. John's wort, do not interact with selective serotonin reuptake inhibitors.

2. _____ Tyramine-rich foods include aged cheese, yogurt, and soy sauce.

3. _____ Monoamine oxidase inhibitors (MAOIs) are considered first-line therapy for depression.

4. _____ Amitriptyline is considered a selective norepinephrine reuptake inhibitor (SNRI).

5. _____ Causes of depression include decreased circulating neurotransmitter levels or the occurrence of major stressors such as the recent death of a family member.

Complete the following.

6. Clinical response of tricyclic antidepressants (TCAs) occurs after _____ of drug therapy.

7. TCAs _____ mood, _____ interest in daily living, and _____ insomnia.

8. Herbal supplements that can be used to treat mild depression include _____.

9. Atypical antidepressants or _____ _____ affect one or two of the three neurotransmitters: _____, _____, and _____.

10. Any drugs that _____ the _____ can cause a hypertensive crisis when taken with an MAOI.

11. _____ was the first drug used to treat _____ _____ disorder.

12. Lithium's therapeutic index has a _____ range from _____.

13. Nonsteroidal antiinflammatory drugs (NSAIDs) can _____ lithium level whereas _____ and _____ diuretics can _____ lithium levels.

14. SNRIs are used for major depression, _____, and _____.

15. Many antidepressants interact with _____ _____ that can lead to _____.

Match the drugs in Column I with the neurotransmitters affected in Column II. The neurotransmitters in Column II may be used more than once.

Column I

_____ 16. Amitriptyline

_____ 17. Fluoxetine

_____ 18. Venlafaxine

_____ 19. Doxepin

_____ 20. Citalopram

_____ 21. Duloxetine

_____ 22. Selegiline

Column II

a. Dopamine
b. Norepinephrine
c. Serotonin

Match the drugs in Column I with their drug classification in Column II. The drug classifications in Column II may be used more than once.

Column I

_____ 23. Trazodone

_____ 24. Maprotiline

_____ 25. Citalopram

_____ 26. Amitriptyline

_____ 27. Tranylcypromine

_____ 28. Paroxetine

Column II

a. Atypical antidepressants
b. Selective serotonin reuptake inhibitors (SSRIs)
c. Monoamine oxidase inhibitors (MAOIs)
d. Tricyclic antidepressants (TCAs)

NCLEX REVIEW QUESTIONS

Select the best response.

29. The 12-year-old patient has been evaluated for enuresis. After home remedies and other alternatives have been explored, which drug does the nurse know may be prescribed to treat this condition?
    a. Citalopram
    b. Fluvoxamine
    c. Imipramine
    d. Sertraline

30. The patient has been taking phenelzine for several months and his depression have not improved. What is the maximum daily dose for this drug?
    a. 15 mg/day
    b. 45 mg/day
    c. 60 mg/day
    d. 90 mg/day

31. The patient has been prescribed amitriptyline as an adjunct to therapy for depression. What information will the nurse include in the health teaching regarding this drug?
    a. "Check your heart rate daily. It may become very slow."
    b. "Stand up slowly because your blood pressure can drop suddenly."
    c. "You should start to feel less depressed within 12 hours."
    d. "Take your drug in the morning because it will make you alert."

32. Which food(s) or beverage(s) is/are contraindicated in a patient prescribed isocarboxazid? *(Select all that apply.)*
    a. Bananas
    b. Chocolate
    c. Chicken
    d. Milk
    e. Wine

33. The patient has a history of depression and is taking fluoxetine. The patient presents to the emergency department complaining of a severe headache. She is diaphoretic and is unable to sit still. Her family tells the nurse that the patient has been taking "some herb." Which herb does the nurse suspect the patient has been taking?
    a. Ephedra
    b. Ginseng
    c. Garlic
    d. St. John's wort

34. Which is an advantage of taking SSRIs over TCAs?
    a. Fewer sexual side effects
    b. Increased appetite
    c. Less sedation
    d. Less tachycardia

35. Which nursing intervention is most important for a patient taking lithium?
    a. Advising the patient that he or she can stop taking the drug when not in a manic phase
    b. Emphasizing the importance of patient-adjusted dosage
    c. Monitoring for excessive thirst, weight gain, and increased urination
    d. Teaching the patient to limit fluid intake to prevent weight gain

36. The patient has been diagnosed with bipolar disorder and is acutely manic. The patient is currently taking lithium. What laboratory value causes particular concern in the nurse?
    a. BUN
    b. Blood glucose
    c. INR
    d. Platelet count

37. The patient has been taking lithium 1800 mg/day in three divided doses for 10 days. He remains agitated and hyperactive, with a lithium level of 0.7 mEq/L. He complains of feeling slow and thirsty. What does the nurse suspect is occurring?
    a. The patient is experiencing lithium toxicity.
    b. The patient's lithium level is subtherapeutic.
    c. The patient's lithium level is therapeutic.
    d. The patient is allergic to lithium.

38. The nurse is teaching the patient about lithium. Which statement by the patient indicates a need for more education?
    a. "I can stop my drug if I have not been manic for 2 weeks."
    b. "I should avoid caffeine products that may aggravate the manic phase."
    c. "I should take my drug with food."
    d. "It is important that I wear or carry ID indicating that I am taking lithium."

39. The patient has been prescribed venlafaxine for generalized anxiety disorder. Which statement by the patient indicates the need for further health teaching?
    a. "I need to take my drug even if I am not feeling anxious."
    b. "I need to wear sunscreen when I am outdoors."
    c. "If I have any issues with my sexual performance, I can ask my health care provider."
    d. "It is OK if I keep taking my herbal drugs for my depression and anxiety."

40. The patient has a history of bipolar disorder and takes lithium. She tells her health care provider that she would like to become pregnant in the near future. What is/are the concern(s) with taking lithium while pregnant? *(Select all that apply.)*
    a. Congenital anomaly
    b. Excessive weight gain
    c. Hyperemesis gravidarum
    d. Heart defects
    e. Multiple gestation

CASE STUDY

Read the scenario, and answer the following questions on a separate sheet of paper.

F.K., 53 years old, has recently relocated to start a new job after the position she held for 20 years was eliminated. She was prescribed fluoxetine 20 mg at bedtime for complaints of insomnia, sadness, tearfulness, and inability to concentrate. She tells the nurse, "I can't believe I lost my job and have to start over. I feel like such a failure." She is postmenopausal and has a history of hypertension and migraines.

1. Discuss SSRIs and their mechanism of action.

2. What questions should the nurse ask in the initial interview?

3. What discharge health education regarding fluoxetine should the nurse provide?

24 Antiinflammatories

STUDY QUESTIONS

Match the term in Column I with the definition in Column II.

Column I

_____ 1. Acetylsalicylic acid (ASA)

_____ 2. Indomethacin

_____ 3. Ketorolac

_____ 4. Fenamates

_____ 5. Oxicams

_____ 6. Immunomodulators

_____ 7. Colchicine

_____ 8. Allopurinol

_____ 9. Celecoxib

Column II

a. Disrupts the inflammatory process and delays disease progression

b. Indicated for long-term arthritic conditions

c. One of the first nonsteroidal antiinflammatory drugs (NSAIDs) introduced

d. Oldest antiinflammatory agent

e. The first injectable NSAID

f. The first drug used to treat gout

g. Drug of choice for patients with chronic tophaceous gout

h. Potent class of NSAID used for acute and chronic arthritic conditions

i. Cyclooxygenase inhibitor

Complete the following.

10. Inflammation is a response to tissue _____ and _____.

11. The five cardinal signs of inflammation are _____, _____, _____,
     _____, and _____.

12. Leukocyte infiltration of the inflamed tissue occurs during the _____ phase of inflammation.

13. The half-life of each NSAID (does/does not) differ greatly. *(Circle correct answer.)*

14. When using NSAIDs for inflammation, the dosage is generally _____ than that for pain relief.

15. The half-life of corticosteroids is greater than _____ hours.

NCLEX REVIEW QUESTIONS

Select the best response.

16. What occurs during the vascular phase of inflammation?
     a. Leukocyte and protein infiltration into inflamed tissue
     b. Vasoconstriction with leukocyte infiltration into inflamed tissue
     c. Vasoconstriction and fluid influx into the interstitial space
     d. Vasodilation with increased capillary permeability

17. A patient who is taking NSAIDs for arthritis complains of persistent heartburn. What further question(s) should the nurse ask the patient about the heartburn? *(Select all that apply.)*
     a. "Do you take your drug with food?"
     b. "Have you been drinking an increased amount of water?"
     c. "Have you noticed a change in the color of your bowel movements?"
     d. "What dosage of the NSAID are you taking?"
     e. "Where is the heartburn located?"

18. When preparing discharge teaching for a patient who has been prescribed ibuprofen for arthritis, how does the nurse explain the mode of action?
    a. "Ibuprofen is a COX-2 inhibitor, so it blocks prostaglandin synthesis."
    b. "Ibuprofen inhibits prostaglandin synthesis."
    c. "Ibuprofen binds with opiate receptor sites."
    d. "Ibuprofen promotes vasodilation to increase blood flow."

19. A patient with a complicated medical history including hypertension, atrial fibrillation, and arthritis calls the health care provider's office to speak with a nurse about "all of these bruises I have all of a sudden." Which potential drug interaction should concern the nurse with these symptoms?
    a. Aspirin and warfarin
    b. Sulfasalazine and acetaminophen
    c. Tolmetin and propranolol
    d. Meloxicam and amlodipine

20. A father presents to the emergency department with his 4-year-old son. The father explains that his son had a fever, so he gave the child baby aspirin to decrease the fever and it has not worked. What should concern the nurse about a 4-year-old receiving aspirin?
    a. Aspirin has the potential to cause gastrointestinal (GI) bleeding in children.
    b. Aspirin has the potential to cause ringing in the ears in children.
    c. Aspirin has the potential to cause hyperglycemia in children.
    d. Aspirin has the potential to cause Reye's syndrome in children.

21. The patient with a history of asthma has been prescribed sulfasalazine for arthritis. What can salicylic acid and salicylate derivatives cause that should concern the nurse?
    a. Tachycardia
    b. Increased secretions
    c. Bronchospasm
    d. Fluid retention

22. Ibuprofen is a frequently prescribed antiinflammatory, analgesic, and antipyretic. What is a positive aspect of this drug in relation to other NSAIDs?
    a. It tends to cause less GI irritation.
    b. It may be taken between meals.
    c. It has a long half-life of 20–30 hours.
    d. It has no drug-drug interactions.

23. A 35-year-old female patient has been prescribed ibuprofen 400 mg tid for arthritis. What statement by the patient would indicate a need for further education?
    a. "This drug may cause GI upset."
    b. "Now I won't have to drink so much water."
    c. "I know this drug might cause some diarrhea."
    d. "I will need to stop taking this drug if I get pregnant."

24. What advantage does piroxicam have over other NSAIDs?
    a. No GI irritation
    b. Few drug-drug interactions
    c. Long half-life
    d. Rapid onset

25. By which action does colchicine relieve the symptoms of gout?
    a. It inhibits the migration of leukocytes to the inflamed area.
    b. It blocks reabsorption of uric acid.
    c. It blocks prostaglandin release.
    d. It inhibits uric acid synthesis.

26. Uricosuric agents such as probenecid are used in the treatment of gout. What is the mechanism of action?
    a. Retention of urate crystals in the body
    b. Inhibition of the reabsorption of uric acid
    c. Promotion of uric acid removal in the ureters
    d. Increased release of uric acid

27. A patient has been switched to the immunomodulator etanercept for severe rheumatoid arthritis. What is the mechanism of action for etanercept?
    a. It neutralizes tumor necrosis factor (TNF), thereby altering the inflammatory response.
    b. It inhibits IL-1 from binding to interleukin receptor sites in cartilage and bone.
    c. It blocks COX-2 receptors, which are needed for biosynthesis of prostaglandins.
    d. It promotes uric acid reabsorption.

28. When discontinuing steroid therapy, how long of a period should the dosage should be tapered?
    a. No tapering is necessary
    b. 1–4 days
    c. 5–10 days
    d. More than 10 days

29. A patient has started taking corticosteroids for an arthritic condition. What information should the nurse include in a health teaching plan? *(Select all that apply.)*

    a. Corticosteroids are used to control arthritic flare-ups in severe cases.

    b. Corticosteroids have a short half-life.

    c. Corticosteroids are usually administered once a day.

    d. Corticosteroids are tapered over the course of 5–10 days.

    e. Corticosteroids may not be taken with prostaglandin inhibitors.

30. The nurse is planning teaching regarding antigout drug. What information should be included? *(Select all that apply.)*

    a. Include large doses of vitamin C supplements.

    b. Increase fluid intake.

    c. Avoid alcoholic beverages.

    d. Avoid foods high in purine.

    e. Take the drug with food.

    f. Avoid direct sunlight.

31. The patient has been prescribed infliximab for severe rheumatoid arthritis. Her spouse calls the clinic and states his wife has a fever of 101.9° F, chills, nausea, vomiting and is very dizzy. What will the nurse advise the patient's spouse to do?

    a. Nothing. These are common side effects of infliximab.

    b. Have the patient take a cool bath.

    c. Wait 24 hours and, if symptoms continue, call back.

    d. Bring the patient to the emergency department or clinic for further evaluation.

CASE STUDY

Read the scenario, and answer the following questions on a separate sheet of paper.

F.E., 54 years old, comes to the clinic for treatment of an inflammatory condition. He reports that he has been taking 975 mg of aspirin combined with 65 mg of caffeine q4h for the past week. He states that his joint pain is getting worse, and he now has noticed some blood in his stools. F.E.'s vital signs are blood pressure 90/62 mm Hg, heart rate 118 beats/min, respiratory rate 24 breaths/min, temperature 37.8° C, and pulse oximetry 98% on room air. His skin is pale and cool.

1. What is the therapeutic dosage range for aspirin? What is the maximum dose?

2. What are the common side effects of aspirin?

3. What are the signs and symptoms of aspirin overdose?

4. Discuss the possible causes for the patient's abnormal vital signs.

25 Analgesics

Complete the following.

1. The _____ theory proposes tissue injury activates _____ and causes the release of chemical mediators.

2. Opioids such as morphine activate the same receptors as _____ to reduce pain.

3. Nonsteroidal antiinflammatory drugs (NSAIDs) control pain at the _____ level by blocking pain-sensitizing chemicals and interfering with the production of _____.

4. As a result of unrelieved pain, a patient may develop glucose intolerance and _____ respiratory rate, heart rate, blood pressure, and stress response.

Match the term in Column I to its definition in Column II.

Column I

_____ 5. Pain threshold

_____ 6. Pain tolerance

_____ 7. Neuropathic pain

_____ 8. Endorphins

_____ 9. Analgesics

_____ 10. Nociceptors

Column II

a. Neurohormones that naturally suppress pain conduction
b. Class of drugs that relieve pain
c. Level of stimulus needed to create a painful sensation
d. Sensory receptors for pain
e. Pain due to disease or injury of the PNS or CNS
f. Amount of pain a person can endure without interfering with normal functioning

Complete the following.

11. Opioids act primarily on the _____ and nonopioid analgesics act on the _____ at the pain receptor sites.

12. In addition to suppressing pain impulses, opioids also suppress _____ and _____.

13. In addition to pain relief, many opioids have _____ and _____ effects.

14. Opioids are contraindicated for use in patients with _____ and _____.

15. The patient taking meperidine reports blurred vision. The nurse knows this is a(n) _____ and would report this finding to the _____.

16. Pentazocine, an opioid agonist-antagonist, is classified as a Schedule _____ drug.

Match the term in Column I to its definition in Column II.

Column I

_____ 17. Acute pain

_____ 18. Cancer pain

_____ 19. Somatic pain

_____ 20. Visceral pain

_____ 21. Chronic pain

_____ 22. Superficial pain

_____ 23. Vascular pain

Column II

a. Originates from smooth muscle and organs
b. Occurs from pressure on nerves and organs
c. Occurs suddenly and is usually less than 3 months in duration
d. Contributes to headaches or migraines
e. Originates in skeletal muscle, ligaments, and joints
f. Persists for more than 3 months and is difficult to treat
g. Originates on surface areas such as skin and mucous membranes

NCLEX REVIEW QUESTIONS

Select the best response.

24. The patient has returned to the floor from surgery after a hip arthroplasty. For the first 48 hours postoperatively, meperidine is ordered for pain control. Which of the following is a major side effect of meperidine?
    a. Decreased blood pressure
    b. Decreased pulse rate
    c. Decreased temperature
    d. Decreased urine output

25. The nurse is assessing a patient for a possible overdose of opioids. Which of the following is an indication of opioid overdose?
    a. Dilated pupils
    b. Increased urinary output
    c. Pinpoint pupils
    d. Diarrhea

26. Which nursing assessment would be least important when monitoring a patient who is receiving hydromorphone?
    a. Bowel sounds
    b. Fluid intake
    c. Pain scale
    d. Vital signs

27. What information should the nurse include in a teaching plan for a patient who is being discharged home after knee surgery with a prescription for an opioid? *(Select all that apply.)*
    a. Dietary restrictions while taking hydrocodone
    b. Instructions not to exceed recommended dosage
    c. Instructions not to use alcohol or central nervous system depressants while taking hydrocodone
    d. Instructions on how to prevent constipation
    e. Side effects to report

28. Which factor is most relevant to the relief of chronic pain?
    a. Administration of drugs at patient's request
    b. Use of opioid analgesics
    c. Use of injectable drugs
    d. Use of drugs with long duration of action

29. The patient is brought to the emergency department with a reported overdose of morphine. Which drug does the nurse anticipate will be prescribed?
    a. Butorphanol
    b. Naloxone
    c. Flumazenil
    d. Pentazocine

30. Mixed opioid agonist-antagonists were developed in hopes of decreasing what problem?
    a. Chronic pain
    b. Opioid abuse
    c. Renal failure
    d. Respiratory depression

31. The patient has been taking an opioid for 8 weeks for a back injury he sustained at work. He has stopped taking his drug. How many hours after he last takes his medication does the nurse anticipate his withdrawal symptoms will begin?
    a. 6–12 hours
    b. 24–48 hours
    c. 48–72 hours
    d. 72–96 hours

32. The patient has breast cancer and is in hospice care. She has been taking morphine for pain control. What is the duration of pain relief for controlled-release morphine?
    a. 1–2 hours
    b. 4–5 hours
    c. 8–12 hours
    d. 24–48 hours

33. What will the nurse do to be more successful in treating pain in an 8-year-old patient who fell from a tree and broke his arm? *(Select all that apply.)*
   a. Assume the child hurts and administer pain drug.
   b. Discuss the child's typical responses with the caregivers.
   c. Only utilize nonpharmacologic pain control methods.
   d. Use a pain scale appropriate for children such as the Ouch Scale.
   e. Utilize developmentally appropriate communication techniques.

34. The nurse is completing the medication reconciliation for the patient who will be discharged home with a prescription for oxycodone and acetaminophen. Which drug that the patient is currently taking raises a concern for the nurse?
   a. Ampicillin
   b. Cholestyramine
   c. Furosemide
   d. Propranolol

35. The nurse is concerned that the patient is experiencing side effects of opioid agonist-antagonists. What would be priorities for the nurse to assess if this patient is experiencing side/adverse effects? *(Select all that apply.)*
   a. Constipation
   b. Dysuria
   c. Hypertension
   d. Nausea and vomiting
   e. Respiratory depression

36. The patient is taking morphine after a procedure. The patient has made his third request for pain medication in the past 4 hours. The patient's vital signs are temperature 97.5° F, heart rate 88 beats/min, respiratory rate 12 breaths/min, blood pressure 104/60 mm Hg, and oxygen saturation 98% on room air. He rates his pain as an 8 on a scale of 1 to 10. Assuming that a dose of the drug is due, what is the nurse's best action?
   a. Administer the dose and contact the health care provider about his respiratory rate.
   b. Administer the dose and contact the health care provider about his pain control.
   c. Hold the dose and contact the health care provider regarding his respiratory rate.
   d. Hold the dose and contact the health care provider about his pain control.

37. The older adult patient has a fentanyl patch 50 mg for chronic pain from an injury. What does the nurse know regarding this drug for this patient?
   a. This patient should not have a fentanyl patch for chronic pain.
   b. The dose may be too low.
   c. The dose may be too high for this patient.
   d. The dose is appropriate.

38. The patient is taking a combination drug of hydrocodone and ibuprofen after reconstructive knee surgery. Which statement by the patient indicates the need for more teaching?
   a. "I must take only what is prescribed for my pain."
   b. "I may need to take a laxative if I get constipated while I am taking this drug."
   c. "Having a few beers on the weekend will help me relax and ease the pain."
   d. "I should not take anything with ibuprofen in it while I am taking this drug."

39. The patient has had major surgery and has been prescribed oral ketorolac. What is the maximum length of time this drug can be taken?
   a. 24 hours
   b. 3 days
   c. 5 days
   d. 2 weeks

40. The patient has fallen off his mountain bike and sustained multiple abrasions to both of his knees. Which would be appropriate drug(s) for pain management for this patient? *(Select all that apply.)*
   a. Acetaminophen
   b. Aspirin
   c. Hydrocodone
   d. Ibuprofen
   e. Morphine

Read the scenario and answer the following questions on a separate sheet of paper.

G.F., 25 years old, presents to the emergency department with a severe headache on the left side of her head. She states that she has had the headache for the last day and "it just won't go away." She is nauseated and is vomiting. G.F. states that lights hurt her eyes and "everything sounds loud." Her vital signs are temperature 98.2° F, heart rate 92 beats/min, respiratory rate 18 breaths/min, blood pressure 142/76 mm Hg, and oxygen saturation 100% on room air. She rates her pain as a "13 on a scale of 1–10." The health care provider diagnoses her with a migraine headache.

1.   What is the mechanism behind the pain associated with a migraine?

2.   What is the difference between the two types of migraine and a cluster headache?

3.   What treatment options are available for this patient?

26 Antibacterials

SECTION 26A: PENICILLINS AND CEPHALOSPORINS

STUDY QUESTIONS

Match the antibiotic in Column I to its category in Column II.

Column I

_____ 1. Penicillin G

_____ 2. Amoxicillin

_____ 3. Oxacillin

_____ 4. Piperacillin/tazobactam

_____ 5. Cefazolin

_____ 6. Cefaclor

_____ 7. Cefdinir

_____ 8. Cefepime

_____ 9. Ceftolozane/tazobactam

Column II

a. First-generation cephalosporin
b. Second-generation cephalosporin
c. Third-generation cephalosporin
d. Fourth-generation cephalosporin
e. Fifth-generation cephalosporin
f. Basic penicillin
g. Penicillinase-resistant penicillins
h. Broad-spectrum penicillin
i. Extended-spectrum penicillins

NCLEX REVIEW QUESTIONS

Select the best response.

10. A 28-year-old female patient presents to the clinic with complaints of severe vaginal itching and discharge. She tells the nurse that she is usually very healthy but has been taking antibiotics for an ear infection. What does the nurse recognize as a possible cause of her vaginal itching and discharge?
    a. Anaphylaxis
    b. Hypersensitivity
    c. Nephrotoxicity
    d. Superinfection

11. A patient is scheduled to receive ceftriaxone for *Klebsiella pneumoniae.* What will the nurse teach the patient about this drug?
    a. It is given IM or IV only.
    b. There is no cross-reaction to penicillins.
    c. Ceftriaxone is safe to take with anticoagulants.
    d. There is no effect on lab values.

12. A 40-year-old patient with renal dysfunction is suffering from a *Staphylococcus aureus* infection. He is prescribed cefprozil monohydrate. What is the maximum dose the nurse would anticipate?
    a. 250 mg/d
    b. 500 mg/d
    c. 750 mg/d
    d. 1 g/d

13. A 24-year-old comes to the emergency department with difficulty breathing and fever. The patient is admitted to the intensive care unit with a severe lower respiratory tract infection and is started on aztreonam. Which of the following doses would be appropriate for an adult?
    a. 500 mg q8h
    b. 500 mg q6h
    c. 1500 mg q8h
    d. 2000 mg daily

125

Copyright © 2018, Elsevier Inc. All rights reserved.

Chapter **26** Antibacterials

14. Which class of drug would increase the risk of nephrotoxicity in a patient taking ceftriaxone?

    a. Angiotensin-converting enzyme (ACE) inhibitors
    b. Antidysrhythmics
    c. Loop diuretics
    d. Nonsteroidal antiinflammatory drugs (NSAIDs)

15. The patient has been started on ceftriaxone. Her family is concerned regarding her recent weight loss. What can the nurse tell the family regarding side effects of ceftriaxone?
    a. Loss of appetite is a common side effect.
    b. Gastrointestinal bleeding may occur frequently.
    c. Ceftriaxone causes nutrient absorption problems.
    d. She will eat more when the infection is cured.

16. What statement by a parent indicates more discharge teaching is necessary for care of a 5-year-old child who has been prescribed dicloxacillin for otitis media?
    a. "Abdominal pain can be a side effect."
    b. "She needs to drink plenty of orange juice with this medication."
    c. "My child must take all of the drug until it is gone."
    d. "If my child develops a rash, I should bring her back to the doctor."

17. What category of drugs is known to increase the serum levels of cephalosporins?
    a. Antacids
    b. Laxatives
    c. Opioids
    d. Uricosurics

18. How does penicillin V potassium work?
    a. Alteration in membrane permeability
    b. Inhibition of cell-wall synthesis
    c. Inhibition of protein synthesis
    d. Interference with cellular metabolism

19. A 35-year-old patient presents to the clinic with a complaint of sore throat. Vital signs are temperature 101° F, blood pressure 132/60 mm Hg, heart rate 98 beats/min, respiratory rate 18 breaths/min. She is allergic to dextromethorphan and takes oral contraceptives, vitamin C, and fexofenadine. She is diagnosed with strep throat and prescribed amoxicillin/clavulanate potassium. What instruction should the nurse include in the discharge teaching regarding this drug?
    a. "Increase calcium intake."
    b. "Wear sunscreen at all times."
    c. "Use an alternate method of birth control."
    d. "Stop the fexofenadine."

20. Which specific nursing intervention(s) should be performed for a patient taking ceftazidime? (Select all that apply.)
    a. Obtain a culture.
    b. Administer IV dose over 20 minutes every day.
    c. Assess for allergic reaction.
    d. Monitor urine output.
    e. Restrict oral fluid intake.

21. Which patient should not be taking amoxicillin?
    a. 10-year-old patient with a staphylococcal infection of the skin
    b. 21-year-old pregnant patient
    c. 38-year-old patient with asthma
    d. 62-year-old diabetic patient

22. A patient has been prescribed cefaclor for otitis media. What order will the nurse question?
    a. IR, 250 mg q8h
    b. IR, 500 mg q8h
    c. IR, 750 mg q8h
    d. ER, 375 mg q12h

SECTION 26B: MACROLIDES, OXAZOLIDINONES, LINCOSAMIDES, GLYCOPEPTIDES, KETOLIDES, TETRACYCLINES, AND GLYCYLCYCLINES

STUDY QUESTIONS

Match the drug in Column I with the category in Column II. Categories in Column II may be used more than once.

Column I

_____ 1. Clindamycin

_____ 2. Tigecycline

_____ 3. Erythromycin

_____ 4. Telithromycin

_____ 5. Azithromycin

_____ 6. Doxycycline

_____ 7. Clarithromycin

Column II

a. Macrolides
b. Lincosamides
c. Ketolides
e. Tetracyclines
f. Glycylcyclines

NCLEX REVIEW QUESTIONS

Select the best response.

8. Which laboratory test is influenced by tetracycline?
   a. White blood count
   b. Serum calcium level
   c. Blood urea nitrogen level
   d. Serum sodium levels

9. The patient has been prescribed doxycycline. What statement(s) by the patient indicate(s) that the nurse needs to provide more discharge teaching? *(Select all that apply.)*
   a. "It is best if I take this with meals."
   b. "I should drink milk."
   c. "I have to take this drug on an empty stomach."
   d. "I should wait a half-hour after meals to take the medication."
   e. "I cannot eat eggs when I take this drug."

10. What will the nurse include in the teaching for a patient taking tetracycline for a respiratory tract infection? *(Select all that apply.)*
    a. Outdated tetracycline breaks down into toxic by-products and must be discarded.
    b. Observe for superinfection like vaginitis or gastritis.
    c. Avoid tetracycline during first and third trimesters of pregnancy.
    d. Anticipate urinary urgency.
    e. Wear sunscreen and limit outdoor exposure during peak daylight hours.

11. Which drug(s), if prescribed for a patient taking doxycycline, will the nurse question? *(Select all that apply.)*
    a. Prenatal vitamins
    b. Antacids
    c. Warfarin
    d. Morphine
    e. Omeprazole

12. Which specific nursing intervention(s) should be implemented for a patient taking doxycycline for chlamydia? *(Select all that apply.)*
    a. Restricting fluids
    b. Storing the drug away from light
    c. Ordering renal and liver profiles
    d. Obtaining a specimen for culture and sensitivity
    e. Advising the patient to use additional contraceptives when taking this drug

13. The nurse is performing a morning assessment on a 65-year-old patient who is receiving vancomycin. The patient states that her ears have been ringing all night. What does the nurse know about vancomycin and ringing in the ears?
    a. Only low-pitched sounds are affected by vancomycin.
    b. Tinnitus is a sign of vancomycin allergy.
    c. Ototoxicity is caused by damage to cranial nerve VIII.
    d. Only female patients have ringing in their ears.

14. The nurse is noting the intake and output for a 70-year-old patient receiving vancomycin and sees that the patient's urine output has decreased to 500 mL/day. What is the best action by the nurse?
   a. Increase the patient's oral fluid intake.
   b. Increase the patient's IV rate.
   c. Contact the health care provider.
   d. Document this in the patient's chart.

15. The patient has been prescribed azithromycin for an upper respiratory tract infection. What statement by the patient indicates understanding of side effects of the drug?
   a. "I need to stay out of the sun or wear sunscreen."
   b. "I have to take it on an empty stomach to prevent nausea."
   c. "If my eyes get red and itchy, I shouldn't wear my contacts."
   d. "I cannot take anything for pain if I get a headache."

16. Quinupristin/dalfopristin is marketed for IV use against life-threatening infection caused by which bacteria?
   a. Vancomycin-resistant *Enterococcus faecium*
   b. *Escherichia coli*
   c. *Proteus mirabilis*
   d. *Klebsiella pneumoniae*

SECTION 26C: AMINOGLYCOSIDES, FLUOROQUINOLONES, AND LIPOPEPTIDES

Complete the following.

1. Streptomycin sulfate was the first _____ available against the bacterium *Streptomyces griseus*.

2. Aminoglycosides cross the blood-brain barrier in (adults/children). *(Circle the correct answer.)*

3. An increased risk for ototoxicity can occur when taking aminoglycosides concurrently with _____.

4. Fluoroquinolones interfere with the enzyme _____ _____, which is needed to synthesize bacterial _____.

5. Patients taking fluoroquinolones should (increase/decrease) fluid intake. *(Circle the correct answer.)*

Match the drug in Column I with its category in Column II. Categories in Column II may be used more than once.

Column I

_____ 6. Amikacin

_____ 7. Moxifloxacin

_____ 8. Gentamicin

_____ 9. Ciprofloxacin

_____ 10. Daptomycin

_____ 11. Tobramycin

Column II

a. Aminoglycosides
b. Fluoroquinolones
c. Lipopeptides

12. Which fluoroquinolone order will the nurse question?
   a. Levofloxacin 750 mg IV q12h
   b. Ofloxacin 200 mg PO q12h
   c. Moxifloxacin 400 mg PO q day
   d. Ciprofloxacin 250 mg PO bid

13. The nurse assesses a patient who is taking gentamicin. What assessment finding(s) should be cause for serious concern? *(Select all that apply.)*
   a. Nausea
   b. Ototoxicity
   c. Headache
   d. Photosensitivity
   e. Elevated renal function tests

14. The patient is taking gentamicin for a postsurgical infection, and the nurse needs to draw a peak level. The patient takes the drug at 0900 and at 2100. When is the correct time to draw a drug peak level?
    a. 0930
    b. 1000
    c. 2045
    d. 2130

15. The trough level that the nurse drew for a patient taking gentamicin is 3.5 mcg/mL. What is the best action by the nurse?
    a. Administer the medication at the correct time.
    b. Hold the drug and contact the health care provider.
    c. Repeat the trough level after the next dose of medication.
    d. Give the patient Benadryl to decrease the risk of a reaction.

16. The patient tells the nurse that she has developed vaginal discharge since she began taking gentamicin. What does the nurse suspect may be occurring?
    a. The patient has been exposed to other infectious agents.
    b. The patient is experiencing an allergic reaction.
    c. A superinfection has developed.
    d. A drug-drug interaction is taking place.

17. What will the nurse routinely monitor in a 65-year-old patient taking gentamicin? *(Select all that apply.)*
    a. Hearing loss
    b. Color and clarity of urine
    c. AST/ALT
    d. Blood glucose
    e. Visual acuity

18. A patient is receiving daptomycin for a gram-positive microorganism. The nurse is reviewing the trough level. Which of the following trough levels is appropriate?
    a. 5 mcg/mL by the second dose
    b. 5.9 mcg/mL by the third dose
    c. 6 mg/mL by the third dose
    d. 6.5 mg/mL by the fourth dose

SECTION 26D: SULFONAMIDES AND NITROIMIDAZOLES

STUDY QUESTIONS

Complete the following.

1. Sulfonamides inhibit bacterial synthesis of _____ _____.

2. Clinical use of sulfonamides has decreased because of the availability and effectiveness of _____.

3. The antibacterial drug that has a synergistic effect with sulfonamides is _____.

4. Sulfonamides (are/are not) effective against viruses and fungi. *(Circle correct answer.)*

5. Anaphylaxis (is/is not) common with the use of sulfonamides. *(Circle correct answer.)*

6. Sulfonamide drugs are metabolized in the _____ and excreted by the _____.

7. Sulfonamides are (bacteriostatic/bactericidal). *(Circle correct answer.)*

8. The use of warfarin with sulfonamides (increases/decreases) the anticoagulant effect. *(Circle correct answer.)*

Match the drug in Column I with its duration of action in Column II. Duration of action in Column II may be used more than once.

Column I

_____ 9. Trimethoprim-sulfamethoxazole

_____ 10. Sulfasalazine

_____ 11. Sulfadiazine

Column II

a. Short-acting

b. Intermediate-acting

129

Select the best response.

12. The patient has sustained partial-thickness and full-thickness burns over 20% of his body in a house fire. Which medication would be useful for treatment?
    a. Sulfadiazine
    b. Sulfasalazine
    c. Sulfacetamide sodium
    d. Silver sulfadiazine

13. The patient has her first postnatal visit with her obstetrician. She is complaining of frequency and burning on urination. She has been diagnosed with a urinary tract infection (UTI) and is started on TMP-SMZ. What important question(s) should the nurse ask when teaching the patient? *(Select all that apply.)*
    a. "What kind of juice do you like to drink?"
    b. "Are you breastfeeding?"
    c. "Are you allergic to any medications?"
    d. "Do you have a history of kidney stones?"
    e. "What drugs do you take regularly?"

14. What intervention(s) should the nurse implement in a 50-year-old patient with bronchitis who is receiving TMP-SMZ and lisinopril? *(Select all that apply.)*
    a. Encourage fluids.
    b. Monitor urinary output.
    c. Observe for undesired side effects.
    d. Assess lung sounds.
    e. Administer laxatives.

15. What is the usual adult dose of TMP-SMZ?
    a. 160 mg TMP/800 mg SMZ q6h
    b. 160 mg TMP/800 mg SMZ q12h
    c. 40 mg TMP/60 mg SMZ q6h
    d. 40 mg TMP/60 mg SMZ q12h

16. Why are sulfonamides not classified as antibiotics?
    a. They do not inhibit cell-wall growth.
    b. They are only bacteriostatic, not bactericidal.
    c. They were not obtained from biological sources.
    d. They are only effective against viruses and fungi.

17. The patient has been started on TMP-SMZ for otitis. The nurse will advise the patient about which side effect?
    a. Confusion
    b. Constipation
    c. Fever
    d. Insomnia

18. The 28-year-old patient is taking sulfasalazine for Crohn disease. What is the maintenance dose?
    a. 500 mg q6h
    b. 1000 mg q6h
    c. 1250 mg per day
    d. 1500 mg per day

CASE STUDY

Read the scenario and answer the following questions on a separate sheet of paper.

D.T., 72 years old, presents to the emergency department from a long-term acute care facility (LTAC) with complaints of fever, shaking chills, flank pain, and burning on urination. Vital signs are temperature 100.3° F, heart rate 94 beats/min, respiratory rate 16 breaths/min, and blood pressure 102/70 mm Hg. His medical history is positive for adult-onset diabetes and cerebrovascular accident with residual left-sided weakness. His current drugs include glyburide, warfarin, and a daily multivitamin. He is allergic to all cephalosporins.

He is been diagnosed with an *E. coli* urinary tract infection and was prescribed oral trimethoprim-sulfamethoxazole (TMP-SMZ).

1. What is the mechanism of action and standard dosage for oral TMP-SMZ?

2. What will the nurse discuss with the patient and his family regarding the plan of care as it relates to TMP-SMZ?

3. What adverse reactions will the nurse monitor?

27 Antituberculars, Antifungals, and Antivirals

Complete the following.

1. *Mycobacterium* species is an _____ bacillus that can cause _____.

2. Multidrug-resistant tuberculosis (MDRTB) continues to be a problem because people (do/do not) complete the drug regimen. *(Circle correct answer.)*

3. Tuberculosis is transmitted by droplets when people _____, _____, or _____

   and people in close contact _____ the particles.

4. A person who had _____ _____ _____ can develop TB disease.

5. Since isoniazid is metabolized through the liver and excreted by the kidneys, isoniazid is contraindicated in

   persons with severe _____ and _____ disease. List the other contraindications for
   receiving isoniazid.

6. Psychotic behavior (is/is not) a side effect of isoniazid. *(Circle correct answer.)*

7. (Single/combination) therapy against TB disease is more effective in eradicating infection. *(Circle correct answer.)*

8. A common adverse effect with isoniazid is peripheral neuropathy. A supplement with _____ is usually taken concomitantly to prevent neuropathy.

9. Children who have latent TB infection should be treated with _____ for _____ months.

Match the drug in Column I with its type in Column II. Answers may be used more than once.

Column I

_____ 10. Ethambutol

_____ 11. Rifapentin

_____ 12. Pyrazinamide

_____ 13. Capreomycin

_____ 14. Isoniazid

_____ 15. Aminosalicylate

_____ 16. Ethionamide

_____ 17. Streptomycin

_____ 18. Rifampin

Column II

a. First-line drug
b. Drug-resistant TB

Complete the following.

19. Overgrowth of fungus usually occurs in persons who are immunocompromised and is classified as an _____ infection.

20. Rapid IV infusion of echinocandins can cause _____ reactions.

21. Herpes virus type 1 (HSV-1) is usually associated with _____, and herpes virus type 2 (HSV-2) is associated with _____.

22. Varicella-zoster virus that has lain dormant in nerve root ganglia can be reactivated as _____. Painful vesicular rash occurs along the _____.

23. Currently, hepatitis _____ and hepatitis _____ are vaccine preventable.

24. Specific therapy (does/does not) exist for acute hepatitis B. *(Circle correct answer.)*

25. Hepatitis _____ and hepatitis _____ can develop into chronic hepatitis.

NCLEX REVIEW QUESTIONS

Select the best response.

26. Which outcome is a life-threatening adverse effect of isoniazid?

    a. Crystalluria
    b. Hepatotoxicity
    c. Ototoxicity
    d. Palpitations

27. Which person should not receive prophylactic treatment for tuberculosis with isoniazid?
    a. 29-year-old concurrently taking theophylline
    b. 46-year-old with alcoholism
    c. 57-year-old taking warfarin
    d. 65-year-old with parkinsonism

28. The patient has just started taking rifapentine. The nurse knows that this drug will be taken how often?
    a. Twice per day
    b. Daily
    c. Twice per week
    d. Every other day

29. The patient is immunocompromised and has recently been diagnosed with histoplasmosis. The patient has been started on amphotericin B. Which of the following would the nurse anticipate administering to alleviate side effects? *(Select all that apply.)*
    a. Diphenhydramine
    b. Acetaminophen
    c. Diazepam
    d. Hydrocortisone

30. Which of the following would be ordered for a patient with hepatitis C viral infection?

a.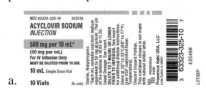

b.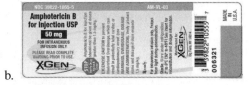

c.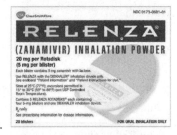

d.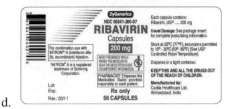

31. During the admission interview, which information will the nurse seek to obtain from a 69-year-old patient taking isoniazid? *(Select all that apply.)*
    a. Blood glucose level
    b. Drug allergies
    c. History of TB exposure
    d. Date of last purified protein derivative (PPD) and chest x-ray

32. The 28-year-old patient has been diagnosed with TB disease. The patient weighs 80 kg. What is the initial dose of INH?
    a. 2 mg/kg/day for 2 months
    b. 5 mg/kg/day for 2 months
    c. 7.5 mg/kg/day for 2 months
    d. 10 mg/kg/day for 2 months

33. Why is it important to monitor liver function tests in a patient who is taking INH?
    a. INH is excreted by the liver.
    b. INH causes liver cancer.
    c. INH can be hepatotoxic.
    d. INH cannot be metabolized by patients who have liver disease.

34. The patient has just been prescribed INH for active tuberculosis. Which drug taken by the patient would be of concern to the nurse?
    a. Cetirizine
    b. Lisinopril
    c. Maalox
    d. Metformin

35. What priority health teaching should the nurse include for the patient who has just started a course of INH? *(Select all that apply.)*
    a. The patient may need to take vitamin B_6 supplements.
    b. Alcohol should be avoided.
    c. Fluid intake should be restricted.
    d. Body fluids including urine and tears may turn a brownish-orange color.
    e. Daily weights should be monitored.

36. How should rifampin be taken to decrease the incidence of resistance?
    a. Daily
    b. In conjunction with another antitubercular drug
    c. Once a week
    d. Only if patient is symptomatic

37. An immunocompromised patient has aspergillosis and has been prescribed amphotericin B. How is this medication administered?
    a. Intramuscularly
    b. Intravenously
    c. Orally
    d. Rectally

38. A 40-year-old patient has coccidioidomycosis and is in the intensive care unit. He has been prescribed amphotericin B, and the nurse is preparing his first dose. How should the nurse administer the drug?
    a. Dilute and infuse over 30 minutes while monitoring vital signs every 5 minutes.
    b. Dilute, protect from light, and infuse slowly using an in-line filter.
    c. Administer 300 mg by intravenous push slowly over 15 minutes.
    d. Prepare the drug in a solution and have the patient drink it slowly.

39. The patient is being treated with amphotericin B for histoplasmosis. What statement by the patient would be concerning to the nurse?
    a. "I know I can only get this drug by having an IV."
    b. "This drug may make me feel flushed."
    c. "I should not eat for 12 hours before receiving the drug."
    d. "I should let my health care provider know if I am not urinating as much."

40. The patient has been prescribed acyclovir. What priority information should be part of the teaching plan for this patient? *(Select all that apply.)*
    a. Be sure to drink plenty of water to maintain hydration.
    b. Be sure to use spermicide to prevent infecting others.
    c. Drug can be taken at mealtime.
    d. Arise slowly because of the risk for orthostatic hypotension.
    e. Report any decreased urinary output, dizziness, or confusion.

41. A patient is being treated with peginterferon. Which symptom(s) will the nurse advise the patient taking peginterferon to report to the health care provider? *(Select all that apply.)*
    a. Mood changes
    b. Fever
    c. Vision changes
    d. Photophobia
    e. Urinary urgency

42. Available:

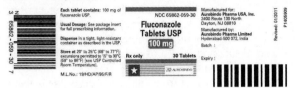

The patient's prescription is for a maintenance dose of fluconazole, 150 mg/day. How many tablets should the patient take per dose?
a. 1 tablet
b. 1.5 tablets
c. 2 tablets
d. 2.5 tablets

43. Which laboratory value(s) must be frequently monitored in the patient taking fluconazole? *(Select all that apply.)*
a. AST
b. ALT
c. BUN
d. Glucose
e. Potassium
f. PT

CASE STUDY

Read the scenario and answer the following questions on a separate sheet of paper.

C.J., 22 years old, has presented to the clinic complaining of "white spots in my mouth." She has been taking multiple antibiotics during the past month for a severe lower respiratory tract infection. Nystatin suspension is ordered, 5 mL oral swish and swallow qid.

1. What questions should the nurse ask in the assessment?

2. What is the likely source of the patient's symptoms?

3. What specific instructions will the nurse include in health teaching regarding nystatin?

28 Peptides, Antimalarials, and Anthelmintics

STUDY QUESTIONS

Match the term in Column I with the appropriate definition in Column II.

Column I

_____ 1. Tissue phase

_____ 2. Erythrocyte phase

_____ 3. Prophylaxis

_____ 4. Helminthiasis

_____ 5. Trichinosis

_____ 6. Drug-resistant infection

_____ 7. Peptides

Column II

a. Prevention
b. Worm infection
c. Invasion of the body tissue
d. Infection caused by eating raw or undercooked pork
e. Invasion of the blood cells
f. Provides the ability to kill a range of parasites and viruses
g. When microbes are not sensitive to antimicrobials

NCLEX REVIEW QUESTIONS

Select the best response.

8. Which is the most common site for helminthiasis?
   a. Blood
   b. Intestines
   c. Liver
   d. Urinary tract

9. What is the causative agent for malaria?
   a. Bacterium
   b. Fungus
   c. Protozoan
   d. Virus

10. The patient has recently returned from an archeology dig in Belize. She presents to the emergency department with complaints of fever, chills, and body aches. She has been diagnosed with malaria. What drug does the nurse anticipate she may be prescribed?
    a. Acyclovir
    b. Chloroquine HCl
    c. Delavirdine
    d. Tobramycin

11. Which laboratory value(s) is/are affected by chloroquine usage? *(Select all that apply.)*
    a. Creatinine
    b. Glucose
    c. Hemoglobin
    d. Hematocrit
    e. Red blood cell count
    f. Aspartate aminotransferase (AST)

12. The patient is planning a mission trip to Haiti, and her health care provider has prescribed chloroquine as prophylaxis for malaria. What statement by the patient indicates the need for more health education by the nurse?
    a. "I may have some abdominal cramping and nausea."
    b. "I only need to take my medication before my trip."
    c. "If my ears start ringing, I should contact my health care provider."
    d. "I should avoid taking any antacid while I am taking this drug."

13. The patient has been diagnosed with malaria and has been treated with chloroquine. He returns to his health care provider after he has finished his drug and states, "I still feel awful. This isn't getting any better." Vital signs are temperature 104.5° F, heart rate 120 beats/min, respiratory rate 22 breaths/min, blood pressure 138/82 mm Hg, and oxygen saturation 99% on room air. What does the nurse anticipate the next treatment will be?
    a. Continue 5 more days of chloroquine.
    b. Change medication to artemether/lumefantrine.
    c. Start thiabendazole.
    d. Start zidovudine.

135

14. What priority(ies) should be included in the patient teaching for anthelmintics? *(Select all that apply.)*
    a. Bathing in hot water instead of showering
    b. Changing clothing, linen, and towels daily
    c. Taking the drug on an empty stomach to aid in absorption
    d. Understanding the importance of hand hygiene
    e. Thoroughly cooking all foods containing pork

15. The 18-year-old patient has been diagnosed with cysticercosis, which is caused by pork tapeworm. He is being treated with praziquantel. Which possible side effect(s) should the nurse include in patient teaching? *(Select all that apply.)*
    a. Blurred vision
    b. Difficulty hearing
    c. Dizziness
    d. Headache
    e. Weakness

16. An 18-year-old is being treated with an antibiotic. Which of the following statements by the patient would concern the nurse about a potential risk for antibiotic resistance? *(Select all that apply.)*
    a. "If I run out of my antibiotic, I can use my leftovers from a previous infection."
    b. "I will take the antibiotics as prescribed."
    c. "Sometimes my friends ask me if I have any antibiotics. If I feel better, I will give my friends my leftovers."
    d. "When I stop having a fever I can stop taking the drug."

CASE STUDY

Read the scenario and answer the following questions on a separate sheet of paper.

J.C., 25 years old, helped his friend with his farm and ranch. Several days later, he noticed some abdominal pain and anal itching. He was diagnosed with helminths.

1. What are helminths?

2. What are the common helminths causing infection in humans and how do they infect humans?

3. How are helminths treated?

29 HIV- and AIDS-Related Drugs

STUDY QUESTIONS

Match the drug in Column I to its drug classification of antiretroviral therapy in Column II. Answers may be used more than once.

Column I

_____ 1. Didanosine

_____ 2. Enfuvirtide

_____ 3. Raltegravir

_____ 4. Maraviroc

_____ 5. Idinavir

_____ 6. Ritonavir

_____ 7. Efavirenz

_____ 8. Tenofovir

_____ 9. Nevirapine

_____ 10. Zidovudine

Column II

a. Nucleoside/nucleotide reverse transcriptase inhibitors
b. Protease inhibitors
c. Integrase strand transfer inhibitors
d. Fusion inhibitors
e. Nonnucleoside reverse transcriptase inhibitors
f. CCR5 antagonists

Complete the following.

11. The phases of the HIV life cycle include _____, _____, reverse transcription, integration, _____, _____, and budding.

12. Individuals who fail antiretroviral therapy (ART) (should/should not) be tested for drug-resistance testing. (Circle correct answer.)

13. Patients on HIV medication therapy should strive for _____ percent adherence.

14. Drug-drug interactions can occur when drugs are metabolized by the _____ system.

15. _____ is the only NNRTI that penetrates cerebrospinal fluid.

16. Selection of a protease inhibitor–based regimen should consider _____. (List at least three considerations.)

17. _____ is a syndrome that is related to a disease- or pathogen-specific inflammatory response in patients on antiretroviral therapy.

Select the best response.

18. A nurse is teaching a patient who is positive for HIV. Which of the following statements by the patient indicates a need for further teaching on HIV transmission? *(Select all that apply.)*
    a. "It is okay to share my razor."
    b. "I need to wear a condom with any type of sexual intercourse."
    c. "I can spread HIV by sharing my toothbrush."
    d. "I can donate my sperm."

19. Which of the following laboratory tests is used to monitor the efficacy of HIV drug therapy?
    a. White blood cell count
    b. CD41 T-cell count
    c. Plasma B-cells
    d. Complete blood count

20. What is the goal of combination antiretroviral therapy?
    a. Decrease the viral load and decrease the CD41 count
    b. Decrease the CD41 count and increase the viral load
    c. Increase the CD41 count and decrease the viral load
    d. Replace the memory cells within the immune system

21. If therapy is to be initiated, the selection of ART should be based on which of the following? *(Select all that apply.)*
    a. Patient's other comorbid conditions
    b. Patient's age and support system
    c. Patient's willingness to accept therapy
    d. Probability of adherence to therapy
    e. Pregnancy status

22. Drug adherence has improved since the advent of ART. Which of the following advancements to ART helped in increasing adherence?
    a. More pill burden
    b. Increased potency of newer ART
    c. Improved side effect profile
    d. Decreased potency of newer ART to reduce side effects

23. An adult patient is scheduled to begin taking zidovudine 300 mg by mouth. How frequently is zidovudine generally scheduled to be taken?
    a. Daily
    b. q12h
    c. q6h
    d. q8h

24. The patient, 8 weeks old, has been diagnosed with HIV and will be receiving zidovudine orally. He weighs 4.5 kg. What would the nurse anticipate would be the dose for this patient?
    a. 9 mg/kg/dose bid
    b. 12 mg/kg/dose bid
    c. 120 mg/kg/dose bid
    d. 300 mg/kg/dose bid

25. During the time that a patient is taking zidovudine, frequent monitoring of which laboratory value(s) is required? *(Select all that apply.)*
    a. ALT/AST
    b. Complete blood count (CBC) with differential
    c. Creatinine
    d. Serum sodium
    e. Urine sedimentation rate

26. The nurse is assessing a patient taking zidovudine. What should the nurse expect to see if the patient is experiencing side effects? *(Select all that apply.)*
    a. Constipation
    b. Headache
    c. Myalgia
    d. Rash
    e. Seizures

27. Which of the following nonnucleoside reverse transcriptase inhibitors (NNRTIs) penetrates the blood-brain barrier?
    a. Rilpivirine
    b. Delavirdine
    c. Efavirenz
    d. Nevirapine

28. Efavirenz is initially scheduled to be taken at which of the following intervals?
    a. 600 mg q6h
    b. 600 mg q8h
    c. 600 mg q12h
    d. 600 mg daily

29. During the time that a patient is taking efavirenz, periodic monitoring of which laboratory value(s) is required?
    a. BUN/creatinine
    b. CBC and platelets
    c. Electrolytes
    d. Liver panel

30. What will the nurse assess in a patient taking efavirenz if he appears to be experiencing side effects? *(Select all that apply.)*
    a. Diarrhea
    b. Difficulty swallowing
    c. Dizziness
    d. Rash
    e. Seizures

31. A patient is being discharged on efavirenz. What priority teaching point(s) will the nurse provide to this patient? *(Select all that apply.)*
    a. "Avoid alcohol while taking this drug."
    b. "Be sure to drink 2500 mL of fluid a day."
    c. "Don't take St. John's wort with this drug, as it will decrease its effectiveness."
    d. "This drug can cause convulsions and possibly liver failure."
    e. "Vomiting is a serious adverse reaction to efavirenz."

32. What laboratory value(s) is/are high priority for the nurse to monitor in a patient taking tenofovir? *(Select all that apply.)*
    a. Blood glucose
    b. Cholesterol
    c. Liver enzymes
    d. Triglycerides
    e. Potassium

33. The patient is being discharged on tenofovir. What priority teaching information should this patient receive? *(Select all that apply.)*
    a. "You cannot take St. John's wort while taking this drug."
    b. "You can take this drug with or without food."
    c. "You will need to learn to measure your blood glucose level."
    d. "Side effects may include nausea, vomiting, and diarrhea."
    e. "You will not be able to drive until you stop taking this drug."

34. What is the standard of care for prophylactic treatment for the asymptomatic pregnant patient?
    a. Combination drug therapy
    b. No therapy since all ART is contraindicated during pregnancy
    c. Single drug therapy with zidovudine only
    d. No therapy since the patient is asymptomatic

35. What side effect(s) would the nurse expect to see in a patient taking atazanavir? *(Select all that apply.)*
    a. Diarrhea
    b. Nausea
    c. Rash
    d. Urinary retention
    e. Vomiting

36. Which of the following can help increase HIV drug adherence? *(Select all that apply.)*
    a. Pill organizers
    b. Drug charts
    c. Scheduled pill holidays
    d. Alarms on cell phone or watch
    e. Taking drugs at the same time each day, such as after brushing teeth.

CASE STUDY

Read the scenario and answer the following questions on a separate sheet of paper.

D.D., 28 years old, works as a registered nurse in the trauma unit. He sustains a needle stick from a patient with HIV.

1. What should the nurse do first?

2. What is involved in postexposure prophylaxis (PEP), and how long does treatment last?

3. What are potential side effects associated with PEP?

30 Transplant Drugs

STUDY QUESTIONS

Complete the following.

1. Transplanation of a healthy organ at the time of the donor's death is called _____.

2. A critical component of the cellular immune response is the _____ activation of lymphocytes.

3. Taking cyclosporine with HMG-CoA reductase inhibitors, such as _____, can cause rhabdomyolysis.

4. Patients on belatacept are at increased risk for _____ _____ _____ if they do not have immunity to _____ _____.

5. Sirolimus is in the class of _____ drugs that block _____ and _____ activation.

6. Combining corticosteroids with potassium-wasting diuretics increases the risk of _____.

7. Patients taking trimethoprim-sulfamethoxazole should protect their _____ from the _____.

Make the following false statements into true statements.

8. Induction therapy includes transplant drugs that provide improved immunity.

9. An example of a living-donor transplantation is when a kidney donated by a living person is transplanted into the body with severe kidney disease.

10. Transplant recipients receiving immunosuppressive drugs can receive live vaccines.

11. Sirolimus is primarily excreted by the kidneys.

12. Antithymocyte globulin alters B-cell function and prolongs T-cell addition.

Match the drug in Column I to the correct drug classes in Column II. Answers may be used more than once.

Column I

_____ 13. Tacrolimus

_____ 14. Everolimus

_____ 15. Basiliximab

_____ 16. Cyclosporine

_____ 17. Belatacept

_____ 18. Sirolimus

_____ 19. Azathioprine

_____ 20. Mycophenolate mofetil

_____ 21. Prednisone

Column II

a. Purine antimetabolites
b. Corticosteroids
c. Calcineurin inhibitors
d. Inosine monophosphate dehydrogenase inhibitors
e. Mammalian target of rapamycin inhibitors
f. T-cell costimulation blocker
g. Monoclonal antibody

Select the best response(s).

22. A 27-year-old is receiving basiliximab before renal transplant surgery. The nurse monitoring the patient believes cytokine release syndrome is occurring. Which of the following are signs and symptoms of cytokine release syndrome? *(Select all that apply.)*
     a. Hypotension
     b. Bradycardia
     c. Dyspnea
     d. Hypothermia
     e. Headache

23. A nurse should anticipate administering which of the following drugs to reduce the symptoms from cytokine release syndrome?
     a. Corticosteroid
     b. Diltiazem
     c. Furosemide
     d. Naloxone

24. Cyclosporine oral solution should not be mixed in which of the following types of fluids?
     a. Apple juice
     b. Orange juice
     c. Grape juice
     d. Grapefruit juice

25. Which of the following statements by the patient demonstrates an understanding of cyclosporine?
     a. "If I get an infection, I can take any antibiotics."
     b. "I can take cimetidine if I get an upset stomach."
     c. "If I have a fever, I need to call my doctor."
     d. "If I get mild muscle aches, I can take ibuprofen."

26. A patient is scheduled to receive a maintenance dose of belatacept post renal transplant. The provider ordered belatacept 10 mg/kg IV starting at week 10. What is the best action by the nurse?
     a. Call the provider who ordered the drug.
     b. Give the drug since the order is correct.
     c. Give the drug; the provider wanted the lower dose.
     d. Give the drug but at the correct recommended dose.

27. Which of the following patients is appropriate to treat with mammalian target of rapamycin inhibitors?
     a. A patient who had a lung transplant
     b. A patient who had a heart transplant
     c. A patient who had a liver transplant
     d. A patient who had a kidney transplant

28. Which of the following organ transplants is/are appropriate for mycophenolate mofetil? *(Select all that apply.)*
     a. Heart transplant
     b. Pancreas transplant
     c. Liver transplant
     d. Kidney transplant
     e. Corneal transplant

29. A patient is taking high doses of corticosteroids for acute transplant rejection. The nurse teaches the patient to avoid abrupt discontinuation of the drug, knowing that
     a. corticosteroids prevent infections by promoting leukocytes.
     b. corticosteroids promote the inflammatory response that suppresses the immune system.
     c. corticosteroids suppress adrenal function.
     d. corticosteroids promote leukocyte activation.

30. Before receiving antithymocyte globulin, the patient should receive which of the following drugs to decrease the incidence and severity of adverse reactions?
     a. Corticosteroid and antibiotic
     b. Antihistamine and antibiotic
     c. Antibiotic and diuretic
     d. Corticosteroid and antihistamine

31. A 34-year-old female post heart transplant is to receive immunosuppressive drugs to prevent rejection. Which of the following nursing interventions is a priority in this patient?
     a. Advise the patient to avoid anyone with an active infection.
     b. Instruct the patient to take blood pressure and temperature measurements each day.
     c. Instruct the patient that exercising places undue stress on the body, further suppressing the immune system.
     d. Promote proper nutrition by cooking all foods, including fruits and vegetables.

CASE STUDY

Read the scenario and answer the following questions on a separate sheet of paper.

J.R., a 64-year-old male, is scheduled to receive a liver transplant. Several hours before the surgery, J.R. is to receive cyclosporine and methylprednisolone sodium succinate.

1. What types of drugs are cyclosporine and methylprednisolone sodium succinate, and what are their general mechanisms of action?

2. What are some of the common side effects and adverse effects of cyclosporine and methylprednisolone sodium succinate?

3. Explain why patients receiving immunosuppressive drugs should not receive live vaccines.

31 Vaccines

Match the term in Column I to its definition in Column II.

Column I

_____ 1.   Seroconversion

_____ 2.   Pathogen

_____ 3.   Vaccine

_____ 4.   Antibody

_____ 5.   Attenuated viruses

_____ 6.   Passive immunity

_____ 7.   Toxoids

Column II

a.   Transient immunity
b.   Weakened microorganisms
c.   Another term for *immunoglobulins*
d.   Acquisition of detectable levels of antibodies
e.   A small amount of antigen that is administered to stimulate the immune response
f.   Bacteria, viruses, and fungi that invade the body
g.   Inactivated toxins to stimulate antitoxins

Complete the following.

8.   In the United States, there are more than _____ infectious diseases that may be prevented with vaccination.

9.   The Advisory Committee on Immunizations identified recommended _____, _____ to vaccinate, _____, and _____.

10. Yellow fever is transmitted by _____.

11. Adverse effects to vaccines must be reported through a surveillance system called _____.

12. _____ zoster is the reactivation of _____ zoster, usually settling in a dorsal root ganglion and causing severe pain.

NCLEX REVIEW QUESTIONS

Select the best response.

13. Which is the term used for vaccines made from the inactivated toxic substances produced by some microorganisms?
     a. Attenuated vaccines
     b. Conjugate vaccines
     c. Recombinant subunit vaccines
     d. Toxoids

14. In which situation(s) is/are acquired passive immunity important? *(Select all that apply.)*
     a. In fetuses in utero
     b. When time does not permit active vaccination alone
     c. When the exposed individual is at high risk for complications of the disease
     d. When a woman is pregnant
     e. When a person suffers from an immune system deficiency that renders the person unable to produce an effective immune response

145

15. What is the process by which antibodies are received by an individual, used for protection against a particular pathogen, and acquired from another source?
    a. Active immunity
    b. Childhood immunity
    c. Passive immunity
    d. Toxoids

16. What occurs when there is an acquisition of detectable levels of antibodies in the bloodstream after receiving vaccines?
    a. Passive immunity
    b. Acquired natural immunity
    c. Immunization
    d. Seroconversion

17. A mother of a newborn is scheduling her baby's 2-month checkup. The nurse advises her that at that time some vaccinations will be given. The mother states, "I'm not really sure I want to have her vaccinated. What do most vaccines really do?" What is the nurse's best response?
    a. "Vaccines are perceived by the body as antibodies."
    b. "Vaccines cause an allergic reaction."
    c. "Vaccines produce a mild form of the disease."
    d. "Vaccines stimulate an immune response."

18. The 45-year-old patient had measles as a child. What is the type of immunity that usually persists for the remainder of the individual's life after being infected with a disease?
    a. Natural acquired
    b. Humoral
    c. Active acquired artificial
    d. Passive natural

19. When is a child's first vaccine usually administered?
    a. At birth
    b. 2 months of age
    c. 4 months of age
    d. 6 months of age

20. What is rubella commonly known as?
    a. German measles
    b. Hard measles
    c. Herpes zoster
    d. Smallpox

21. Susceptible individuals age 13 years or older receive two doses of varicella vaccine spaced how long apart?
    a. At least 4 weeks
    b. 3 months
    c. 6 months
    d. 1 year

22. In the event of an adverse reaction to a vaccine, to whom should a health care provider report the details?
    a. Centers for Disease Control and Prevention (CDC)
    b. His or her immediate supervisor
    c. Vaccine Adverse Events Reporting System
    d. Vaccine manufacturer

23. Which type of immunity is conferred by the Td vaccine?
    a. Active
    b. Inactive
    c. Natural
    d. Passive

24. Which immunizations are examples of live, attenuated vaccines?
    a. Influenza and hepatitis B
    b. Measles-mumps-rubella (MMR) and poliomyelitis
    c. MMR and varicella
    d. Varicella and Td

25. The patient presents to his health care provider and states, "I think I have the flu." What are the signs and symptoms of influenza?
    a. Abdominal pain, cough, and nasal congestion
    b. Fever, diarrhea, and dizziness
    c. Fever, myalgia, and cough
    d. Vomiting, diarrhea, and headache

26. When the MMR vaccine is not given the same day as the varicella vaccine, what should be the minimum interval between administrations?
    a. 1 week
    b. 2 weeks
    c. 3 weeks
    d. 4 weeks

27. A 4-month-old patient's parent reports that after her first dose of DTaP, the patient experienced some redness and tenderness at the injection site in her left thigh. With this in mind, what should the nurse administer?
    a. DTaP again, because these are common side effects, not contraindications
    b. DT in the right thigh
    c. DTaP subcutaneously instead of intramuscularly to prevent muscle soreness
    d. Half the usual dose of DTaP to reduce the likelihood of a reaction

28. What information should the nurse provide the parent of a 4-month-old patient who just received her immunizations before the parent leaves the clinic today? *(Select all that apply.)*
    a. Appointment card for the next immunization clinic visit
    b. Immunization record
    c. List of side effects to observe
    d. Report of adverse reaction form
    e. Vaccine Information Statements (VIS) for all vaccines administered

29. What is a good source of health and immunization information for nurses assisting patients before international travel?
    a. Centers for Disease Control and Prevention
    b. No source is necessary because there are no special immunization needs for travelers
    c. The patient's travel agent
    d. U.S. embassy in the destination country

30. In the case of an anaphylactic reaction to a vaccine, which drug should the nurse have readily available?
    a. Acetaminophen
    b. Diphenhydramine
    c. Epinephrine
    d. Ranitidine

CASE STUDY

Read the scenario and answer the following questions on a separate sheet of paper.

M.E., 62 years old, was working in the garden and stepped on a garden tool. She sustained a deep puncture wound to her right foot. She presents to the clinic with a localized redness and swelling to her foot. She tells the nurse that she takes "only aspirin for my arthritis because I don't really like coming to the doctor much." She has no allergies. She receives an annual influenza vaccine at a local flu shot clinic but has received no other vaccinations in more than 20 years. Vital signs are blood pressure 118/80 mm Hg, heart rate 70 beats/min, respiratory rate 16 breaths/min, and temperature 37.8° C. M.E. weighs 53 kg.

1. What is the concern for a patient who has sustained a puncture wound?

2. What are the signs and symptoms of this disease process?

3. Which vaccines should be administered to the patient at this time?

32 Anticancer Drugs

Match the chemotherapy drugs/terms in Column I with the most appropriate description in Column II.

Column I

_____ 1. Alkylating drugs

_____ 2. Aromatase inhibitors

_____ 3. Cyclophosphamide

_____ 4. Doxorubicin

_____ 5. Palliative chemotherapy

_____ 6. Fluorouracil

_____ 7. Hormonal agents

_____ 8. Methotrexate

_____ 9. Personal protective equipment (PPE)

_____ 10. Vincristine

Column II

a. Associated with hemorrhagic cystitis
b. Leucovorin rescue
c. Stomatitis is early sign of toxicity
d. Associated with cardiotoxicity
e. Associated with neurotoxicity
f. Powder-free gloves, mask, impermeable gown
g. Mask cancer cells and prevent them from using hormones
h. Cause cross-linking of DNA strands, abnormal base pairing, or DNA strand breaks
i. Used to relieve symptoms associated with advanced disease
j. Block conversion of androgens to estrogen

Identify the environmental influences on cancer.

11. _____ Acute myelogenous leukemia

12. _____ Ultraviolet rays

13. _____ Epstein-Barr virus

14. _____ Animal fat

15. _____ Alcohol

NCLEX REVIEW QUESTIONS

Select the best response.

16. The nurse is caring for a patient receiving combination chemotherapy. The patient asks why she has to take more than one drug. What is the nurse's best response?
    a. "It has better response rates than single-drug chemotherapy."
    b. "It has fewer side effects than when given alone."
    c. "It is always more effective than surgery or radiation."
    d. "Survival rates are always better."

17. The nurse is teaching a community group about factors that influence the development of cancer in humans. Which information will the nurse include in this teaching?
    a. Aflatoxin is associated with cancer of the lung.
    b. Benzene is associated with cancer of the tongue.
    c. Epstein-Barr virus is associated with cancer of the stomach.
    d. Human papillomavirus is associated with cancer of the cervix.

149

18. A patient is receiving chemotherapy and asks the nurse about side effects. What should the nurse know concerning the side effects of chemotherapy?
   a. Side effects are minimal because chemotherapy drugs are highly selective.
   b. Side effects usually only occur during the first cycle of treatment.
   c. Side effects are caused by toxicities to normal cells.
   d. Side effects of chemotherapy are usually permanent.

19. The 65-year-old patient has metastatic cancer. He is scheduled to receive palliative chemotherapy. He states that he does not understand why he should receive palliative chemotherapy if it will not kill the cancer cells. What is the best response?
   a. "It is done to help improve your quality of life."
   b. "It is given to limit further growth of the cancer."
   c. "It is given to slow the growth of the cancer."
   d. "It will shrink the tumors throughout your body."

20. The patient will be receiving chemotherapy that will lower her white blood cell count. Monitoring for which finding will be a nursing priority?
   a. Change in temperature
   b. Evidence of petechiae
   c. Increase in diarrhea
   d. Taste changes

21. The patient has thrombocytopenia secondary to chemotherapy. Which nursing actions would be the most appropriate?
   a. Apply pressure to the injection site and assess for occult bleeding.
   b. Help the patient conserve energy by scheduling care.
   c. Monitor breath sounds and vital signs.
   d. Provide small, frequent meals and monitor loss of fluids from diarrhea.

22. The patient has diarrhea secondary to chemotherapy. What important information should be included in patient teaching about chemotherapy-related diarrhea?
   a. Eat only very hot or very cold foods.
   b. Increase intake of fresh fruits and vegetables.
   c. Increase intake of high-fiber foods.
   d. Limit caffeine intake.

23. The 70-year-old patient is to receive cyclophosphamide for treatment of his lymphoma. His medical history is also positive for atrial fibrillation, arthritis, and cataracts. He takes digoxin 0.125 mg daily and naproxen 500 mg at bedtime. What should the nurse be aware of when giving these drugs?
   a. Cyclophosphamide increases digoxin levels.
   b. Cyclophosphamide decreases digoxin levels.
   c. Digoxin increases cyclophosphamide levels.
   d. These drugs cannot be given together.

24. The patient is in the outpatient oncology clinic for treatment of her colon cancer. She is receiving fluorouracil (5-FU) as part of her treatment and has recently been started on metronidazole for treatment of trichomoniasis. What should concern the nurse about this order?
   a. 5-FU may decrease the effectiveness of metronidazole.
   b. 5-FU cannot be given with metronidazole.
   c. Metronidazole may increase the side effects of 5-FU.
   d. Metronidazole may increase 5-FU toxicity.

25. The patient, 61 years old, is to receive doxorubicin as part of his chemotherapy protocol. Which assessment is the most important before administering the drug?
   a. Cardiac status
   b. Liver function
   c. Lung sounds
   d. Neurologic status

26. The patient, 69 years old, is receiving cyclophosphamide, doxorubicin, and methotrexate (CAM) for the treatment of prostate cancer. During morning rounds, the patient complains of feeling short of breath. Physical assessment reveals crackles in both lungs. What is the most likely cause of this clinical manifestation?
   a. Anxiety
   b. Cyclophosphamide
   c. Doxorubicin
   d. Methotrexate

27. A patient is to receive fluorouracil (5-FU) intravenously as part of a treatment protocol for colon cancer. He is to receive an antiemetic. When should the nurse administer the antiemetic?
   a. 1 day after administering 5-FU
   b. 1 day before administering 5-FU
   c. 30–60 minutes before administering 5-FU
   d. 4 hours before administering 5-FU

28. A patient has reached the lowest level of his blood counts secondary to chemotherapy. Which nursing diagnosis is the most appropriate?
   a. Risk for cardiac failure
   b. Risk for dehydration
   c. Risk for infection
   d. Risk for malnutrition

29. Which nursing outcome would be most appropriate as part of the planning for a patient scheduled to receive cyclophosphamide?
   a. Patient will be free from symptoms of stomatitis.
   b. Patient will maintain cardiac output.
   c. Patient will show no signs of hemorrhagic cystitis.
   d. Patient will show no signs of syndrome of inappropriate antidiuretic hormone secretion (SIADH).

30. The patient is to receive cyclophosphamide as part of her cancer treatment. Which nursing intervention should the nurse expect to complete?
   a. Assess for signs of hematuria, urinary frequency, or dysuria.
   b. Decrease fluids to reduce the risk of calculus formation.
   c. Hydrate the patient with IV fluids only after administration of cyclophosphamide.
   d. Medicate with an antiemetic only after the patient complains of nausea.

31. The nurse is teaching a 29-year-old patient about cyclophosphamide, which will be given as part of her treatment protocol for cancer. Which priority information should be included in the teaching?
   a. Hair loss has never been reported with the use of cyclophosphamide.
   b. Menstrual irregularities and sterility are not expected with this drug.
   c. No special isolation procedures are needed when receiving this chemotherapy.
   d. Pregnancy should be prevented during treatment with cyclophosphamide.

32. The nurse is administering IV fluorouracil (5-FU) to a patient in the outpatient oncology clinic. Which nursing intervention would be most appropriate?
   a. Assess for severe pain and signs of infiltration at the IV site.
   b. Apply heat to the IV site if extravasation occurs.
   c. Assess for tissue necrosis at the IV site attributable to extravasation.
   d. Encourage mouth rinses once every 8 hours during chemotherapy.

33. A patient receiving cyclophosphamide, epirubicin, and fluorouracil (5-FU) (CEF) has experienced severe nausea, vomiting, and diarrhea over the past week. He has lost 5.5 pounds in 3 days. Which nursing diagnosis would be most appropriate?
   a. Knowledge deficit related to chemotherapeutic regimen
   b. Pain secondary to diarrhea
   c. Risk for altered nutrition
   d. Risk for infection secondary to low WBC counts

34. The nurse is teaching a patient about doxorubicin, which she will receive as part of her treatment for breast cancer. Which statement made by the patient indicates that she needs additional teaching?
   a. "Doxorubicin is a severe vesicant."
   b. "My blood counts will be checked."
   c. "My cardiac status will be closely monitored."
   d. "This drug may make my urine turn blue."

35. The nurse is administering doxorubicin to a patient in the outpatient oncology clinic. What is priority information to include in the patient teaching?
   a. Blood counts will most likely remain normal.
   b. Complete alopecia rarely occurs with this drug.
   c. Report any shortness of breath, palpitations, or edema to your health care provider.
   d. Tissue necrosis usually occurs 2–3 days after administration.

36. The nurse is administering doxorubicin to a patient diagnosed with cancer. What should the nurse keep in mind with regard to tissue necrosis associated with this drug?
   a. Tissue necrosis may occur 3–4 weeks after administration.
   b. Tissue necrosis occurs immediately after administration.
   c. Tissue necrosis occurs 2–4 days after administration.
   d. Tissue necrosis rarely occurs with this drug.

37. One week ago in the outpatient oncology clinic, a patient received his first cycle of chemotherapy consisting of cyclophosphamide, doxorubicin, and fluorouracil (5-FU) (CAF). He returns to the clinic today for follow-up. Which nursing intervention would be most appropriate at this time?
   a. Culture the IV site and send a specimen to the laboratory for analysis.
   b. Monitor blood counts and laboratory values.
   c. Offer analgesics for pain and evaluate effectiveness.
   d. Teach the patient about good skin care.

38. The nurse is preparing IV vinblastine, bleomycin, and cisplatin (VBP) for administration to a patient on the nursing unit. Which precaution should the nurse take when hanging IV chemotherapy?
    a. Wear a clean cotton gown.
    b. Wear shoe covers.
    c. Wear a hair net.
    d. Wear two pairs of gloves.

39. A patient is being discharged after receiving IV chemotherapy. Which statement made by the patient indicates a need for additional teaching?
    a. "Chemotherapy is excreted in my bodily fluids."
    b. "I will not need to know how to check my temperature."
    c. "My spouse should wear gloves when emptying my urinal."
    d. "The chemotherapy will remain in my body for 2–3 days."

40. The nurse is preparing to administer chemotherapy, which can cause severe nausea and vomiting, to a patient in the outpatient clinic. Which nursing action would be most appropriate?
    a. Give an antiemetic before administering the chemotherapy.
    b. Withhold any antiemetic drugs until the patient complains of nausea.
    c. Give an antiemetic only after the patient has vomited.
    d. Offer the patient a glass of ginger ale to prevent nausea.

41. A patient is admitted to the hospital 1 week after receiving teniposide in the outpatient oncology clinic. On physical assessment, the nurse notes the presence of petechiae, ecchymoses, and bleeding on the toothbrush when the patient brushes his teeth. Which nursing diagnosis would be most appropriate?
    a. Risk for fatigue
    b. Risk for infection
    c. Risk for bleeding
    d. Risk for falls

42. A patient with breast cancer is scheduled to receive anastrozole, an aromatase inhibitor. Which information should be included in the patient teaching?
    a. Aromatase inhibitors block the peripheral conversion of androgens to estrogens.
    b. Aromatase inhibitors are used to treat tumors that are not hormonally sensitive.
    c. Aromatase inhibitors are used only in premenopausal women with breast cancer.
    d. Aromatase inhibitors are used only in postmenopausal women with breast cancer.

43. A patient is scheduled to receive vincristine as part of treatment for cancer. The medication record for the patient indicates that he is receiving phenytoin to control a seizure disorder. What should the nurse monitor in this patient?
    a. Headaches
    b. Increased blood pressure
    c. Renal failure
    d. Seizures

44. A patient is scheduled to receive vincristine as part of her treatment for non-Hodgkin's lymphoma. She reports that she likes to "rely on nature" for complementary therapy. Which herbal/supplement(s) should be avoided by this patient? (Select all that apply.)
    a. St. John's wort
    b. Daily multivitamin
    c. Periwinkle
    d. Echinacea
    e. Valerian

45. A patient in the outpatient oncology clinic has developed stomatitis secondary to cancer therapy. Which statement made by the patient would indicate that she needs additional teaching about stomatitis?
    a. "I will rinse my mouth out frequently with normal saline."
    b. "I will try using ice pops or ice chips to help relieve mouth pain."
    c. "I will use a mouthwash that has an alcohol base."
    d. "I will use a soft toothbrush."

46. A patient presents with neutropenia secondary to cancer therapy. Which nursing diagnosis would be the most appropriate?
    a. Risk for cardiac failure
    b. Risk for dehydration
    c. Risk for infection
    d. Risk for malnutrition

CASE STUDY

Read the scenario, and answer the following questions on a separate sheet of paper.

C.Z., 25-years-old, is being treated for multiple myeloma with cyclophosphamide.

1. To which class of drugs does cyclophosphamide belong, and how does it work?

2. What are major side effects?

3. What are key factors in the nursing assessment for this patient?

4. What are priority teaching points for this patient with regards to her drug regimen?

33 Targeted Therapies to Treat Cancer

STUDY QUESTIONS

Complete the following.

1. The _____ _____ binding to cell receptors on the cell membrane can activate tyrosine kinases, which then turn on signal transduction pathways promoting cell division.

2. _____ _____ and _____ _____ are methods of communication by way of signal molecules for cells to maintain homeostasis, regulate cell growth and division, develop into tissues, and coordinate cellular functions.

3. Tyrosine kinases are a family of enzymes that activate other substances by adding a phosphate molecule, a process known as _____.

4. _____ _____ for cell division are substances that enter the nucleus and signal the cell that mitosis is needed.

5. _____ are part of a family of proteins that, when active, stimulate the cell to move through the cell cycle.

6. _____ are multienzyme complexes that degrade proteins intracellularly.

7. Intracellular homeostasis is maintained through _____, a process that involves _____ degradation and _____ of unnecessary or damaged cellular components.

8. Targeted therapies _____ signal transduction, which blocks the _____ and _____ of cancer cells.

9. The largest class of targeted therapy drugs that attack one particular molecular target is _____ inhibitor.

10. _____ are enzymes that activate other proteins, including signal transduction pathways.

Match the class of targeted therapy drug in Column I to the mechanism of action in Column II.

Column I

_____ 11. mTOR kinase inhibitor

_____ 12. EGFR inhibitor

_____ 13. Angiogenesis inhibitor

_____ 14. Monoclonal antibody

_____ 15. Tyrosine kinase inhibitor

Column II

a. Prevents formation of new blood vessels
b. Binds to different areas of EGFR, blocking its activity
c. Primarily affects BCR-ABL kinase enzyme
d. Lead to G_1 arrest and cell death
e. Targets cell-membrane surface antigens

Select the best response.

16. During the first dose of trastuzumab, the patient complains of shortness of breath and pruritus. What is the best action by the nurse?
    a. Decrease the infusion rate by 50% and notify the health care provider.
    b. Disconnect the IV and attach a 0.22-micron filter.
    c. Review the pretreatment multigated acquisition (MUGA) scan.
    d. Stop the infusion and manage the reaction.

17. What is the rationale for administering bevacizumab in a patient with metastatic colon cancer?
    a. To enhance the patient's immune response
    b. To increase apoptosis
    c. To inhibit tumor's microvascular growth
    d. To modulate an inflammatory response

18. Gefitinib most frequently causes which side/adverse effect?
    a. Hypocalcemia
    b. Diarrhea
    c. Myelosuppression
    d. Seizures

19. An oncology patient is to begin treatment for non–small-cell lung cancer (NSCLC) with administration of gefitinib. The nurse notes on his medical record that the patient is also taking warfarin daily for atrial fibrillation. What should concern the nurse about the patient taking gefitinib and warfarin?
    a. Gefitinib increases the effects of warfarin.
    b. Gefitinib may require a dose increase when taken with warfarin.
    c. Gefitinib is never given to a patient taking anticoagulants.
    d. Gefitinib may reach toxic levels when given concurrently with warfarin.

20. A patient in the outpatient oncology clinic is receiving sunitinib as part of his treatment for gastrointestinal stromal tumors (GIST). The health care provider prescribes ketoconazole to treat a fungal infection. What should concern the nurse about taking these drugs concurrently?
    a. Ketoconazole may decrease the effectiveness of sunitinib.
    b. Ketoconazole may potentiate sunitinib toxicity.
    c. Sunitinib may decrease the effectiveness of ketoconazole.
    d. Sunitinib may lead to toxic levels of ketoconazole.

21. A patient is beginning therapy with the epidermal growth factor/receptor inhibitor (EGFRI) erlotinib for non-small cell lung cancer (NSCLC). Which is the most important status for the nurse to assess before beginning therapy with this targeted drug?
    a. Cardiac status
    b. Hearing function
    c. Lung sounds
    d. Mental status

22. A patient is admitted to the hospital 1 week after receiving imatinib. On physical assessment, the nurse notes the presence of petechiae, ecchymoses, and bleeding gums. Which nursing diagnosis would be most appropriate?
    a. Bleeding, risk for
    b. Falls, risk for
    c. Fatigue, risk for
    d. Altered nutrition, risk for

23. A patient is to start ziv-aflibercept, in addition to 5-fluorouracil (5-FU), leucovorin, and irinotecan. Which of the following statements made by the patient indicates a lack of understanding for receiving ziv-aflibercept?
    a. "The new drug is going to starve cancer cells."
    b. "I will need to stay indoors because medicine will make my skin more sensitive to the sun."
    c. "The drug will allow my good cells to grow new vessels."
    d. "The drug will prevent the cells from dividing."

24. Which of the following are types of monoclonal antibodies? *(Select all that apply.)*
    a. Fully human antibodies
    b. Chimeric antibodies
    c. Equine antibodies
    d. Porcine antibodies
    e. Murine antibodies

25. A patient who is to receive rituximab has a blood pressure of 90/52 mm Hg and a heart rate of 82 beats/min. Upon reviewing the patient's routine medications, the nurse notes antihypertensives. What is the best action by the nurse?
    a. Start the infusion. The blood pressure and heart rate are within the parameters.
    b. Notify the health care provider.
    c. Infuse 250 mL of 0.9% sodium chloride over 2 hours before infusing rituximab.
    d. Retake the blood pressure in the other arm.

CASE STUDY

Read the scenario and answer the following questions on a separate sheet of paper.

S.M., 32 years old, has been diagnosed with ovarian cancer and presents to the outpatient oncology clinic for treatment. She is being treated with bevacizumab for metastatic disease.

1. How is bevacizumab administered?

2. What is the mechanism of action?

3. What are potential side effects and adverse effects?

4. What teaching should be provided by the nurse in relation to bevacizumab therapy?

34 Biologic Response Modifiers

STUDY QUESTIONS

Complete the following.

1. Immunotherapies, also called _____ _____ _____, enhance, direct, or _____ the body's immune system.

2. Two advances in biologic therapies include _____ _____ and _____ _____.

3. Biologic response modifiers assist the immune system through _____ and prevent cancer cells from _____.

4. Macrophages are considered mature _____.

5. Erythropoietin stimulates the production of _____ _____ _____ in the bone marrow.

6. Granulocyte colony–stimulating factor is produced by macrophages, _____, and other immune cells and stimulates the synthesis of _____.

7. Many adverse effects of exogenous interleukins are due to _____ _____ _____.

Match the description in Column II with the appropriate term in Column I.

Column I

_____ 8. Colony-stimulating factors (CSFs)

_____ 9. Erythropoietin

_____ 10. Granulocyte colony–stimulating factor (G-CSF)

_____ 11. Granulocyte-macrophage colony–stimulating factor (GM-CSF)

Column II

a. Glycoprotein that stimulates the production of neutrophils

b. Proteins that stimulate growth and maturation of bone marrow stem cells

c. Glycoprotein produced by the kidneys in response to low oxygen (hypoxia)

d. Supports survival, proliferation, and differentiation of hematopoietic progenitor cells

NCLEX REVIEW QUESTIONS

Select the best response.

12. What is/are the primary function(s) of biologic response modifiers (BRMs)? *(Select all that apply.)*
    a. To slow tumor cell's growth
    b. To enhance host's normal immunologic function
    c. To improve liver functioning
    d. To promote differentiation of bone marrow stem cells
    e. To replicate red blood cells

13. A patient is receiving GM-CSF therapy. Which system will the nurse focus attention on, both during and after these infusions?
    a. Cardiac system
    b. Central nervous system
    c. Musculoskeletal system
    d. Respiratory system

14. Before administering erythropoietin, what is a priority assessment for the nurse?
    a. Renal function
    b. Hemoglobin level
    c. Liver function
    d. Chest x-ray

15. A patient is being treated with interferon for chronic myelogenous leukemia. When should the nurse anticipate stopping treatment? *(Select all that apply.)*
    a. Severe depression
    b. Hepatic decompensation
    c. Absolute neutrophil count $<500/mm^3$
    d. Platelets $>140,000/mm^3$

16. A 70-year-old patient has hairy cell leukemia that is being treated with interferon. The patient reports neurologic side effects. What will the nurse tell the patient about the side effects?
    a. "These side effects are common and will subside after the drug is stopped."
    b. "These side effects rarely occur."
    c. "These side effects will diminish as treatment goes on."
    d. "The worst effect is mild confusion."

17. For which dermatologic effect(s) should the nurse assess in a patient taking interferon? *(Select all that apply.)*
    a. Alopecia
    b. Bruising
    c. Xerostomia
    d. Rash

18. Which of the following statements are priority health teaching information for a patient who has hairy cell leukemia and is being treated with interferon alpha? *(Select all that apply.)*
    a. Report any unusual weight loss.
    b. Teach information on the effect of BRM-related fatigue on activities of daily living
    c. Side effects from a BRM disappear within 12–24 hours after discontinuation of therapy.
    d. Persistent headache or blurred vision should be reported to the health care provider.

19. For which condition(s) may GM-CSF be administered to patients? *(Select all that apply.)*
    a. Absolute neutrophil count $>1500/mm^3$
    b. Autologous bone marrow transplant (BMT) recipient
    c. Allogeneic BMT recipient
    d. 12 hours after high-dose chemotherapy administration
    e. Kaposi sarcoma

20. The patient is to start aldesleukin for metastatic renal cell cancer. Which of the following would the nurse monitor to determine dose interruption or discontinuation? *(Select all that apply).*
    a. New irregular cardiac rhythm
    b. Oxygen saturation less than 95%
    c. Stool positive for blood
    d. Existing skin rash that was present before starting aldesleukin
    e. Hypoglycemia

CASE STUDY

Read the scenario, and answer the following questions on a separate sheet of paper.

K.U., 38-years-old, has been diagnosed with acute myelogenous leukemia (AML) and will be undergoing treatment. She is scheduled to receive G-CSF and wants to know what this drug will do to cure her cancer. She will be receiving 75 mcg/kg/day IV.

1. What type of medication is G-CSF, and how does it work?

2. What are the potential side effects K.U. may experience with this drug?

3. What priority teaching will the nurse provide to the patient and her significant others?

35 Upper Respiratory Disorders

Match the term in Column I to the description in Column II.

Column I

_____ 1. Antihistamines

_____ 2. Antitussives

_____ 3. Decongestants

_____ 4. Expectorants

Column II

a. Act on the cough-control center in the medulla
b. Loosen bronchial secretions so they can be removed by coughing
c. H_1 blockers or H_1 antagonists
d. Stimulate the alpha-adrenergic receptors, producing vascular constriction in the nasal capillaries

Complete the following.

5. Antihistamines are _____ antagonists that have effects on the _____ muscles.

6. Many over-the-counter (OTC) cold remedies contain a _____ _____antihistamine that can cause side effects such as ____ _____ and _____.

7. Second-generation antihistamines are considered _____ and have fewer _____ symptoms.

8. Frequent use of nasal decongestants can result in _____and _____ _____ _____, which can occur in as little as ___ _____.

9. Nasal decongestants stimulate the _____ receptors that cause _____, which can also cause _____.

Match the antihistamine in Column I to the correct generation in Column II. The generation in Column II may be used more than once.

Column I

_____ 10. Diphenhydramine

_____ 11. Cetirizine

_____ 12. Loratadine

_____ 13. Chlorpheniramine

_____ 14. Azelastine

_____ 15. Clemastine fumarate

Column II

a. First generation
b. Second generation
c. Other antihistamine

NCLEX REVIEW QUESTIONS

Select the best response.

16. Antihistamines are another group of drugs used for the relief of cold symptoms. What properties of these drugs result in decreased secretions?
    a. Analgesic
    b. Anticholinergic
    c. Antitussive
    d. Cholinergic

17. Compared to first-generation antihistamines, second-generation antihistamines have a lower incidence of which side effect?
    a. Drowsiness
    b. Headache
    c. Tinnitus
    d. Vomiting

159

18. The U.S. Food and Drug Administration has ordered removal of all cold remedies containing which drug?
    a. Dextromethorphan
    b. Guaifenesin
    c. Histamine
    d. Phenylpropanolamine

19. The patient has environmental allergies and asks the student health nurse about the appropriate dose of diphenhydramine. What is the recommended dosage of diphenhydramine?
    a. 25–50 mg q6–8h
    b. 25–50 mg daily
    c. 50–100 mg q4–6h
    d. 100 mg daily

20. What is one of the effects of diphenhydramine?
    a. Anticoagulant
    b. Anticonvulsant
    c. Antihypertensive
    d. Antitussive

21. Diphenhydramine blocks histamine receptors. Which histamine receptors does it block?
    a. H_1
    b. H_2
    c. B_1
    d. B_2

22. A patient taking diphenhydramine breastfeeds her infant daughter. What advice will the nurse give her?
    a. Breastfeeding provides allergy relief to the infant.
    b. Large amounts of the drug pass into breast milk; breastfeeding is not recommended.
    c. Small amounts of the drug pass into breast milk; breastfeeding is not recommended.
    d. The drug does not affect breastfeeding.

23. The health teaching plan for a patient taking diphenhydramine should include the side effects of the drug. What might the nurse assess in a patient experiencing a side effect? *(Select all that apply.)*
    a. Disturbed coordination
    b. Drowsiness
    c. Hypertension
    d. Nausea
    e. Urinary retention

24. What is the advantage of systemic decongestants over nasal sprays and drops?
    a. Fewer side effects
    b. Less costly
    c. Preferred by older patients
    d. Provide longer relief

25. Which expectorant is frequently an ingredient in cold remedies?
    a. Dextromethorphan
    b. Ephedrine
    c. Guaifenesin
    d. Promethazine

26. What group(s) of drugs is/are used to treat cold symptoms? *(Select all that apply.)*
    a. Antihistamines
    b. Antitussives
    c. Decongestants
    d. Expectorants
    e. Xanthines

27. Decongestants are contraindicated or to be used with extreme caution for patients with which condition(s)? *(Select all that apply.)*
    a. Cardiac disease
    b. Diabetes mellitus
    c. Hypertension
    d. Hyperthyroidism
    e. Obesity

28. Which priority information should be included in teaching a patient who is taking drugs for a common cold and also has a history of atrial fibrillation and depression? *(Select all that apply.)*
    a. Administer 4 puffs of nasal spray for a full 10 days.
    b. Antibiotics are also needed to fight a common cold virus.
    c. Do not drive during initial use of a cold remedy containing an antihistamine.
    d. Read labels of over-the-counter drugs for any interactions with current drugs.
    e. Take cold remedies with a decongestant for a better night's sleep.

CASE STUDY

Read the scenario, and answer the following questions on a separate sheet of paper.

G.H., 53 years old, is preparing to fly across the country for a conference. He presents to his health care provider with nasal stuffiness. He states, "I hate to fly when my nose is this way. It just makes the trip all that much longer." A decongestant, oxymetazoline, is ordered.

1. What is the purpose of oxymetazoline, and how does it work?

2. What is the standard dosage for this drug?

3. What is rebound congestion? What other side effects might be expected, and how can they be prevented? Are there any other options for a decongestant?

36 Lower Respiratory Disorders

Match the drug in Column I with its category in Column II. Drugs may belong to more than one category.

Column I

_____ 1. Acetylcysteine

_____ 2. Zafirlukast

_____ 3. Albuterol

_____ 4. Ipratropium bromide

_____ 5. Dexamethasone

_____ 6. Epinephrine

_____ 7. Arformoterol tartrate

_____ 8. Tiotropium

Column II

a. Alpha-adrenergic agonist
b. Beta-adrenergic agonist
c. Glucocorticoid
d. Mucolytic
e. Leukotriene receptor antagonist
f. Anticholinergic

Complete the following.

9. The substance responsible for maintaining bronchodilation is _____ _____.

10. In an acute bronchospasm caused by anaphylaxis, the nonselective sympathomimetic drug administered subcutaneously to promote bronchodilation and elevate the blood pressure is _____.

11. The first line of defense in an acute asthmatic attack are the drugs categorized as _____ _____.

12. Sympathomimetics cause dilation of the bronchioles by increasing _____.

13. Theophylline (increases/decreases) the risk of digitalis toxicity. *(Circle correct answer.)*

14. When theophylline and beta$_2$-adrenergic agonists are given together, a(n) _____ effect can occur.

15. The half-life of theophylline is (shorter/longer) for smokers than for nonsmokers. *(Circle correct answer.)*

16. Aminophylline, theophylline, and caffeine are _____ derivatives used to treat _____.

17. The drugs commonly prescribed to treat unresponsive asthma are _____.

18. Cromolyn is used as a _____ treatment for bronchial asthma. It acts by inhibiting the release of _____.

19. A serious side effect of cromolyn is _____ _____.

20. The newer drugs for asthma are more selective for _____ receptors.

21. The leukotriene receptor antagonist (is/is not) considered safe for use in children 6 years and older. *(Circle correct answer.)*

22. The preferred time of day for the administration of leukotriene receptor antagonists is _____.

23. The usual dose of montelukast for an adult is _____ and for a child 6 to 14 years old is

    _____.

24. A group of drugs used to liquefy and loosen thick mucous secretions is _____.

25. With infection resulting from retained mucous secretions, a(n) _____ may be prescribed.

NCLEX REVIEW QUESTIONS

Select the best response.

26. The patient is being treated for chronic obstructive pulmonary disease (COPD). His medication is delivered via a metered-dose inhaler. Related health teaching would include which priority information?
    a. Hold the inhaler upside down.
    b. Refrigerate the inhaler.
    c. Shake the inhaler well just before use.
    d. Test the inhaler each time to see if the spray works.

27. When compared to oral drugs for asthma, what information regarding a drug administered by a metered-dose inhaler should be aware to the nurse? *(Select all that apply.)*
    a. The inhaled dose will deliver more of the drug directly to the lungs.
    b. There are fewer side effects with an inhaled drug.
    c. Inhaled drug is longer-lasting.
    d. Inhaled drug has a more rapid onset.
    e. Some oral and inhaled drugs can be taken together.

28. The patient has been prescribed both ipratropium and cromolyn. How many minutes should the patient wait between using the two drugs?
    a. 1
    b. 5
    c. 10
    d. It does not matter

29. The patient is taking an inhaled beta agonist and a steroid for his asthma. He states, "I don't have time to wait between taking drugs. I'm very busy. Why do I have to do this?" What is the nurse's best response to the patient?
    a. "The inhaled drug will allow the bronchioles to dilate so the steroid works better."
    b. "This is done so you remember which one comes first."
    c. "The inhaled medication will make your heart circulate the steroid faster."
    d. "The steroid may make your nose stuffy, so you take the inhaled drug first."

30. What is/are the side effect(s) of long-term use of glucocorticoids? *(Select all that apply.)*
    a. Impaired immune response
    b. Insomnia
    c. Hyperglycemia
    d. Vomiting
    e. Weight loss

31. Which of the following anticholinergic drugs has few systemic effects and is administered by aerosol?
    a. Albuterol
    b. Ipratropium
    c. Isoproterenol
    d. Tiotropium

32. Drug selection and dosage in older adults with conditions of the lower respiratory tract need to be considered. The use of large, continuous doses of a beta$_2$-adrenergic agonist may cause which side effect(s) in the older adult? *(Select all that apply.)*
    a. Bronchoconstriction
    b. Constipation
    c. Tachycardia
    d. Tremors
    e. Urinary retention

33. The 40-year-old patient has been taking theophylline for long-term treatment of his asthma. He has also been taking ephedra to stay alert while finishing a project at work. The patient presents to the clinic with complaints of feeling ill. Vital signs are temperature 36.4° C oral, heart rate 124 beats/min, respiratory rate 18 breaths/min, blood pressure 170/90 mm Hg, and oxygen saturation 99% on room air. Fingerstick blood glucose is 210 mg/dL. His theophylline level is 26 mcg/mL. What does the nurse suspect may be the cause of the patient's symptoms?
    a. Acute allergic reaction
    b. Asthma attack
    c. Stevens-Johnson syndrome
    d. Theophylline toxicity

34. The patient has exercise-induced bronchospasm and is being treated with a short-acting beta$_2$ agonist. Which priority information will the nurse include in a review of inhaler administration for this patient? *(Select all that apply.)*
   a. "Cleanse all washable parts of inhaler equipment daily."
   b. "Hold your breath for a few seconds, remove mouthpiece, and exhale slowly."
   c. "Keep your lips secure around the mouthpiece and inhale while pushing the top of the canister once."
   d. "Monitor your heart rate while taking this medication."
   e. "Wait 5 minutes and repeat the procedure if a second inhalation is needed."

35. The 68-year-old patient has been diagnosed with COPD. When providing health teaching for this patient, the nurse discusses the side effects that may occur with the use of bronchodilators. Which possible clinical manifestation(s) should concern the patient? *(Select all that apply.)*
   a. Bradycardia
   b. Dry eyes
   c. Lethargy
   d. Nervousness
   e. Palpitations

36. Which medication(s) when prescribed with theophylline will concern the nurse? *(Select all that apply.)*
   a. Beta blockers
   b. Digitalis
   c. Lithium
   d. Stool softeners
   e. Phenytoin

37. Which of the following is/are side effect(s) of theophylline? *(Select all that apply.)*
   a. Cardiac dysrhythmias
   b. Diarrhea
   c. Gastrointestinal bleeding
   d. Headache
   e. Seizures

38. The patient has asthma and takes cromolyn. Which statement by the patient indicates the need for more education?
   a. "I must take this drug every day."
   b. "It will stop an asthma attack when taken immediately."
   c. "I can rinse my mouth out with water to get rid of the taste."
   d. "It is important for me to take this exactly as directed."

39. A patient presents to the health care provider's office for a follow-up visit. The patient is taking theophylline, and the nurse is reviewing the lab results. What level of theophylline would fall in the therapeutic range?
   a. 2 mcg/mL
   b. 8 mcg/mL
   c. 14 mcg/mL
   d. 23 mcg/mL

CASE STUDY

Read the scenario, and answer the following questions on a separate sheet of paper.

H.K., 35 years old, has recently been diagnosed with asthma and has been prescribed albuterol, montelukast sodium, and fluticasone propionate/salmeterol 100/50.

1. To which classes of drugs do each of these drugs belong? How does each medication work?

2. What are priority teaching points for this patient with a new diagnosis of asthma?

37 Cardiac Glycosides, Antianginals, and Antidysrhythmics

Match the ECG waveform in Column I to its definition in Column II.

Column I

_____ 1. P wave

_____ 2. QRS complex

_____ 3. T wave

_____ 4. PR interval

_____ 5. QT interval

Column II

a. Ventricular action potential duration
b. Atrial activation (depolarization)
c. Ventricular repolarization
d. AV conduction time
e. Ventricular depolarization

Complete the following.

6. Heart failure occurs when the myocardium (strengthens/weakens) and (shrinks/enlarges), which causes the heart to lose its ability to pump blood through the heart and circulatory system. *(Circle correct answers.)*

7. With heart failure there is a(n) (increase/decrease) in preload and afterload. *(Circle correct answer.)*

8. Cardiac glycosides are also called _____, _____ which _____ the sodium-potassium pump.

9. The action of antianginal drugs is to increase blood flow and to (increase/decrease) oxygen supply or to (increase/decrease) oxygen demand by the myocardium. *(Circle correct answers.)*

10. Name three of the four effects digitalis preparations have on the heart muscle (myocardium): _____,

     _____, and _____.

11. Beta blockers and calcium channel blockers (decrease/increase) the workload of the heart. *(Circle correct answer.)*

12. To prevent thromboembolus in patients with atrial dysrhythmias, _____ is prescribed concurrently with antidysrhythmics.

13. Electrolyte imbalances such as _____, _____, and _____ can increase digitalis toxicity.

14. ACE inhibitors help patients with heart failure by _____ venules and _____, which

     improves _____ blood flow and _____ blood fluid volume.

15. Nitroglycerin (NTG) is not swallowed because it undergoes _____, thereby decreasing its effectiveness.

16. NTG acts directly on the _____, causing relaxation and dilation.

17. NTG sublingually acts within _____ minutes. Administration may be repeated _____ times.

18. The most common side effect of NTG is _____.

19. The two drug groups that may be used as an antianginal, antidysrhythmic, and antihypertensive are _____ _____ and _____ _____ _____.

20. Calcium channel blockers that are effective in the long-term treatment of angina, dysrhythmia, and hypertension and have the side effect of bradycardia are _____ and chest _____.

21. Beta blockers and calcium channel blockers should not be discontinued without health care provider approval. Withdrawal symptoms may include _____ _____ and _____.

22. Classic angina occurs when the patient is _____.

23. Unstable angina (preinfarction) has the following pattern of occurrence: _____.

24. Variant angina (Prinzmetal's angina) occurs when the patient _____.

25. Prinzmetal's angina is due to _____ of the vessels.

26. The major systemic effect of nitrates is _____.

27. Cardiac dysrhythmias can result from (hypoxia/hyperoxia) and (hypocapnia/hypercapnia). *(Circle correct answers.)*

28. Examples of antidysrhythmics include _____, _____, and _____.

29. Patients with heart failure should avoid _____ and _____.

The nurse should obtain a history of herbs the patient is taking. This is especially true for patients taking digoxin. Match the herbs in Column I with their effects on digoxin in Column II. Answers may be used more than once.

Column I

_____ 30. St. John's wort

_____ 31. Ephedra

_____ 32. Aloe

_____ 33. Goldenseal

_____ 34. Ginseng

Column II

a. Increased risk of digitalis toxicity
b. Decreased digoxin absorption
c. Decreased effects of digoxin
d. Falsely elevated digoxin levels

NCLEX REVIEW QUESTIONS

Select the best response.

35. What are digitalis preparations effective for treating?
    a. Asthma
    b. Heart failure (HF)
    c. Thrombophlebitis
    d. Vascular insufficiency

36. Phosphodiesterase inhibitors are used to treat HF by inhibiting phosphodiesterase enzyme. What do these agents promote?
    a. Increased serum sodium and potassium levels
    b. Negative inotropic action
    c. Positive inotropic action
    d. Vasoconstriction

37. What is an example of a phosphodiesterase inhibitor?
    a. Amlodipine
    b. Digoxin
    c. Milrinone
    d. Isosorbide dinitrate

38. The 64-year-old patient has a history of atrial flutter. His health care provider has prescribed quinidine. The patient asks the nurse how this medication will help his heart. What is the nurse's best response?
    a. "It will help your heart pump stronger."
    b. "It will prevent you from having chest pain."
    c. "It will decrease myocardial oxygen consumption."
    d. "It will slow down the speed of your heart so that it will work more effectively."

39. What type of drug is propranolol?
    a. Calcium channel blocker
    b. Cardioselective beta blocker
    c. Fast sodium blocker
    d. Nonselective beta blocker

40. The 61-year-old patient is in cardiac arrest. His ventricular fibrillation is refractory to other treatment. What drugs is the drug of choice when other agents are ineffective?
    a. Amiodarone
    b. Atropine
    c. Acebutolol HCl
    d. Propafenone HCl

41. What is/are the action(s) of antidysrhythmics? *(Select all that apply.)*
    a. Block adrenergic stimulation to the heart
    b. Decrease conduction velocity
    c. Decrease preload
    d. Increase heart rate
    e. Increase force of myocardial contraction

42. What is lidocaine primarily used to treat?
    a. Atrial fibrillation
    b. Bradycardia
    c. Complete heart block
    d. Ventricular dysrhythmias

43. The patient has been diagnosed with angina and has been prescribed verapamil. What priority teaching point(s) should the nurse include regarding this drug? *(Select all that apply.)*
    a. "Eat lots of fiber to avoid constipation."
    b. "High blood pressure can be caused by verapamil."
    c. "This drug is taken three times per day."
    d. "Wear sunscreen due to photosensitivity."
    e. "You should not take this drug if you are diabetic."

44. Which is the most potent calcium channel blocker?
    a. Diltiazem
    b. Nicardipine
    c. Nifedipine
    d. Verapamil

45. The patient has been prescribed amlodipine to help control his hypertension. What laboratory values must be monitored carefully?
    a. Arterial blood gasses
    b. Blood glucose
    c. Complete blood count
    d. Liver enzymes

46. Abnormal levels of atrial natriuretic peptide (ANP) and brain natriuretic peptide (BNP) indicate which disease process?
    a. Aneurysm
    b. Cerebrovascular accident
    c. Heart failure
    d. Myocardial infarction

47. An 80-year-old patient is taking digoxin daily along with several other drugs. Her BNP is 630 pg/mL. What concerns the nurse about this level?
    a. It is below the normal/reference range for her age.
    b. Nothing. It is within the normal range.
    c. It is slightly elevated.
    d. It is markedly elevated.

48. The patient presents to the emergency department and states he feels dizzy. He takes digitalis but he is unable to tell you why he is taking the drug. The nurse knows that this drug is usually prescribed for what abnormal rhythm?
    a. Atrial fibrillation
    b. Paroxysmal atrial tachycardia
    c. Second-degree heart block
    d. Ventricular tachycardia

49. What is the usual maintenance dose of digoxin?
    a. 3.4–5.1 mcg/kg/d
    b. 1–1.75 mcg/kg/d
    c. 1.75–3 mcg/kg/d
    d. 6–10 mcg/kg/d

50. The patient presents to her health care provider's office for a follow-up visit. She has been taking digoxin for approximately 2 weeks. What is a therapeutic digitalis level?
    a. 0.15–0.5 ng/mL
    b. 0.8–2 ng/mL
    c. 2–3.5 ng/mL
    d. 3.5–4 ng/mL

51. The 76-year-old patient has a history of heart failure and is taking digoxin 0.125 mg/day. He calls his health care provider's office with complaints of vision changes, fatigue, headache, and a heart rate of 42 beats/min. He states, "I have an appointment in 2 weeks. Is it OK to wait until then?" What is the nurse's best response?
    a. "It is fine to wait until your next appointment."
    b. "You may just have the flu. Stay in bed until you are not dizzy."
    c. "Just take your digoxin every other day."
    d. "You need to be seen either here or in the emergency department today."

Chapter **37** **Cardiac Glycosides, Antianginals, and Antidysrhythmics**

52. What is the antidote for digitalis toxicity?
   a. Cardizem
   b. Digoxin immune Fab
   c. Gamma globulin
   d. Protamine

53. The nurse is reviewing the patient's medication administration record (MAR). Which drug(s) on the MAR will concern the nurse, given that the patient is taking digitalis? *(Select all that apply.)*
   a. Cortisone
   b. Furosemide
   c. Hydrochlorothiazide
   d. Nitroglycerin
   e. Potassium supplement

54. How often should the pulse be checked for a patient taking digoxin?
   a. Daily before taking dose
   b. Once per week
   c. Only when dosage is changed
   d. Only if the patient has symptoms

55. The patient has been prescribed digoxin for treatment of heart failure. The nurse is providing health teaching for this patient. With regards to diet, what food(s) should the patient avoid? *(Select all that apply.)*
   a. Apples
   b. Celery
   c. Hot dogs
   d. Lettuce
   e. Potatoes

56. Which class of drug(s) may be used to treat heart failure? *(Select all that apply.)*
   a. Angiotensin-converting enzyme (ACE) inhibitors
   b. Beta blockers
   c. Calcium channel blockers
   d. Sodium channel blockers
   e. Diuretics
   f. Vasodilators

57. What common side effects are seen in a patient who is taking nitroglycerin (NTG)? *(Select all that apply.)*
   a. Dizziness
   b. Headache
   c. Nausea
   d. Weakness

58. What priority health teaching should be given to a patient taking sublingual (SL) nitroglycerin (NTG)? *(Select all that apply.)*
   a. Sips of water may be taken before placing NTG SL to aid in absorption.
   b. NTG should be stored in its original container and away from light.
   c. The tablet is to be chewed and swallowed.
   d. Notify your health care provider if chest pain is not relieved after three tablets.
   e. Patients should not take vitamin C supplements while taking NTG.

59. What is the duration of action of a nitroglycerin transdermal patch?
   a. 6–8 hours
   b. 10–12 hours
   c. 18–24 hours
   d. 36–48 hours

60. The patient has been prescribed atenolol 50 mg/d. What type of drug is this?
   a. Adrenergic stimulant
   b. Beta blocker
   c. Calcium channel blocker
   d. Cardiac glycoside

61. The patient has been prescribed acebutolol for treatment of ventricular dysrhythmia. What is the *initial* proper dose for this medication?
   a. 200 mg q12h
   b. 200 mg daily
   c. 600 mg bid
   d. 1200 mg daily

62. What type of drug is acebutolol?
   a. Antianginal
   b. Calcium channel blocker
   c. Cardioselective beta blocker
   d. Fast sodium channel blocker

63. What priority teaching should the nurse provide to a patient who has just started taking acebutolol?
   a. "Do not abruptly stop this drug, or you risk your heart rate beating very fast or irregularly."
   b. "Drowsiness is a common side effect."
   c. "No laboratory work will be required while taking this drug."
   d. "Fluid intake should be increased to prevent dehydration."

64. What possible side effect(s) should be discussed with a patient who is beginning acebutolol? *(Select all that apply.)*
   a. Diarrhea
   b. Edema
   c. Hypertension
   d. Erectile dysfunction
   e. Vomiting

65. Which herbal preparation(s) must be avoided when taking digitalis preparations? *(Select all that apply.)*
   a. Aloe
   b. Feverfew
   c. *Ginkgo biloba*
   d. Ginseng
   e. Ma-huang

66. What condition(s) can directly lead to cardiac dysrhythmias? *(Select all that apply.)*
   a. Electrolyte imbalances
   b. Excess catecholamines
   c. Hepatitis
   d. Hypocapnia
   e. Hypoxia

CASE STUDY

Read the scenario and answer the following questions on a separate sheet of paper.

P.E., 43 years old, has a history of hypertension, diet-controlled diabetes, and vasospastic angina. He presents to the emergency department with severe left-sided chest pain, nausea, shortness of breath, and diaphoresis. Vital signs are temperature 97.7° F, heart rate 102 beats/min, respiratory rate 20 breaths/min, blood pressure 164/100 mm Hg, and oxygen saturation on room air of 99%. After administering one sublingual nitroglycerin tablet, his vital signs are heart rate 120 beats/min, respiratory rate 22 breaths/min, and blood pressure 110/60 mm Hg. He feels lightheaded and nauseated, but his chest pain persists. A nitroglycerin drip is started, and he is admitted to critical care.

1. What are the three different types of angina?

2. Describe nonpharmacologic and pharmacologic treatments for vasospastic angina.

3. What medications other than nitroglycerin can be used to treat angina?

4. Why did this patient's blood pressure drop?

Chapter **37** Cardiac Glycosides, Antianginals, and Antidysrhythmics

38 Diuretics

Labeling Diagram

1. **Label the different segments of the renal tubules, its major class of diuretics, and the primary electrolytes influenced by the diuretic.**

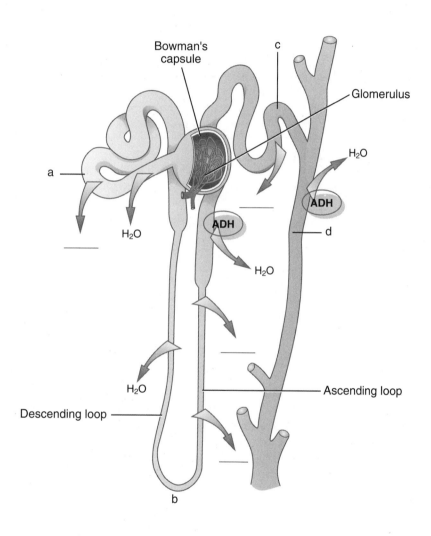

Identify the normal levels of the chemistry panel, and list the possible abnormal results (hypo- or hyper-) associated with thiazide diuretics.

Laboratory Test	Normal Levels	Abnormal Results
2. Potassium		
3. Magnesium		
4. Ionized calcium		
5. Chloride		
6. Bicarbonate		
7. Uric acid		
8. Blood sugar		
9. Blood lipids		

SHORT ANSWER QUESTIONS

Answer the following in one to two sentences.

10. What are the two main purposes for diuretics?

11. How do diuretics have antihypertensive properties?

NCLEX REVIEW QUESTIONS

Select the best response.

12. Which group(s) of diuretics is/are frequently prescribed to treat hypertension and congestive heart failure? *(Select all that apply.)*
    a. Carbonic anhydrase inhibitors
    b. Loop diuretics
    c. Osmotic diuretics
    d. Potassium-sparing diuretics
    e. Thiazide diuretics

13. When compared with thiazides, how do loop (high-ceiling) diuretics differ?
    a. They are more effective as antihypertensives.
    b. They promote potassium absorption.
    c. They cause calcium reabsorption.
    d. They are more potent as diuretics.

14. The patient has been prescribed hydrochlorothiazide (HCTZ) for her hypertension. When she comes to the office for a follow-up appointment, the nurse observes her drinking an energy drink. Which herb, commonly found in some energy drinks, can increase blood pressure when taken with thiazide diuretics?
    a. Ginger
    b. Ginkgo
    c. Licorice
    d. St. John's wort

15. What is the pharmacologic action of spironolactone?
    a. Increase potassium and sodium excretion
    b. Promote potassium retention
    c. Promote potassium and calcium retention
    d. Promote potassium excretion and sodium retention

16. What is the classification of furosemide?
    a. Loop diuretic
    b. Osmotic diuretic
    c. Potassium-sparing diuretic
    d. Thiazide diuretic

17. The 65-year-old patient had an acute myocardial infarction 6 months ago and has been prescribed spironolactone 100 mg/day to treat an irregular heart rate. What statement by the patient indicates that he understands the medication teaching the nurse has provided?
    a. "I need sodium so my heart beats regularly."
    b. "This drug is dangerous if you have had a heart attack."
    c. "It helps keep potassium so my heart does not get irregular."
    d. "I need to take it with lots of bananas to keep my potassium up."

172

18. The nurse has received an order to administer 40 mg of furosemide IV to the patient. What does the nurse know about how this drug should be administered?
    a. It must be mixed in 50 mL of normal saline.
    b. It can only be given in a central line.
    c. The patient must be on a cardiac monitor.
    d. It should be given over 1–2 minutes.

19. Which lab value(s) should a nurse monitor for a patient receiving chlorothiazide? *(Select all that apply.)*
    a. Potassium
    b. Sodium
    c. Bicarbonate
    d. Calcium
    e. AST/ALT

20. A patient who has had an acute myocardial infarction has been started on spironolactone 50 mg/day. When evaluating routine laboratory work, the nurse discovers the patient has a potassium level of 5.8 mEq/L. What is the priority intervention to be implemented?
    a. The spironolactone dose should be held and the intake of foods rich in potassium should be restricted.
    b. The spironolactone dose should be continued and the patient should be encouraged to eat fruits and vegetables.
    c. The spironolactone dose should be increased and the patient instructed to decrease foods rich in potassium.
    d. Instruct the patient to continue with the current dose of spironolactone and report any signs or symptoms of hypokalemia.

21. Which individual is the best candidate to take acetazolamide?
    a. A 50-year-old with open-angle glaucoma
    b. A 58-year-old with acute heart failure
    c. A 60-year-old with narrow-angle glaucoma
    d. A 75-year-old with acute glaucoma

22. What type of acid-base imbalance could occur if a patient is taking high doses of acetazolamide or uses the drug constantly?
    a. Metabolic acidosis
    b. Metabolic alkalosis
    c. Respiratory acidosis
    d. Respiratory alkalosis

23. The 70-year-old patient has heart failure and has been prescribed hydrochlorothiazide. What statement by the patient indicates understanding of the dosing regimen?
    a. "I need to take it on an empty stomach for it to work."
    b. "I really only need to take my medicine when I am having a hard time breathing."
    c. "It may take several weeks before it starts to work."
    d. "I should take it in the morning so I don't have to go to the bathroom at night."

24. The patient has a complicated medical history including heart failure, cardiac arrhythmias, arthritis, and depression. He is taking furosemide for his heart failure. Which of his other medications would be of major concern to the nurse?
    a. Amiodarone
    b. Acetaminophen
    c. Amitriptyline
    d. Zolpidem

25. The 62-year-old patient has been taking ethacrynic acid for severe edema. The family calls to report that the patient is very weak and unable to ambulate and is complaining of severe leg cramps. Knowing the mechanism of action of ethacrynic acid, the nurse is concerned the patient may be experiencing which electrolyte imbalance?
    a. Hyponatremia
    b. Hypermagnesemia
    c. Hypokalemia
    d. Hyperchloremia

26. What is the optimal time to administer diuretics?
    a. At bedtime
    b. After arising for the day
    c. On an empty stomach
    d. With meals

27. The nurse assesses the patient who is taking hydrochlorothiazide (HCTZ) for hypertension. What might the nurse expect to see if the patient is experiencing undesired side effects? *(Select all that apply.)*
    a. Diarrhea
    b. Dizziness
    c. Headache
    d. Hypocalcemia
    e. Vomiting

28. Which drug–lab value interaction is caused by thiazide diuretics?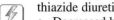
    a. Decreased blood glucose level
    b. Elevated lithium level
    c. Elevated BUN
    d. Decreased calcium level

29. The patient is taking furosemide 80 mg/day. She has a history of hypertension and heart failure. She presents to the emergency department after sustaining a fall at a local sports bar. She has a laceration to her posterior scalp. Vital signs are temperature 38° C, heart rate 98 beats/min, respiratory rate 16 breaths/min, and blood pressure 94/62 mm/Hg. Her electrolytes are within normal limits. Her blood alcohol is 0.06, and her toxicology screen is negative. What does the nurse know about possible drug interactions?
    a. Furosemide can cause severe hypoglycemia and headache.
    b. Furosemide can cause hyperkalemia and dizziness.
    c. Furosemide can cause orthostatic hypotension when consumed with alcohol.
    d. Furosemide can lead to elevated uric acid levels, causing the patient to faint.

30. In which patient are loop diuretics contraindicated?
    a. The patient with anuria
    b. The patient with asthma
    c. The patient with allergy to ceftriaxone
    d. The patient with gastric ulcers

31. The patient has been diagnosed with hypertension and diabetes and has been started on hydrochlorothiazide. What statement by the patient indicates understanding of the drug teaching the nurse has provided?
    a. "It will start working within minutes."
    b. "I don't need to monitor my blood sugar."
    c. "I should take my drug on an empty stomach so it works better."
    d. "I need to keep track of my weight and blood pressure at home."

CASE STUDY

Read the scenario, and answer the following questions on a separate sheet of paper.

J.S., 21 years old, was involved in a motorcycle collision and has a severe traumatic brain injury. While preparing to take the patient to surgery, the neurosurgeon orders mannitol to be administered. Vital signs are temperature 37.6° C, heart rate 62 beats/min, respiratory rate controlled on a ventilator at 18 breaths/min, and blood pressure 194/132 mm Hg. The patient has an increased intracranial pressure (ICP) of 36 mm Hg. He weighs 80 kg.

1. What class of diuretic is mannitol, and how does it work?

2. What is the standard dosage range for mannitol? How is mannitol administered?

3. What would the correct dose be for this patient?

39 Antihypertensives

Complete the following.

1. When hypertension cannot be controlled nonpharmacologically, antihypertensive drugs may be prescribed. Three of the five sympatholytic groups are _____, _____, and _____.

2. Two categories of antihypertensives in addition to the sympatholytics are _____ and _____.

3. The Joint National Committee on Prevention, Detection, Evaluation, and Treatment of High Blood Pressure (JNC-8) uses three classifications for defining elevated systolic blood pressure (SBP): _____, _____, and _____.

4. Thiazide diuretics may be combined with other antihypertensive drugs. Examples of other antihypertensives include _____ and _____.

5. Many antihypertensive drugs can cause fluid retention. To decrease body fluid, the drug group often administered with antihypertensive drugs is _____.

6. A patient with a blood pressure of 182/105 mm Hg has what stage of hypertension according to JNC-7? _____

7. Beta-adrenergic blockers reduce cardiac output by diminishing the sympathetic nervous system response. With continued use of beta blockers, vascular resistance is (increased/diminished) and blood pressure is (lowered/increased). *(Circle correct answers.)*

8. Atenolol and metoprolol are examples of (cardioselective/noncardioselective) antihypertensive drugs. *(Circle correct answer.)*

9. The alpha blockers are useful in treating hypertensive patients with lipid abnormalities. The effects they have on lipoproteins include (decrease/increase) VLDL and LDL; and (decrease/increase) HDL. *(Circle the correct answer.)*

Match the generic drug name in Column I with the category of antihypertensive in Column II.

Column I

_____ 10. Captopril

_____ 11. Verapamil

_____ 12. Prazosin

_____ 13. Atenolol

_____ 14. Methyldopa

_____ 15. Hydralazine

_____ 16. Candesartan

_____ 17. Carvedilol

Column II

a. Cardioselective beta blocker
b. Selective alpha blocker
c. Angiotensin-converting enzyme (ACE) inhibitor
d. Calcium channel blocker
e. Centrally acting alpha$_2$ agonist
f. Direct-acting vasodilator
g. Angiotensin II–receptor antagonist (A-II blocker)
h. Nonselective beta$_1$ and beta$_2$ blocker

175

Select the best response.

18. The patient presents to the health care provider for his annual checkup. His vital signs are blood pressure 136/82 mm Hg, heart rate 72 beats/min, respiratory rate 16 breaths/min, and temperature 97.5° F. According to JNC-8, to which hypertension category does this patient belong?
    a. Normal
    b. Prehypertension
    c. Stage 1
    d. Stage 2

19. A cardioselective beta-adrenergic blocker is also known by which other term?
    a. Alpha-beta blocker
    b. Alpha blocker
    c. Beta-angiotensin agent
    d. Beta blocker

20. Which patient would be most suited for treatment with a nonselective alpha-adrenergic blocker?
    a. A 45-year-old patient with mild to moderate renal failure
    b. A 46-year-old patient with hypertension associated with pheochromocytoma
    c. A 50-year-old patient with hyperlipidemia
    d. A 55-year-old patient with type 2 diabetes

21. Where in the body do direct-acting vasodilators act to decrease blood pressure?
    a. Cardiac valves
    b. Dopaminergic receptors in kidneys
    c. Renal tubules
    d. Smooth muscles of the blood vessels

22. With use of direct-acting vasodilators, sodium and water are retained and peripheral edema occurs. Which category of drugs should be given to avoid fluid retention?
    a. Anticoagulants
    b. Antidysrhythmics
    c. Cardiac glycosides
    d. Diuretics

23. Which is/are action(s) of angiotensin II–receptor blockers (ARBs)? *(Select all that apply.)*
    a. Block angiotensin II
    b. Cause vasodilation
    c. Decrease peripheral resistance
    d. Increase sodium retention
    e. Slow heart rate

24. An ARB can be combined with the thiazide diuretic hydrochlorothiazide. What is the purpose of combining these two drugs?
    a. To decrease rapid blood pressure drop
    b. To enhance the antihypertensive effect by promoting sodium and water loss
    c. To increase sodium and water retention for controlling blood pressure
    d. To promote potassium retention

25. ARBs may be prescribed for hypertensive patients instead of an ACE inhibitor. What is the most limiting factor in the use of ACE inhibitors?
    a. Coughing
    b. Dizziness
    c. Shortness of breath
    d. Sneezing

26. Which orders should the nurse question if the patient was prescribed an ACE inhibitor as a monotherapy?
    a. A 45-year-old Hispanic man
    b. A 48-year-old Asian woman
    c. A 50-year-old Caucasian woman
    d. A 55-year-old African American man

27. The patient, a 48-year-old African American female, presents to her health care provider. Her blood pressure is 164/88 mm Hg, and a decision is made to start antihypertensive drug. What group of drugs would be more effective than ACE inhibitors for this patient?
    a. Angiotensin II blockers
    b. Beta blockers
    c. Calcium blockers
    d. Direct renin inhibitor

28. Herb-drug interactions may occur if the patient is taking certain herbal supplements. An herb history should be obtained. What may occur in an individual who also uses ma-huang (ephedra) with an antihypertensive drug?
    a. A decrease or counteraction of the effects of the antihypertensive drug
    b. A decrease in the hypertensive state
    c. An increase in the hypotensive effects of the antihypertensive drug
    d. No effect on the action of the antihypertensive drug

29. Captopril is from which group of antihypertensives?
   a. ACE inhibitor
   b. Beta blocker
   c. Calcium blocker
   d. Direct-acting vasodilator

30. What is the action of captopril?
   a. Dilation of the arteries
   b. Increase in sodium and water excretion
   c. Inhibition of the formation of angiotensin II
   d. Inhibition of the alpha receptors

31. The patient has essential hypertension. He is taking captopril 25 mg tid. If the patient takes captopril with another highly protein-bound drug, what might occur?
   a. Captopril and the highly protein-bound drug will compete for protein sites.
   b. The concentration of captopril will be increased.
   c. There will be moderate drug displacement of captopril, which is moderately to highly protein-bound.
   d. There will be no drug displacement, because captopril is not highly protein-bound.

32. If a patient takes captopril with nitrates, diuretics, or adrenergic blockers, what might the nurse assess in this patient?
   a. Hypoglycemic reaction
   b. Hypotensive reaction
   c. Hyperkalemic reaction
   d. Hypertensive reaction

33. If a patient takes captopril with a potassium-sparing diuretic, what might occur?
   a. Hypokalemia
   b. Hyperkalemia
   c. Hypocalcemia
   d. Hypercalcemia

34. A patient states that he wishes to stop taking captopril for his hypertension. What is the nurse's best response?
   a. "Blood pressure can be controlled by diet and exercise, so you don't have to take drug."
   b. "It is important to keep taking your drug as directed until you speak with your health care provider."
   c. "Once your blood pressure is normal for one month, you can stop taking your drug."
   d. "Wean yourself off of the drug over a 10-day period."

35. A patient's antihypertensive drug was changed from captopril to nifedipine 30 mg daily. What type of antihypertensive drug is nifedipine?
   a. Angiotensin antagonist
   b. Beta blocker
   c. Calcium channel blocker
   d. Centrally acting sympatholytic

36. What is the protein-binding power of amlodipine?
   a. Highly protein-bound
   b. Moderately to highly protein-bound
   c. Moderately protein-bound
   d. Low protein-bound

37. The nurse is assessing the patient with newly diagnosed essential hypertension following the shift report. What might the nurse assess if the patient were experiencing side effects from metoprolol? *(Select all that apply.)*
   a. Dizziness
   b. Headache
   c. Increased blood pressure
   d. Nausea
   e. Paranoia

38. Aliskiren is in what class of antihypertensives?
   a. ACE inhibitor
   b. Angiotensin II blocker
   c. Calcium channel blocker
   d. Direct renin inhibitor

39. What action does amlodipine have in the vasculature?
   a. Increased peripheral vascular resistance
   b. Peripheral clotting
   c. Thrombolysis
   d. Vasodilation

40. The patient, 62 years old, is taking amlodipine and complains of swelling in her ankles. What is the nurse's best response to her concern?
   a. "Swelling is common when taking amlodipine. You should cut the tablet in half to reduce your dosage."
   b. "Swelling may occur with amlodipine. I will contact your health care provider to determine if the drug should be changed."
   c. "You should not be taking that drug because of your age. I will see what other antihypertensive drug you can take."
   d. "You should stop taking the drug for several days and check that the swelling has decreased."

41. What classification of drug is bisoprolol?
    a. ACE inhibitor
    b. Beta blocker
    c. Calcium blocker
    d. Diuretic

42. What classification of drug is pindolol?
    a. ACE inhibitor
    b. Beta blocker
    c. Calcium blocker
    d. Diuretic

43. What is/are the advantage(s) of using cardioselective beta-adrenergic blockers as an antihypertensive? *(Select all that apply.)*
    a. They can be abruptly discontinued without causing rebound symptoms.
    b. They help prevent bronchodilation.
    c. They increase serum electrolyte levels.
    d. They maintain renal blood flow.
    e. They minimize the hypoglycemic effect.

44. ARBs have gained popularity for treating hypertension. Which is/are example(s) of ARB agents? *(Select all that apply.)*
    a. Irbesartan
    b. Losartan potassium
    c. Valsartan
    d. Lisinopril
    e. Metoprolol

45. Which statement best describes the direct renin inhibitor aliskiren?
    a. It is effective for treating severe hypertension.
    b. It can be combined with another antihypertensive drug.
    c. It can cause hypokalemia when taken as a monotherapy drug.
    d. It is more effective than calcium channel blockers in treating hypertension in African American patients.

CASE STUDY

Read the scenario and answer the following questions on a separate sheet of paper.

J.H., 68 years old, has a history of hypertension. She presents to her health care provider with complaints of headache, epistaxis, and dizziness. Vital signs are blood pressure 232/146 mm Hg, heart rate 62 beats/min, respiratory rate 16 breaths/min, and temperature 98.3° F. J.H.'s electrocardiogram (ECG) reveals normal sinus rhythm with an occasional premature ventricular contraction. The health care provider calls for emergency medical services (EMS) to transport J.H. to the hospital for treatment of a hypertensive emergency. While waiting for EMS, the nurse reviews her drug list and finds that J.H. takes chlorthalidone with clonidine on a daily basis but "sometimes forgets a dose or two."

1. How does chlorthalidone work with clonidine to lower blood pressure?

2. What are the options for J.H. for treatment of a hypertensive emergency?

3. What priority teaching should the nurse provide to J.H. at time of discharge from the hospital?

40 Anticoagulants, Antiplatelets, and Thrombolytics

STUDY QUESTIONS

Complete the following.

1. A thrombus can form in a(n) _____ or in a(n) _____.

2. Anticoagulants are used to inhibit _____ _____. They ____ _____ dissolve clots.

3. Anticoagulants and thrombolytics (have/do not have) the same action. *(Circle correct answer.)*

4. The most frequent use of heparin is to prevent _____.

5. Heparin can be given (orally/subcutaneously/intravenously). *(Circle all the correct answers.)*

6. The low–molecular-weight heparins (LMWHs) are derivatives of ____ _____. The advantage of the use of LMWHs is that they _____ _____.

7. The International Normalized Ratio (INR) is a laboratory test to monitor the therapeutic effect of (warfarin/heparin). *(Circle correct answer.)*

8. Heparin can (decrease/increase) the platelet count, causing thrombocytopenia. *(Circle correct answer.)*

9. A thrombus disintegrates when a thrombolytic drug is administered within _____ hours following an acute myocardial infarction.

10. The action of the thrombolytic drugs streptokinase and urokinase is the conversion of _____ to _____.

11. The major complication with the use of thrombolytic drugs is _____ _____.

12. A synthetic anticoagulant, _____, indirectly inhibits thrombin production and is closely related in structure to heparin and LMWH.

13. **Number the following steps of heparin activity in correct order.**

    _____ a. Inhibits conversion of fibrinogen to fibrin

    _____ b. Inactivates antithrombin III to prevent the formation of thrombin

    _____ c. Clot prevented

    _____ d. Heparin binds with antithrombin III

Match the drug in Column I with its drug group in Column II. Answers may be used more than once.

Column I

_____14. Warfarin

_____15. Aspirin

_____16. Enoxaparin

_____17. Dalteparin sodium

_____18. Protamine sulfate

_____19. Clopidogrel

_____20. Streptokinase

_____21. Bivalirudin

_____22. Alteplase (tissue plasminogen activator [tPA])

Column II

a. Anticoagulant: LMWH
b. Direct thrombin inhibitor (parenteral)
c. Oral anticoagulant
d. Antiplatelet
e. Anticoagulant antagonist
f. Thrombolytic

NCLEX REVIEW QUESTIONS

Select the best response.

23. The patient with a deep vein thrombosis in her lower leg and was started on warfarin. She asks the nurse how warfarin works. What is the nurse's best response?
   a. "Warfarin will help dissolve the blood clots."
   b. "Warfarin is given with thrombolytics to help break up clots."
   c. "Warfarin prevents new clots from forming."
   d. "Warfarin dilates the veins to improve blood flow."

24. The nurse has several patients receiving warfarin. Which INR(s) should concern the nurse? *(Select all that apply.)*
   a. 1.2
   b. 1.4
   c. 1.8
   d. 2.0
   e. 2.4

25. What is one of the primary reasons LMWHs are given?
   a. Enhance the action of warfarin
   b. Prevent cerebrovascular accidents
   c. Prevention of DVTs after hip or knee surgery
   d. Treatment of acute myocardial infarction

26. Which drug is not considered a LMWH? *(Select all that apply.)*
   a. Enoxaparin sodium
   b. Clopidogrel
   c. Dalteparin
   d. Apixaban

27. The patient, 58 years old, has unstable angina and is having an emergent percutaneous transluminal coronary angioplasty (PTCA). The nurse is completing preprocedure teaching and explains that he will be receiving a medication right before the procedure and then for the next 12 hours by IV drip to prevent ischemia. What drug is the nurse teaching the patient about?
   a. Abciximab
   b. Aminocaproic acid
   c. Protamine sulfate
   d. Warfarin

28. The patient weighs 168 pounds and is going to receive abciximab for unstable angina. What is the correct dosage for a continuous infusion?
   a. 9.5 mcg/min
   b. 19 mcg/min
   c. 25 mg/min
   d. 42 mg/min

29. Which statement best describes clopidogrel?
   a. It is the most effective anticoagulant when used with ibuprofen.
   b. It is most effective when prescribed as a single drug to prevent stroke.
   c. It is an inexpensive alternative to warfarin.
   d. It can be used together with aspirin after myocardial infarction (MI) or cerebrovascular accident (CVA) to prevent platelet aggregation.

30. The 72-year-old patient has a history of atrial fibrillation and has been discharged from the hospital on warfarin. He was taking heparin before being changed to warfarin for discharge. With regards to lab monitoring, what is a priority teaching intervention for the nurse?
   a. "INR will be monitored closely."
   b. "Periodic evaluation of your electrolytes is very important."
   c. "Your blood must be monitored for BUN/creatinine values to evaluate for new renal failure."
   d. "You will not need any further lab work while taking this medication."

31. Enoxaparin sodium is an anticoagulant used to prevent and treat deep vein thrombosis and pulmonary embolism. To which category does this drug belong?
   a. Oral anticoagulant
   b. Low–molecular-weight heparin
   c. Standard heparin
   d. Thrombolytic

32. The 3-year-old patient has gotten into a box of rat poison under the sink. The family brings the box to the emergency department, and the main ingredient is warfarin. What priority medication will the nurse prepare to administer?

   a. Anagrelide
   b. Protamine sulfate
   c. Ticlopidine
   d. Vitamin K (phytonadione)

33. What is the protein-binding power of warfarin?
   a. Highly protein-bound
   b. Low protein-bound
   c. Not protein-bound at all
   d. Moderately protein-bound

34. The patient is given heparin for early treatment of deep vein thrombosis. Later, warfarin is prescribed. If the patient is also taking fluoxetine, which is highly protein-bound, what might occur?
   a. Drug displacement of the highly protein-bound drug but not displacement of warfarin
   b. Drug displacement of warfarin
   c. Drug displacement varies from patient to patient
   d. No drug displacement of either drug

35. The patient presents to the emergency department with complaints of gastrointestinal bleeding. She is currently taking fondaparinux at home after having major orthopedic surgery. She has been taking 2.5 mg for the past 5 days. What does the nurse anticipate is occurring?
   a. Adverse reaction
   b. Allergic reaction
   c. Insufficient dose of fondaparinux
   d. Stevens-Johnson syndrome

36. What is one of the benefits of rivaroxaban?
   a. Does not require monitoring of frequent labs
   b. Inexpensive
   c. Long half-life
   d. Minimal drug-drug interactions

37. The patient is in the emergency department (ED) and has been diagnosed with an acute MI. The patient will be receiving alteplase immediately while still in the ED. What might the nurse assess in a patient who is experiencing an allergic reaction to this drug? *(Select all that apply.)*
   a. Bronchospasm
   b. Dyspnea
   c. Hives
   d. Hypotension
   e. Nausea

38. The patient has received alteplase for treatment of a CVA. The patient begins to hemorrhage. What drug does the nurse anticipate will potentially be used as treatment for this hemorrhage?
   a. Reteplase
   b. Aminocaproic acid
   c. Calcium gluconate
   d. Protamine sulfate

Chapter **40** **Anticoagulants, Antiplatelets, and Thrombolytics**

39. What action(s) will the nurse perform when caring for a patient who is receiving tenecteplase? *(Select all that apply.)*
   a. Assess for reperfusion arrhythmias.
   b. Monitor liver panel.
   c. Observe for signs and symptoms of bleeding.
   d. Obtain a type and crossmatch.
   e. Record vital signs and report changes.

40. Which patient(s) would be candidate(s) for anticoagulant use? *(Select all that apply.)*
   a. A 28-year-old with deep vein thrombosis
   b. A 35-year-old with an artificial heart valve
   c. A 45-year-old with migraines
   d. A 52-year-old who has had a knee replacement
   e. A 68-year-old with a CVA

CASE STUDY

Read the scenario, and answer the following questions on a separate sheet of paper.

R.K., 30 years old, has been diagnosed with a pulmonary embolus after having laparoscopic surgery. She is admitted to the intensive care unit and started on a heparin drip. The patient will be discharged home on warfarin and will receive therapy for 3–6 months.

1. How does heparin work in a patient who already has a pulmonary embolus?

2. How does warfarin work to prevent further development of deep vein thrombosis that may lead to pulmonary embolism?

3. What priority teaching information will the nurse need to provide for this patient before discharge?

41 Antihyperlipidemics and Peripheral Vasodilators

STUDY QUESTIONS

Complete the following.

1. The four major categories of lipoprotein are _____, _____, _____, and _____.

2. High-density lipoproteins (HDLs) are the densest lipoproteins and contain more _____ and less _____ than the other lipoproteins.

3. Persons with elevated low-density lipoproteins (LDLs) have the risk of developing _____ _____ and _____ _____.

4. In addition to LDL, _____ (a lipoprotein) is a better indicator of risk for coronary artery disease (CAD).

5. Statin drugs inhibit _____ _____ in cholesterol biosynthesis and are called _____ _____ _____.

6. B vitamins and folic acid can lower serum _____ levels.

7. Primary causes of peripheral arterial disease include _____ and _____.

Match the drug in Column I with its drug group in Column II. Answers may be used more than once.

Column I

_____ 8. Colestipol hydrochloride

_____ 9. Gemfibrozil

_____ 10. Atorvastatin

_____ 11. Simvastatin

_____ 12. Cholestyramine resin

_____ 13. Niacin

_____ 14. Ezetimibe

Column II

a. Statins
b. Bile-acid sequestrants
c. Fibrates
d. Cholesterol absorption inhibitors
e. Nicotinic acid

NCLEX REVIEW QUESTIONS

Select the best response.

15. Which elevated apolipoprotein can be an indication of risk for coronary artery disease (CAD)?
    a. apoA-1
    b. apoA-2
    c. apoB-100
    d. apoC-4

16. The patient is taking atorvastatin 80 mg/day. The patient's partner calls to report that the patient is feeling weak and complaining of muscle pain. What severe side effect of statins does the nurse suspect?
    a. Stevens-Johnson syndrome
    b. Pseudomembranous colitis
    c. Gastric ulcers
    d. Rhabdomyolysis

17. Homocysteine is a protein in the blood that has been linked to cardiovascular disease and stroke. What other negative action may it also promote?
    a. Flushing of skin
    b. Loss of blood vessel flexibility
    c. Photosensitivity and sunburn
    d. Lowering of low-density lipoprotein levels

18. The patient has intermittent claudication and complains of leg pain. He states, "I don't believe in taking all of that medicine stuff. I prefer to use only natural drugs." What herb does the nurse recognize as being used by some patients with intermittent claudication?
    a. Ginger
    b. Ginseng
    c. Ginkgo
    d. Goldenseal

19. The patient presents to the clinic for a complete physical. The patient states, "I have been doing a lot of reading, so I know what my cholesterol should be." What does the nurse know is the desired range for total cholesterol?
    a. 50–100 mg/dL
    b. 100–150 mg/dL
    c. 150–200 mg/dL
    d. 200–250 mg/dL

20. Low-density lipoproteins (LDLs) are the so-called "bad" lipoproteins. Why are high levels of LDL considered unhealthy?
    a. There is an increased risk of hyperthyroidism.
    b. There is the possibility of digestive problems.
    c. There is an increased risk of rhabdomyolysis.
    d. There is an increased risk of heart disease.

21. What is the standard preferred level of LDL?
    a. Less than 250 mg/dL
    b. Less than 200 mg/dL
    c. Less than 150 mg/dL
    d. Less than 100 mg/dL

22. The patient has a lipid profile drawn as part of an annual physical exam. What does the nurse know about a high-density lipoprotein (HDL) level of 22 mg/dL?
    a. This value puts the patient in a high-risk category.
    b. An HDL level of 22 mg/dL places the patient in a moderate-risk category.
    c. The HDL level must be compared with all other levels before a decision can be made.
    d. This value is within the standard preferred range.

23. The patient had a total cholesterol level of 228 mg/dL. After 2 months of a low-fat, low-cholesterol diet, the total cholesterol level is 212 mg/dL. Why is this level not lower?
    a. The patient most likely did not adhere to the diet.
    b. Diet modification usually decreases cholesterol levels by only 10–30%.
    c. The patient lost less than 10 pounds on the diet.
    d. The patient's exercise program was not rigorous enough.

24. The patient is prescribed simvastatin. She asks if she can eat whatever she wants now that she is taking Zocor. What is the nurse's best response?
    a. "Yes, you may eat whatever you want as long as you are taking simvastatin."
    b. "Diet is not an important factor if you are compliant with your drugs."
    c. "You should maintain a low-fat, low-cholesterol diet and exercise as well."
    d. "With simvastatin, you must lose weight as well as exercise."

25. What is a usual dose of cilostazol?
    a. 100 mg q12h
    b. 200 mg q12h
    c. 250 mg q12h
    d. 300 mg q12h

26. What priority information should the nurse include in the health teaching plan for a patient taking cilostazol? (Select all that apply.)
    a. Take medications with meals.
    b. Avoid drinking grapefruit juice.
    c. Do not take acetaminophen.
    d. Monitor for side effects such as headache and abdominal pain.
    e. Monitor blood pressure.

27. Which drug(s), other than the statins, is/are prescribed for reducing cholesterol and LDL levels? (Select all that apply.)
    a. Bile-acid sequestrants
    b. Alpha-adrenergic agents
    c. Direct thrombin inhibitors
    d. Nicotinic acid
    e. Antiplatelets
    f. Cholesterol absorption inhibitors

28. What type of drug is rosuvastatin?
    a. HMG-CoA reductase inhibitor
    b. Cholesterol absorption inhibitor
    c. Bile-acid sequestrant
    d. Combination of two antilipidemics

184

Chapter **41** Antihyperlipidemics and Peripheral Vasodilators

Copyright © 2018, Elsevier Inc. All rights reserved.

CASE STUDY

Read the scenario and answer the following questions on a separate sheet of paper.

S.S., 39 years old, has a family history of coronary artery disease and has recently been having intermittent chest pain. Her cholesterol level is 267 mg/dL; her LDL level is 146 mg/dL; and her HDL level is 44 mg/dL. She was initially prescribed atorvastatin 10 mg/day. The dosage has now been increased to 20 mg/day. Her medical history is positive for type 2 diabetes. She has no allergies, and she tells the nurse that she is "starting to think about getting pregnant."

1. Discuss the mode of action for atorvastatin and the purpose of this drug.

2. What are the implications of atorvastatin and pregnancy?

3. What should be monitored during drug therapy, and how long will the drug therapy last?

4. What teaching points should be included in patient education for S.S.?

42 Gastrointestinal Tract Disorders

Match the words in Column I with the description they are most associated with in Column II.

Column I

_____ 1. Adsorbents

_____ 2. Cannabinoids

_____ 3. Chemoreceptor trigger zone (CTZ)

_____ 4. Emetics

_____ 5. Opiates

_____ 6. Osmotics

_____ 7. Purgatives

Column II

a. Harsh cathartics that cause a watery stool with abdominal cramping
b. Induce vomiting (used after poisoning)
c. Hyperosmolar laxatives
d. Relieve chemotherapy-induced nausea/vomiting
e. Lies near the medulla
f. Adsorb bacteria or toxins that cause diarrhea
g. Decrease intestinal motility, thereby decreasing peristalsis

Complete the following.

8. The _____ lies near the medulla, and the vomiting center is located in the _____.

9. Nonprescription drugs for emesis include _____, _____, and _____ solution.

10. Antihistamine antiemetics have similar side effects to those of _____.

11. Antiemetic drugs in the classes of anticholinergics and antihistamines should not be used in patients with _____ because of the drugs' side effects.

12. Phenothiazines and benzodiazepines are classified as _____ _____ that suppresses emesis by blocking dopamine receptors in the chemoreceptor trigger zone.

13. Serotonin antagonists suppress _____ and _____ by blocking the _____ receptors.

14. A drug to alleviate nausea and vomiting, such as a _____, can also be used as an appetite stimulant.

15. _____ promote a soft stool, whereas _____ result in a soft to watery stool.

16. Saline osmotic laxative products consists of _____ or _____.

17. Laxative abuse can cause fluid volume _____ and _____ losses.

SHORT ANSWER

18. List the eight classes of prescription antiemetics.

19. List at least five common causes of constipation.

20. What instructions should be given to the patient who is prescribed psyllium, a bulk-forming laxative?

ANSWER THE FOLLOWING QUESTIONS AS TRUE OR FALSE.

_____ 21. Prescription or nonprescription antiemetics are safe for pregnant women to take.

_____ 22. A person should have one bowel movement per day to be "normal."

_____ 23. Chronic use of laxatives can cause laxative dependence.

_____ 24. Because castor oil is a natural substance, it is safe for woman in early pregnancy to use castor oil for occasional constipation.

NCLEX REVIEW QUESTIONS

Select the best response.

25. Which area(s) in the brain cause(s) vomiting when stimulated? *(Select all that apply.)*
    a. Chemoreceptor trigger zone
    b. Nausea center
    c. Medulla
    d. Vertigo center
    e. Vomiting center

26. Of the following groups of drugs, which can be used as antiemetics? *(Select all that apply.)*
    a. Anticholinergics
    b. Antihistamines
    c. Cannabinoids
    d. Opioids
    e. Phenothiazines

27. The patient has severe nausea and vomiting and has been prescribed promethazine 25 mg PO q4-6h. The patient asks how the drug works. What is the nurse's best response?
    a. "It stimulates the dopamine receptors in the brain associated with vomiting."
    b. "It blocks the histamine receptor sites and inhibits the CTZ."
    c. "It blocks the acetylcholine receptors associated with vomiting."
    d. "It prohibits the muscle contraction in the abdominal wall, preventing vomiting."

28. The 16-year-old patient has been vomiting since last night. His mother calls the health care provider for an appointment but will be unable to come in for several hours. What nonpharmacologic method(s) can the nurse suggest to decrease nausea and vomiting? *(Select all that apply.)*
    a. "Drink weak tea."
    b. "Takes sips of flat soda."
    c. "Eat small amounts of gelatin if tolerated."
    d. "Crackers may be helpful."
    e. "Breathe deeply in and out through your nose."

29. The patient has a history of seasickness but is going boating this weekend. How far in advance should the nurse advise her to apply a scopolamine patch?
    a. Immediately
    b. 1 hour
    c. 4 hours
    d. 24 hours

30. The nurse is taking care of a newly pregnant patient who is complaining of morning sickness. She asks the nurse what she can do to help stop the nausea. How will the nurse respond? *(Select all that apply.)*
    a. "Ask your health care provider for a prescription for hydroxyzine."
    b. "Take over-the-counter antiemetics like bismuth subsalicylate."
    c. "Try drinking flat soda or weak tea."
    d. "Consider some dry toast or crackers."
    e. "This will just go away in a few months. There is nothing to do."

31. Which nonprescription drugs are most commonly used to treat motion sickness?
    a. Anticholinergics
    b. Antihistamines
    c. Cannibinoids
    d. Osmotics

32. What is the goal behind giving activated charcoal?
    a. Absorb poison
    b. Cause diarrhea
    c. Promote vomiting
    d. Stop nausea

33. What drug(s) is/are classified as antidiarrheal? *(Select all that apply.)*
    a. Adsorbents
    b. Anticholinergics
    c. Opioids
    d. Proton pump inhibitors
    e. Selective serotonin reuptake inhibitors

34. The patient is receiving diphenoxylate with atropine for treatment of diarrhea. What side effect(s) might the nurse expect to see during treatment? *(Select all that apply.)*
    a. Headache
    b. Drowsiness
    c. Hypertension
    d. Hypoglycemia
    e. Urinary retention

35. The patient has recently had surgery and has been taking opioids for pain control. He has become constipated and has been prescribed a laxative. When providing health care teaching for this patient, what type of stool should the nurse tell the patient to expect?
    a. Hard and dry
    b. Liquid
    c. Soft
    d. Soft with hard pieces

36. Which is/are a type of laxative/cathartic? *(Select all that apply.)*
    a. Adsorbents
    b. Bulk-forming
    c. Emetics
    d. Emollients
    e. Stimulants

37. The patient is scheduled for a barium enema and has a prescription for bisacodyl the day before the procedure. She asks the nurse to explain how this drug works to prepare her for her test. What is the nurse's best response?
    a. "Bisacodyl increases peristalsis by irritating the lining of the intestines."
    b. "By stimulating more smooth muscle contraction, bisacodyl will cause your bowel to empty."
    c. "Bisacodyl increases water in the gut."
    d. "Bisacodyl is an emetic, so you will vomit and your stomach will be empty for the test."

38. The 65-year-old patient has recently had a myocardial infarction. His health care provider has ordered docusate sodium 200 mg daily. What is the purpose of this drug for this patient?
    a. Treat diarrhea
    b. Soften stools
    c. Stop vomiting
    d. Prevent nausea

39. The use of saline cathartics should be questioned by the nurse for which patient?
    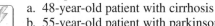
    a. 38-year-old with diabetes
    b. 48-year-old with peripheral vascular disease
    c. 50-year-old with chronic obstructive pulmonary disease (COPD)
    d. 62-year-old with heart failure

40. The patient is taking mineral oil as a laxative. If she continues to take mineral oil for an extended period of time, what should concern the nurse?
    a. Abdominal bloating and flatulence
    b. Decreased absorption of fat-soluble vitamins A, D, E, and K
    c. Dependence on the drug
    d. Excessive fluid loss attributable to diarrhea

41. Which patient should not use a laxative/cathartic?
    a. 48-year-old patient with cirrhosis
    b. 55-year-old patient with parkinsonism
    c. 60-year-old patient with stable angina
    d. 65-year-old patient with bowel obstruction

42. The patient has been prescribed promethazine 25 mg PO for nausea that accompanies her migraines. What side effect(s) should be included in the patient teaching? *(Select all that apply.)*
    a. Blurred vision
    b. Diarrhea
    c. Drowsiness
    d. Dry mouth
    e. Hypotension

43. The patient has cancer and is being treated with dronabinol for nausea and vomiting caused by chemotherapy. When should this drug be administered?
    a. 1–3 hours before chemotherapy
    b. 12 hours before chemotherapy
    c. 6 hours before chemotherapy
    d. Every 4–6 hours as needed

44. The nurse will question an order for antidiarrheal drug for which patient?

    a. 46-year-old with diabetes
    b. 36-year-old with COPD
    c. 60-year-old with heart failure
    d. 65-year-old with hepatitis C

45. The patient is experiencing diarrhea. Which food(s) will the nurse advise the patient to avoid? *(Select all that apply.)*
    a. Bottled water
    b. Clear liquids
    c. Fried foods
    d. Milk products
    e. Gelatin

Read the scenario and answer the following questions on a separate sheet of paper.

L.B., 85 years old, presents to the clinic with complaints of constipation. She lives independently in a senior living center. Approximately 2 months ago, L.B. fell and broke her left hip. She had her hip replaced, received physical therapy, and has returned home. She is currently taking digoxin, a calcium supplement, omeprazole, and hydrocodone PRN for pain. She is prescribed bisacodyl 15 mg PO.

1. What are the potential causes of constipation in L.B.?

2. How does bisacodyl work to treat constipation?

3. Are there any contraindications with any of L.B.'s other drugs? If so, what?

4. What priority teaching instructions are important for this patient regarding her new prescribed drug?

43 Antiulcer

Match the descriptor in Column I with the drug/factor in Column II. Answers may be used more than once.

Column I

_____ 1. Risk factor for the development of peptic ulcer disease (PUD)

_____ 2. Two drug/factor that neutralizes gastric acid

_____ 3. The first proton pump inhibitor marketed

_____ 4. Associated with the development of PUD

_____ 5. Prostaglandin analogue for prevention of NSAID-induced ulcer

_____ 6. Binds with protein to form a protective viscous coat covering the ulcer

_____ 7. Eradication of *H. pylori* requires addition of this antimicrobial

_____ 8. An antacid that can have a diarrheal effect

_____ 9. Over-the-counter (OTC) proton pump inhibitor used in combination to eradicate *H. pylori*

_____ 10. H_2 antagonist with multiple drug interactions

Column II

a. Magnesium hydroxide
b. *Helicobacter pylori*
c. Sucralfate
d. Cimetidine
e. Omeprazole
f. Misoprostol
g. Smoking
h. Antacids
i. Metronidazole

Match the drug in Column I with the category to which it belongs in Column II. Answers may be used more than once.

Column I

_____ 11. Rabeprazole

_____ 12. Ranitidine

_____ 13. Glycopyrrolate

_____ 14. Nizatidine

_____ 15. Esomeprazole magnesium

_____ 16. Sucralfate

_____ 17. Calcium carbonate

_____ 18. Famotidine

_____ 19. Sodium bicarbonate

Column II

a. Anticholinergics
b. Antacid
c. Proton pump inhibitor
d. Histamine$_2$ blocker
e. Pepsin inhibitors

Select the best response.

20. The patient has started taking an OTC antacid for "heartburn." He asks the nurse what is the best time to take it so it is the most effective. What is the best answer?
    a. 1 hour before meals
    b. 1–3 hours after meals and at bedtime
    c. With meals and at bedtime
    d. With meals and 1 hour after

21. With how many ounces of water should a patient take a liquid antacid for best results?
    a. 2–4
    b. 4–6
    c. 6–8
    d. 8 or more

22. Which drug(s) may be used in the prevention of ulcers? *(Select all that apply.)*
    a. Antibiotics
    b. Anticholinergics
    c. Antacids
    d. Histamine$_2$ blockers
    e. Opiates
    f. Proton pump inhibitors

23. The patient presents to the clinic with a sore throat. He tells the nurse, "I just feel like a fire-breathing dragon. It is awful when I go to bed." He has been diagnosed with gastroesophageal reflux disease (GERD). What drug(s) does the nurse know is/are most commonly used to treat GERD? *(Select all that apply.)*
    a. Antacids
    b. Anticholinergics
    c. Histamine$_2$ blockers
    d. Pepsin inhibitors
    e. Proton pump inhibitors

24. What priority information regarding nonpharmacologic treatment can the nurse provide in the health education plan to a patient who has been diagnosed with GERD? *(Select all that apply.)*
    a. Decrease or stop smoking.
    b. Elevate the head of the bed.
    c. Increase fluid intake.
    d. NSAIDs should be taken with food.
    e. Spicy foods should be avoided.

25. The patient has been diagnosed with peptic ulcer disease and has been on propantheline bromide 15 mg tid 30 minutes before meals and 30 mg at bedtime. How does propantheline bromide work?
    a. It blocks H$_2$ receptors.
    b. It coats the lining of the stomach.
    c. It increases gastric motility.
    d. It inhibits gastric secretions.

26. The patient has been diagnosed with an ulcer caused by *H. pylori*. Which drug(s) is/are likely to be used for treatment? *(Select all that apply.)*
    a. Amoxicillin
    b. Clarithromycin
    c. Famotidine
    d. Misoprostol
    e. Omeprazole

27. The patient presents to the clinic with complaints of gnawing abdominal pain that occurs approximately 1 hour after eating. "I have tried everything, and it just won't stop." He has been diagnosed with an ulcer. The health care provider prescribes nizatidine. What priority information should the nurse include in the teaching plan? *(Select all that apply.)*
    a. "Antacids should not be taken within 1 hour of taking your nizatidine."
    b. "Avoid alcoholic beverages and caffeine."
    c. "Eating small, frequent meals may be helpful."
    d. "This drug should be taken with meals and at bedtime."
    e. "You will need to take this for the rest of your life."

28. A patient has been diagnosed with erosive GERD. Which drug is likely to have the highest success rate?
    a. Esomeprazole
    b. Lansoprazole
    c. Omeprazole
    d. Rabeprazole

29. Which side effect(s) of ranitidine will the nurse monitor in the patient? *(Select all that apply.)*
    a. Confusion
    b. Headache
    c. Hypertension
    d. Loss of libido
    e. Nausea

30. Which drug(s) will concern the nurse if prescribed for a patient who is taking esomeprazole? *(Select all that apply.)*
    a. Ampicillin
    b. Digoxin
    c. Ketoconazole
    d. Lisinopril
    e. Propranolol

31. The patient is taking high-dose NSAID therapy for arthritis. She is also taking sucralfate. What laboratory value would concern the nurse?
    a. Hgb 14.1 gm/dL
    b. Potassium 4.2 mEq/L
    c. Blood glucose 185 mg/dL
    d. INR 1.1

192

Read the scenario and answer the following questions on a separate sheet of paper.

S.S., 63 years old, has a high-stress job as a county judge. She complains of abdominal distress after eating. She is currently taking aluminum hydroxide 10 mL with meals and at bedtime. She has been diagnosed with an ulcer.

1. What are the various classes of drugs that can be used to treat ulcers?

2. What drug class does aluminum hydroxide belong to, and how does it work?

3. Is this the proper dose for S.S.?

4. What priority health teaching should the nurse also provide for S.S.?

44 Eye and Ear Disorders

Complete the following.

1. Topical anesthetics (locally/systemically) block the pain signals during selected or ophthalmologic procedures. *(Circle the correct answer.)*

2. Lubricants are used to moisten contact lenses and _____ _____.

3. Classes of ophthalmic antiinflammatories include immunomodulators, _____, and _____.

4. Ophthalmic cyclosporine, an antiinflammatory, allows _____ production.

5. Miotics are used to lower _____ pressure by widening the _____ network to improve drainage of aqueous humor.

6. Ocular decongestants are contraindicated in patients with _____ _____.

7. Carbonic anhydrase inhibitors were developed as _____. They are effective in treating _____.

8. The drug group used to paralyze the muscles of accommodation is _____.

9. Instruct patients with glaucoma to avoid anticholinergic drugs because they (decrease/increase) intraocular pressure. *(Circle the correct answer.)*

10. Antiinfectives are used to treat infections of the eye, including inflammation of the membrane covering the eyeball and inner eyelid known as _____.

11. Drugs that interfere with production of carbonic acid, leading to decreased aqueous humor formation and decreased intraocular pressure, belong to the group _____ _____ _____.

12. Cholinesterase inhibitors can produce systemic _____ effects that include cardiac dysrhythmias, diarrhea, and respiratory depression.

Match the term in Column I with its definition in Column II.

Column I

_____ 13. Otalgia

_____ 14. Optic

_____ 15. Cerumen

_____ 16. Lacrimal duct

_____ 17. Ceruminolytics

_____ 18. Otic

_____ 19. Chalazion

_____ 20. Keratitis

_____ 21. Hordeolum

_____ 22. Acute otitis externa

Column II

a. Also known as tear ducts
b. Drugs that soften or break up earwax
c. Infection of the meibomian glands of the eyelids
d. Ear
e. Swimmer's ear
f. Eye
g. Also known as stye
h. Ear pain
i. Earwax
j. Corneal infection and inflammation

NCLEX REVIEW QUESTIONS

Select the best response.

23. The patient presents to her ophthalmologist for a routine eye examination. Before the exam, eyedrops are used to dilate her eyes. Such drug belongs to which group of drugs?
    a. Carbonic anhydrase inhibitors
    b. Cerumenolytics
    c. Mydriatics
    d. Osmotics

24. A patient is taking acetazolamide for acute closed-angle glaucoma. The nurse will assess for which side effect associated with drugs in the group?
    a. Agitation
    b. Constipation
    c. Electrolyte imbalances
    d. Urinary retention

25. The patient has open-angle glaucoma and is being treated with latanoprost. What is/are priority teaching point(s) for this patient? *(Select all that apply.)*
    a. Permanent brown pigmentation of the iris may occur.
    b. Eyelids may darken.
    c. Blurred vision may occur.
    d. Eyes may feel itchy.
    e. Pupils may get very small.

26. A patient who has frequent cerumen impaction has had his ears irrigated at the clinic. To determine the results of the irrigation, what structure must be visualized?
    a. Auricle
    b. External auditory canal
    c. Semicircular canals
    d. Tympanic membrane

27. The patient has frequent cerumen buildup. Which drug does the nurse anticipate the health care provider will suggest for this patient?
    a. Bimatoprost
    b. Carbamide peroxide
    c. Echothiophate
    d. Proparacaine

28. The patient is receiving pilocarpine eyedrops for treatment of glaucoma. Which side effect(s) is/are most likely to occur? *(Select all that apply.)*
    a. Blurred vision
    b. Cardiac dysrhythmias
    c. Eye pain
    d. Headache
    e. Respiratory depression
    f. Vomiting

29. Which solution(s) is/are commonly used to irrigate the ear? *(Select all that apply.)*
    a. Acetic acid
    b. Boric acid
    c. Cyclopentolate HCl
    d. Hydrogen peroxide 3%
    e. Hypotonic HCl solution 10%

30. The patient has been diagnosed with dry age-related macular degeneration (ARMD). What drug(s) is/are available for treatment? *(Select all that apply.)*
    a. Aflibercept
    b. Bevacizumab
    c. Pegaptanib
    d. Ranibizumab
    e. There is no treatment for dry ARMD.

31. A patient presents to his ophthalmologist with complaints of dry, itching eyes. He works as a landscaper. What option(s) does he have for treatment? *(Select all that apply.)*
    a. Azelastine
    b. Olopatadine
    c. Epinastine
    d. Ketotifen
    e. Tetracaine HCl

32. The most common pathogen in acute otitis media is:
    a. *Staphylococcus aureus.*
    b. *Streptococcus pyrogens.*
    c. *Streptococcus pneumoniae.*
    d. *Lactobacillus.*

33. A patient who has a history of otitis externa presents to the clinic with right ear pain. The ear is painful and swollen. The patient is prescribed ofloxacin otic solution. Before discharge, the nurse inserts a cotton wick into the right external canal. What is the purpose of the wick?
    a. To keep the external auditory canal dry
    b. To allow the drug to reach the external auditory canal
    c. To protect the tympanic membrane from infection
    d. To keep the external auditory canal free of cerumen

CASE STUDY

Read the scenario and answer the following questions on a separate sheet of paper.

Y.G., 80 years old, has chronic open-angle glaucoma and ocular hypertension. She presents to her health care provider for a follow-up appointment. Her medical history is also positive for hypertension, depression, arthritis, and atrial fibrillation. She states that she has been "doing pretty good, I guess." She denies any specific complaints except some blurred vision. She self-administers timolol solution 2 gtt q8h.

1. What is open-angle glaucoma?

2. What kind of a drug is timolol, and how does it work?

3. How are these eyedrops administered?

4. Is this the appropriate dose for this patient? Why or why not?

45 Dermatologic Disorders

Match the term in Column I with the correct description in Column II.

Column I

_____ 1. Macule

_____ 2. Vesicle

_____ 3. Plaque

_____ 4. Papule

Column II

a. Raised, palpable lesion 10 mm in diameter
b. Hard, rough, raised lesion; flat on top, usually >10 mm in diameter
c. Flat, nonpalpable lesion with varying color
d. Raised lesion filled with clear fluid and <1 cm in diameter

Match the condition in Column I to the drug that treats it in Column II. Multiple drugs may be used for a condition.

Column I

_____ 5. Psoriasis

_____ 6. Burns

_____ 7. Acne vulgaris

_____ 8. Verruca vulgaris

Column II

a. Cantharidin
b. Tetracycline
c. Isotretinoin
d. Azelaic acid
e. Adapalene
f. Methotrexate
g. Silver sulfadiazine
h. Calcineurin inhibitors

COMPLETE THE FOLLOWING

9. Tinea pedis is also called _____ _____, and tinea capitis is called _____.

10. _____ are noninflammatory acne lesions that may be _____ (closed) or _____ (open).

11. Isotretinoin is a known _____ and should not be used during pregnancy. Any persons who are to start on isotretinoin must be enrolled in a risk-management program called _____.

12. Psoriasis is a _____ disease affecting predominantly the _____ and _____.

13. Worsening psoriasis with the use of topical corticosteroids is called a _____ effect.

14. Cyclosporine inhibits _____ activation.

15. Salicylic acid promotes _____ when used for verruca vulgaris.

16. Prolonged use of topical corticosteroids is discouraged because it can cause _____ of the skin and _____ of the dermis and epidermis.

Select the best response.

17. The 18-year-old patient has acne. Which type(s) of drug(s) is/are used to treat this condition? *(Select all that apply.)*
    a. Antibiotics
    b. Antifungals
    c. Glucocorticoids
    d. Keratolytics
    e. Nonsteroidal antiinflammatories
    f. T-cell antagonists

18. Psoriasis affects what percentage of the population in the United States?
    a. Less than 1%
    b. Approximately 2%
    c. 5% to 7%
    d. 8% to 10%

19. The patient has psoriasis and presents to her health care provider for treatment. She states that her "lizard skin" is really embarrassing. The health care provider orders calcipotriene. When the patient asks how this drug will work, what is the nurse's best answer?
    a. "This medication will help stop the proliferation of cells."
    b. "It will be very effective against the itching that goes with psoriasis."
    c. "Calcipotriene will cure psoriasis."
    d. "It can be used like makeup to cover up the scales."

20. The patient has psoriasis and is going to be started on a course of infliximab. What does the nurse tell the patient about the dosing regimen he will be following?
    a. "Infliximab is a gel that you will use after bathing."
    b. "Infliximab is a drug that is administered by IV at prescribed intervals."
    c. "You will be able to give yourself an injection once per week."
    d. "This is an oral drug that you will be on for the rest of your life."

21. Which is/are common cause(s) of contact dermatitis? *(Select all that apply.)*
    a. Anesthetics
    b. Cosmetics
    c. Dyes
    d. Peanuts
    e. Sumac

22. The patient has been prescribed tetracycline for acne. What is the initial standard dose?
    a. 125–250 mg q6h
    b. 250–500 mg bid
    c. 500–750 mg q6h
    d. 750–1000 mg daily

23. What is a major side effect of tetracycline to the very young and to pregnant patients?
    a. Cardiac arrhythmias
    b. Glucose intolerance
    c. Hemorrhagic shock
    d. Teeth discoloration

24. What priority information should be provided to the patient taking tetracycline for acne? *(Select all that apply.)*
    a. Alert the health care provider if pregnant or possibly pregnant.
    b. Avoid the use of harsh cleansers.
    c. Eat a high-fiber diet.
    d. It should not be used with isotretinoin.
    e. Use a sunscreen with SPF 2.

25. The patient has male pattern baldness. What drug can be utilized to treat male pattern baldness?
    a. Acitretin
    b. Methotrexate
    c. Minoxidil
    d. Tretinoin

26. The patient presents to his health care provider's office with complaints of severe rash and itching after a hunting trip. He has been diagnosed with contact dermatitis from poison ivy. What antipruritic agent(s) can be utilized for this patient? *(Select all that apply.)*
    a. Triamcinolone
    b. Dexamethasone
    c. Diphenhydramine
    d. Fluconazole
    e. Salicylic acid

CASE STUDY

Read the scenario and answer the following questions on a separate sheet of paper.

C.S., 24 years old, has sustained full-thickness burns over his anterior chest and partial-thickness burns over his forearms bilaterally. Mafenide acetate is ordered to be applied to his burns.

1. What is the difference between full- and partial-thickness burns?

2. What type of drug is mafenide acetate?

3. What other options are available for a topical burn preparation?

4. What are priority nursing interventions for this patient?

46 Pituitary, Thyroid, Parathyroid, and Adrenal Disorders

Match the information in Column I with the correct term in Column II.

Column I

_____ 1. Growth hormone hypersecretion causing excessive growth after puberty

_____ 2. Another name for the anterior pituitary gland

_____ 3. Adrenocorticotropic hormone released by the anterior pituitary gland

_____ 4. Antidiuretic hormone secreted by the posterior pituitary gland

_____ 5. Severe hypothyroidism in children causing delayed physical and mental growth

_____ 6. Growth hormone hypersecretion causing excessive growth during childhood

_____ 7. Cortisol hormone secreted from the adrenal cortex affecting inflammatory response

_____ 8. Another name for the pituitary gland

_____ 9. Aldosterone hormone secreted from the adrenal cortex that regulates sodium, potassium, and hydrogen ions

_____ 10. Severe hypothyroidism in adults causing physical, emotional, and mental changes

_____ 11. Another name for the posterior pituitary gland

_____ 12. Also called Graves disease; caused by hyperfunction of the thyroid gland

_____ 13. T_4 hormone secreted by the thyroid gland

_____ 14. T_3 hormone secreted by the thyroid gland

Column II

a. ADH
b. Gigantism
c. Mineralocorticoid
d. Neurohypophysis
e. Triiodothyronine
f. Acromegaly
g. Myxedema
h. Adenohypophysis
i. ACTH
j. Thyrotoxicosis
k. Thyroxine
l. Glucocorticoid
m. Cretinism
n. Hypophysis

15. **Place the following conditions in the appropriate column.**

hypernatremia	anemia	edema
hypoglycemia	weight loss	delayed wound healing
weight gain	hyperlipidemia	hyperglycemia
fatigue	hirsutism	hyperpigmentation
tachycardia	hypotension	hypokalemia
diarrhea	peptic ulcers	hypertension
buffalo hump	hyponatremia	hyperkalemia

Addison Disease: Adrenal Hyposecretion	Cushing Syndrome: Adrenal Hypersecretion

Match the nursing intervention in Column I with the correct rationale related to glucocorticoid drug administration in Column II.

Column I

_____ 16. Monitor vital signs.

_____ 17. Monitor weight after taking a cortisone preparation for more than 10 days.

_____ 18. Monitor laboratory values, especially blood glucose and electrolytes.

_____ 19. Instruct the patient to take the cortisone with food.

_____ 20. Advise the patient to eat foods rich in potassium.

_____ 21. Instruct the patient not to abruptly discontinue the cortisone preparation.

_____ 22. Teach the patient to report signs and symptoms of potential drug toxicity.

Column II

a. Corticosteroids increase sodium and water retention and increase blood pressure.

b. Adrenal crisis may occur if cortisone is abruptly stopped.

c. Glucocorticoid drugs promote loss of potassium.

d. Weight gain occurs with cortisone use as a result of water retention.

e. Glucocorticoid drugs promote sodium retention, potassium loss, and increased blood glucose.

f. Glucocorticoid drugs may cause moon face, puffy eyelids, edema in the feet, dizziness, and menstrual irregularity at high doses.

g. Glucocorticoid drugs can irritate the gastric mucosa and may cause peptic ulcers.

NCLEX REVIEW QUESTIONS

Select the best response.

23. A 65-year-old patient is being treated for hypothyroidism. The patient is taking levothyroxine 100 mcg/day. What should concern the nurse about the patient's dose of levothyroxine?
   a. It is too low for the patient's age.
   b. It is too high for the patient's age.
   c. Nothing; it is within the normal maintenance dosage range.
   d. Nothing; someone of the patient's age should start at a low dose.

24. How soon after starting levothyroxine should the patient report feeling its effects?
   a. 3–4 days
   b. 4–7 days
   c. 1–2 weeks
   d. 2–4 weeks

25. The nurse assesses the patient for symptoms of hyperthyroidism. Which is/are symptom(s) of hyperthyroidism? *(Select all that apply.)*
   a. Palpitations
   b. Constipation
   c. Excessive sweating
   d. Tachycardia
   e. Tinnitus

26. What time of day should the nurse teach the patient to take levothyroxine?
   a. Before breakfast
   b. With breakfast
   c. After breakfast
   d. With lunch

27. What is priority information to include in the health teaching plan for the patient with hypothyroidism? *(Select all that apply.)*
    a. Avoid over-the-counter (OTC) drugs.
    b. Report numbness and tingling of the hands to the health care provider.
    c. Increase food and fluid intake.
    d. Take the drug with food.
    e. Wear a medical alert identification information device.

28. A patient is taking prednisone for an exacerbation of arthritic knee pain. What is the usual dose of prednisone?
    a. 0.5–6 mg/day
    b. 5–60 mg/day
    c. 60–100 mg/day
    d. 100–125 mg/day

29. While a patient is taking prednisone, which laboratory value should be closely monitored?
    a. Hematocrit
    b. Hemoglobin
    c. Magnesium
    d. Sodium

30. The patient has been started on prednisone for bronchitis to decrease inflammation. When is the best time to take prednisone?
    a. Before meals
    b. With meals
    c. 1 hour after meals
    d. At bedtime

31. Which drug(s) should be used with caution when taking a glucocorticoid? *(Select all that apply.)*
    a. Acetaminophen
    b. Nonsteroidal antiinflammatory drugs (NSAIDs), including aspirin
    c. Digitalis preparations
    d. Phenytoin
    e. Potassium-wasting diuretics

32. What is/are priority nursing intervention(s) to implement in the care of a patient taking prednisone? *(Select all that apply.)*
    a. Follow the physical therapy regimen.
    b. Monitor for signs and symptoms of hyponatremia.
    c. Monitor vital signs.
    d. Obtain a complete medication history.
    e. Record daily weight.

33. Which statement by a patient taking prednisone indicates that she needs more education about her drugs?
    a. "I should wear a medical alert identification device or carry a card."
    b. "I will make sure I force fluids daily."
    c. "I will not abruptly stop taking my drug."
    d. "I will take glucocorticoids only as ordered."

34. When an herbal laxative such as cascara or senna and herbal diuretics such as celery seed are taken with a corticosteroid, what imbalance may occur?
    a. Hypoglycemia
    b. Hypokalemia
    c. Hyponatremia
    d. Hypophosphatemia

35. What changes can occur when ginseng is taken with a corticosteroid?
    a. Central nervous system (CNS) depression
    b. CNS stimulation and insomnia
    c. Counteraction of the effects of the corticosteroid
    d. Electrolyte imbalance

36. Which drug would the nurse anticipate using for a procedure to diagnose adrenal gland dysfunction?
    a. Corticotropin
    b. Ketoconazole
    c. Thyrotropin
    d. Prednisolone

37. The nurse advises a patient to avoid potassium loss by eating which food(s)? *(Select all that apply.)*
    a. Nuts
    b. Meats
    c. Vegetables
    d. Dried fruits
    e. Applesauce

38. 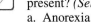 Which drug(s) is/are known to interact with levothyroxine? *(Select all that apply.)*
    a. Anticoagulants
    b. Digitalis
    c. Diuretics
    d. NSAIDs
    e. Oral antidiabetics

39. The nurse assesses a patient for the side effects of prednisone. What assessment finding(s) may be present? *(Select all that apply.)*
    a. Anorexia
    b. Edema
    c. Hypertension
    d. Increased blood sugar
    e. Mood changes

Read the scenario and answer the following questions on a separate sheet of paper.

R.K., 48 years old, has been diagnosed with adrenal insufficiency and is scheduled to start treatment with hydrocortisone.

1. What signs and symptoms are associated with adrenal insufficiency?

2. What is the dosage of hydrocortisone, and how is it administered?

3. What priority teaching is important for this patient?

47 Antidiabetics

STUDY QUESTIONS

Match the term in Column I with its definition in Column II.

Column I

_____ 1.   Diabetes mellitus

_____ 2.   Insulin

_____ 3.   Hypoglycemic reaction

_____ 4.   Ketoacidosis

_____ 5.   Lipodystrophy

_____ 6.   Polydipsia

_____ 7.   Polyphagia

_____ 8.   Polyuria

Column II

a.   Increased hunger
b.   Increased urine output
c.   Use of ketones for energy in diabetics
d.   Disease resulting from deficient glucose metabolism
e.   Increased thirst
f.   Protein secreted from the beta cells of the pancreas
g.   Changes to tissue from frequent insulin injections
h.   Occurs when more insulin is administered than is needed for glucose metabolism

Complete the following.

9.   Hemoglobin A1c (HbA1c) has a life span of approximately _____ or _____ months.

10. Some patients may need higher doses of insulin because of _____, _____, or _____.

11. Subcutaneous injections to the _____ absorb insulin faster than other body sites.

12. Insulin is not administered orally because _____ _____ destroy insulin.

13. Lipoatrophy and lipohypertrophy are terms used to indicate _____ due to not _____ injection sites.

14. Antibody development can cause _____ _____ and _____.

Match the terms in Column I with their definitions in Column II.

Column I

_____ 15.   NPH insulin

_____ 16.   Sulfonylureas

_____ 17.   Regular insulin

_____ 18.   Glucagon

_____ 19.   Insulin lispro

_____ 20.   Insulin glargine

Column II

a.   Oral hypoglycemic drug group
b.   Hyperglycemic hormone that stimulates glycogenolysis
c.   Intermediate-acting insulin
d.   Long-acting insulin
e.   Rapid-acting insulin
f.   Short-acting insulin

Complete the following.

21. All insulins can be administered subcutaneously, but only _____ insulin can be given intravenously.

22. A hypoglycemic event that usually occurs between 2:00 am and 4:00 am followed by an increase in blood glucose level by lipolysis, gluconeogenesis, and glycogenolysis is called the _____.

23. _____ on awakening or the _____ phenomenon is usually controlled by increasing the bedtime dose of insulin.

24. A major side effect of any oral hypoglycemic drug is _____.

25. Metformin, an oral hypoglycemic drug in the _____ class, decreases hepatic production of _____, decreases the _____ from the small intestine, increases insulin _____ sensitivity, and increases _____ glucose uptake at the cellular level.

26. Metformin should be held for _____ _____ before and after administration of IV contrast because _____ _____ or acute renal failure may develop.

27. Incretin mimetics improve glucose control in people with _____ diabetes; they should not be given to people with type 1 diabetes.

NCLEX REVIEW QUESTIONS

Select the best response.

28. What is/are the major symptom(s) that characterize diabetes? *(Select all that apply.)*
    a. Polydipsia
    b. Polyphagia
    c. Polyposia
    d. Polyrrhea
    e. Polyuria

29. Which drug(s) may cause hyperglycemia? *(Select all that apply.)*
    a. Epinephrine
    b. Hydrochlorothiazide
    c. Doxepin
    d. Prednisone
    e. Thiazolidinediones

30. What is the rationale for rotation of insulin injection sites?
    a. It prevents an allergic reaction.
    b. It prevents lipodystrophy.
    c. It prevents polyuria.
    d. It prevents rejection of insulin.

31. What is the only type of insulin that may be administered IV?
    a. Detemir
    b. Lantus
    c. NPH
    d. Regular

32. Which clinical manifestation(s) may be seen in a patient experiencing a hypoglycemic (insulin) reaction? *(Select all that apply.)*
    a. Abdominal pain
    b. Headache
    c. Excessive perspiration
    d. Nervousness
    e. Tremor
    f. Vomiting

33. Which clinical manifestation(s) may be seen in a patient experiencing diabetic ketoacidosis (hyperglycemia)? *(Select all that apply.)*
    a. Bradycardia
    b. Dry mucous membranes
    c. Fruity breath odor
    d. Kussmaul respirations
    e. Polyuria
    f. Thirst

34. The patient has type 1 diabetes. Which medication should the patient not use to control his diabetes?
    a. Insulin glulisine
    b. Insulin lispro
    c. Insulin aspart
    d. Tolazamide

35. Which information should be included in health teaching for patients taking insulin? *(Select all that apply.)*
   a. Adhere to the prescribed diet.
   b. Alter insulin dose based on how you are feeling.
   c. Be sure to exercise.
   d. Monitor blood glucose level.
   e. Recognize signs of hypoglycemic reaction.
   f. Take insulin as prescribed.

36. Which information should be included in health teaching for patients taking oral antidiabetic (hypoglycemic) drugs? *(Select all that apply.)*
   a. Adhere to prescribed diet.
   b. Monitor blood glucose levels.
   c. Monitor weight.
   d. Participate in regular exercise.
   e. Take the drugs based on blood glucose level.

37. Lipoatrophy is a complication that occurs when insulin is injected repeatedly in one site. What is the physiologic effect that occurs?
   a. Depression under the skin surface
   b. Bruising under the skin
   c. Raised lump or knot on the skin surface
   d. Rash at a raised area on the skin surface

38. Where should the patient who takes insulin daily be taught to store the opened insulin?
   a. In a cool place
   b. In the light
   c. In the freezer
   d. Wrapped in aluminum

39. How should the nurse or patient prepare cloudy insulin before administration?
   a. Add diluent to the bottle.
   b. Allow air to escape from the bottle.
   c. Roll the bottle in the hands.
   d. Shake the bottle well.

40. The nurse is preparing to give a patient his daily insulin. The patient receives both NPH and regular insulin. What is the best action by the nurse?
   a. Prepare one injection; draw up both simultaneously and mix well.
   b. Prepare one injection; draw up NPH insulin first.
   c. Prepare one injection; draw up regular insulin first.
   d. Prepare two separate injections.

41. Which type of syringe should be used to administer a patient's daily insulin dose of 6 units of U-100 regular and 14 units of U-100 NPH?
   a. 2-mL syringe
   b. 5-mL syringe
   c. U-40 insulin syringe
   d. U-100 insulin syringe

42. The patient needs to develop a "site rotation pattern" for insulin injections. The American Diabetes Association suggests which action(s)? *(Select all that apply.)*
   a. Choose an injection site for a week.
   b. Change the injection area of the body every day.
   c. Inject insulin each day at the injection site at 1½ inches apart.
   d. Inject insulin IM in the morning and subcut at night.
   e. With two daily injection times, use the right side in the morning and the left side in the evening.

43. When should the nurse expect that the patient may experience a hypoglycemic reaction to regular insulin if administration occurs at 0700 and the patient does not eat?
   a. 0800–0900
   b. 0900–1300
   c. 1300–1500
   d. 1500–1700

44. How long after NPH administration would the nurse expect the patient's insulin to peak?
   a. 1–2 hours
   b. 2–6 hours
   c. 4–12 hours
   d. 12–15 hours

45. Insulin glargine is a long-acting insulin. Which statement(s) best describe(s) insulin glargine? *(Select all that apply.)*
   a. Always combine it with regular insulin for good coverage.
   b. It is given in the evening.
   c. It is safe because hypoglycemia cannot occur.
   d. It is available in a prefilled cartridge insulin pen.
   e. Some patients complain of pain at the injection site.

46. What is a method to determine if the patient has developed an allergy to insulin?
   a. Chemistry laboratory tests
   b. History of other allergies
   c. Skin test with different insulin preparations
   d. Urinalysis to check for glucose

47. The insulin pump, though expensive, has become popular in the management of insulin. What does the nurse know about this method of insulin delivery?
   a. It can be used with intermediate insulin as well as regular insulin.
   b. It can be used with the needle inserted at the same site for weeks.
   c. It is more effective in decreasing the number of hypoglycemic reactions.
   d. It is more effective for use by the type 2 diabetic patient.

48. What is one action of an oral hypoglycemic agent?
    a. It increases the number of insulin cell receptors.
    b. It increases the number of insulin-producing cells.
    c. It replaces receptor sites.
    d. It replaces insulin.

49. The patient asks if repaglinide is oral insulin. What is the nurse's best response?
    a. "No, it is not the same as insulin, and repaglinide can be taken even when the blood sugar remains greater than 250 mg/dL."
    b. "No, it is not the same as insulin. Repaglinide can be used only when there is some beta cell function."
    c. "Yes, it is the same as injected insulin, except it is taken orally."
    d. "Yes, it is similar, but hypoglycemic reactions (insulin shock) do not occur with repaglinide."

50. Which effect(s) is/are representative of second-generation sulfonylureas? *(Select all that apply.)*
    a. Effective doses are less than with first-generation sulfonylureas.
    b. They increase tissue response and decrease glucose production by the liver.
    c. They have less displacement from protein-binding sites by other highly protein-bound drugs.
    d. They have more hypoglycemic potency than first-generation sulfonylureas.

51. The nonsulfonylureas are used to control serum glucose levels after a meal. What best describes their action?
    a. They cause a hypoglycemic reaction.
    b. They decrease hepatic production of glucose from stored glycogen.
    c. They increase the absorption of glucose from the small intestine.
    d. They raise the serum glucose level following a meal.

52. The patient has type 2 diabetes and has just been prescribed pioglitazone HCl. This medication is in the thiazolidinedione group of nonsulfonylureas. How does this group of oral antidiabetics work?
    a. They decrease glucose utilization.
    b. They increase insulin sensitivity for improving blood glucose control.
    c. They increase the uptake of glucose in the liver and small intestine.
    d. They promote absorption of glucose from the large intestine.

53. Herb-drug interaction must be assessed in patients taking herbs and antidiabetic agents. How do ginseng and garlic affect insulin or oral antidiabetic drugs?
    a. They can be taken with insulin without any effect, but they can cause a hypoglycemic reaction with oral antidiabetic drugs.
    b. Ginseng and garlic can lower the blood glucose level.
    c. They decrease the effect of insulin and antidiabetic drugs, causing a hyperglycemic effect.
    d. They may decrease insulin requirements.

54. What is/are the recommended guideline(s) for use of oral antidiabetics in patients with diabetes? *(Select all that apply.)*
    a. Diagnosis of diabetes mellitus for <10 years
    b. Fasting blood sugar <200 mg/dL
    c. Normal renal and hepatic function
    d. Onset at age 40 years or older
    e. Underweight patient

55. Which drug(s) or category(ies) of drug(s) will interact with a sulfonylurea? *(Select all that apply.)*
    a. Antacids
    b. Anticoagulants
    c. Anticonvulsants
    d. Aspirin
    e. Cimetidine

CASE STUDY

Read the scenario and answer the following questions on a separate sheet of paper.

K.C., 25 years old, has type 1 diabetes, which is normally well controlled with daily insulin. He has been under increased stress recently because he has been preparing for defense of his thesis. His friends bring him into the emergency department because "he is acting funny." Before the triage nurse can ask his friends any further questions, they leave. Initially, K.C. is confused, complains of a headache, and has slurred speech. His glucose level in triage reads "low" on the glucometer. While waiting to be taken to a treatment room, he becomes unresponsive.

1. What is a possible cause of his symptoms?

2. How will this be treated before he becomes unconscious?

3. What are the treatment options after he loses consciousness?

48 Urinary Disorders

STUDY QUESTIONS

Match the urinary drug class in Column I to its effect in Column II. Answers may be used more than once.

Column I

_____ 1. Urinary stimulants

_____ 2. Anticholinergics

_____ 3. Urinary antiseptics

_____ 4. Bactericidal

_____ 5. Antimuscarinics

_____ 6. Antiinfectives

_____ 7. Urinary analgesics

_____ 8. Bacteriostatic

_____ 9. Antispasmodics

Column II

a. Inhibits bacterial growth
b. Increases urinary muscle tone
c. Relieves pain and burning
d. Prevents bacterial growth
e. Decreases urgency and urinary incontinence
f. Kills bacteria

Label the infectious processes to the appropriate urinary structures.

10.

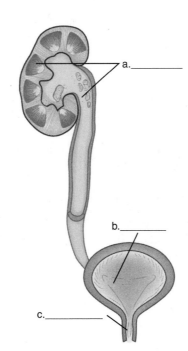

a._____

b._____

c._____

Select the best response.

11. What may occur when methenamine is given with a sulfonamide?
    a. Bleeding
    b. Chest pain
    c. Crystalluria
    d. Intestinal distention

12. The patient has a urinary tract infection and has been advised to increase her fluid intake and decrease her urine pH. What information would the nurse include in discharge teaching to help the patient meet this goal?
    a. "Drinking whole milk will help."
    b. "Cranberry juice will help acidify the urine."
    c. "Be sure to drink 12–14 8-oz glasses of water per day."
    d. "Drink prune juice four times per day to make urine alkaline."

13. A 72-year-old patient has been prescribed flavoxate for urinary spasms. Which diagnosis in the patient's medical history would be of highest concern to the nurse?
    a. Dementia
    b. Glaucoma
    c. Hypoglycemia
    d. Migraines

14. The patient will be receiving ertapenem to prevent recurring UTIs. Which side effect(s) will the nurse include in patient teaching? *(Select all that apply.)*
    a. Visual disturbances
    b. Back pain
    c. Diarrhea
    d. Headache
    e. Nausea

15. Which urinary antiseptic drug–drug interaction(s) is/are correct? *(Select all that apply.)*
    a. Trimethoprim can be combined with sulfamethoxazole.
    b. Antacids increase absorption of ciprofloxacin.
    c. Sodium bicarbonate inhibits the action of methenamine.
    d. Antacids can decrease the absorption of nitrofurantoin.

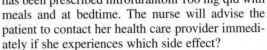

16. The patient is being discharged from the emergency department after being diagnosed with a UTI. She has been prescribed nitrofurantoin 100 mg qid with meals and at bedtime. The nurse will advise the patient to contact her health care provider immediately if she experiences which side effect?
    a. Brown urine
    b. Frequency in urination
    c. Diarrhea
    d. Tingling or numbness of extremities

17. For which condition(s) would the nurse expect to see urinary analgesics prescribed? *(Select all that apply.)*
    a. Burning sensation
    b. Frequency
    c. Hesitation
    d. Retention
    e. Urgency

18. Which drug is commonly prescribed as a urinary analgesic?
    a. Bethanechol
    b. Flavoxate
    c. Phenazopyridine hydrochloride
    d. Trimethoprim

19. The patient has been prescribed an antiinfective and phenazopyridine for a UTI. She calls the clinic and is very concerned that her urine has turned reddish orange. After reviewing the patient's chart and her medications, what will the nurse tell the patient?
    a. "If you do not take the antibiotic with food in your stomach, your urine will turn orange."
    b. "Inadequate liquid intake will cause your urine to turn bright orange."
    c. "This is an indication of an allergic reaction. You need to come back to the clinic."
    d. "Bright reddish-orange urine is to be expected when taking phenazopyridine."

20. What drug is commonly used to treat urinary tract spasms?
    a. Bethanechol
    b. Oxybutynin
    c. Phenazopyridine
    d. Trimethoprim

21. The patient, 68 years old, has a history of environmental allergies, narrow-angle glaucoma, depression, and overactive bladder. Which drug(s) will concern the nurse? *(Select all that apply.)*
   a. Bethanechol
   b. Dimethyl sulfoxide (DMSO)
   c. Nitrofurantoin
   d. Oxybutynin
   e. Tolterodine tartrate

22. Which patient is more likely to benefit from bethanechol chloride?
   a. A 44-year-old patient with prostatitis
   b. A 53-year-old patient with paraplegia
   c. A 65-year-old patient with pyelonephritis
   d. A 70-year-old patient with overactive bladder

CASE STUDY

Read the scenario and answer the following questions on a separate sheet of paper.

G.H., 14 years old, sustained an injury to his urinary tract while playing football and has been prescribed oxybutynin chloride 5 mg bid for spasms.

1. What is the mechanism of action of oxybutynin?

2. Which patients should not take this drug, and why?

3. What are the side effects that can be expected?

4. Are there any dose adjustments that need to be made because of the patient's age?

49 Pregnancy and Preterm Labor

Match the terms in Column I with the definitions in Column II.

Column I

_____ 1.   Preeclampsia

_____ 2.   Gestational hypertension

_____ 3.   HELLP

_____ 4.   L/S (lecithin/sphingomyelin) ratio

_____ 5.   Eclampsia

_____ 6.   Preterm delivery

_____ 7.   Hyperemesis gravidarum

_____ 8.   Surfactant

_____ 9.   Teratogens

_____ 10. Tocolytic therapy

Column II

a.   New onset of seizures with preeclampsia
b.   Prior to 37 gestational weeks
c.   Drug therapy to decrease uterine muscle contractions
d.   Severe nausea and vomiting during pregnancy
e.   Decreases the incidence of respiratory distress syndrome (RDS)
f.   Hypertension during pregnancy without proteinuria
g.   Gestational hypertension with proteinuria
h.   Substances that cause developmental abnormalities
i.   Predictor of fetal lung maturity and risk for neonatal RDS
j.   *H*emolysis, *E*levated *L*iver enzymes, and *L*ow *P*latelet count

Match the letters of the substance in Column II with the associated adverse effects in Column I. Some adverse effects may have more than one cause (substance).

Column I

_____ 11. Increased risk of spontaneous abortion

_____ 12. Smaller head circumference

_____ 13. Hypertonicity, tremulousness beyond infanthood

_____ 14. Abruptio placentae and premature delivery

_____ 15. Degenerative placental lesions

_____ 16. Adverse outcomes to fetus are still unclear

_____ 17. Decreased sucking reflex

_____ 18. Ataxia, syncope, vertigo

_____ 19. Altered facial features, mild to moderate mental retardation

Column II

a.   Alcohol
b.   Caffeine
c.   Cocaine
d.   Heroin
e.   Marijuana
f.   Barbiturates
g.   Tobacco/nicotine
h.   Tranquilizer

Select the best response.

20. What maternal physiologic change(s) is/are seen during pregnancy that affect(s) drug dosing? *(Select all that apply.)*
    a. Decreased urine output
    b. Gastric motility is more rapid, resulting in faster absorption
    c. Increased fluid volume
    d. Increased glomerular filtration rate and rapid elimination of drugs
    e. Increased liver metabolism of drugs

21. The mechanism by which drugs cross the placenta is similar to the way drugs infiltrate which type of body tissue?
    a. Breast
    b. Liver
    c. Subcutaneous
    d. Uterine

22. What is/are the important factor(s) that determine(s) the teratogenicity of any drug ingested during pregnancy? *(Select all that apply.)*
    a. Dosage
    b. Duration of exposure
    c. Gastric motility
    d. Timing
    e. Urinary clearance

23. Surfactant is produced by type II alveolar cells in the lungs. Its purpose is to decrease surface tension and keep the alveoli open. What is the composition of surfactant? *(Select all that apply.)*
    a. Albumin
    b. Lecithin
    c. Progesterone
    d. Sphingomyelin
    e. Thiamine

24. What is the purpose of determining the lecithin/sphingomyelin (L/S) ratio?
    a. Determines the date of delivery
    b. Determines the maturity of the fetal lungs
    c. Determines the ratio of urine output/glomerular filtration rate
    d. Predictor of premature labor

25. The patient is in preterm labor at 28 weeks. The health care provider prescribes betamethasone 12 mg IM q24h for 2 doses. The patient wants to know why she has to receive the drug. What is the nurse's best response?
    a. "Betamethasone will stop your labor."
    b. "It will help the fetus' lungs mature more quickly."
    c. "It will promote closure of a patent ductus arteriosus."
    d. "This drug will promote fetal adrenal maturity."

26. The patient has been diagnosed with gestational hypertension. What is/are the treatment goal(s) for this patient? *(Select all that apply.)*
    a. Decrease the incidence of preterm labor (PTL)
    b. Delivery of an uncompromised infant
    c. Ensure future ability to conceive
    d. Prevention of HELLP syndrome
    e. Prevention of seizures

27. The nurse works in a prenatal clinic. What is/are the most common complaint(s) during pregnancy? *(Select all that apply.)*
    a. Heartburn
    b. Headaches
    c. Nausea
    d. Vomiting
    e. Weakness

28. The patient has iron-deficiency anemia and is pregnant with her first child. Her health care provider has prescribed ferrous sulfate 325 mg bid. Which laboratory value will show the first indication that she is responding to the iron supplement?
    a. Increased BUN
    b. Increased hemoglobin and hematocrit
    c. Increased reticulocyte count
    d. Increased INR

29. The patient is 16 weeks pregnant. She presents to her health care provider with nasal congestion, cough, and headache. She states, "I guess I just have a cold. What can I take for my head to feel better?" What is the nurse's best response?
    a. "A combination of pseudoephedrine, aspirin, and diphenhydramine will work."
    b. "Acetaminophen should be safe to take for your headache."
    c. "Taking 1000 mg of vitamin C will shorten your symptoms."
    d. "Echinacea and garlic should help."

30. The patient presents to the clinic for her first prenatal visit with her entire family. She is a recent immigrant from Mexico and does not speak English. What priority action(s) will the nurse take to ensure culturally competent care? *(Select all that apply.)*
    a. Obtain a trained translator for her visit.
    b. Explain the importance of prenatal vitamins and their safety.
    c. Use a family member to translate.
    d. Hurry through the exam to stay on schedule.
    e. Provide extensive discharge instructions.

31. The patient presents to her health care provider with complaints of morning sickness. "I didn't have it with my first. I'm just not sure what to do." What nonpharmacologic measure(s) can the nurse suggest? *(Select all that apply.)*
    a. Avoid fatty or spicy foods.
    b. Avoid fluids before arising.
    c. Drink flat soda between meals.
    d. Eat crackers, dry toast, cereal, or complex carbohydrates.
    e. Eat a high-protein snack at bedtime.

32. The patient is in her third trimester and presents to her health care provider complaining of severe heartburn. What is/are some nonpharmacologic method(s) the nurse can suggest to help with her symptoms? *(Select all that apply.)*
    a. Avoid citrus juices.
    b. Avoid spicy foods.
    c. Do not recline immediately after eating.
    d. Drink carbonated beverages.
    e. Eat smaller meals.

33. What is/are priority teaching goal(s) for a patient with gestational hypertension? *(Select all that apply.)*
    a. Discuss important symptoms to report to the health care provider.
    b. Explain to the patient the importance of weighing herself daily.
    c. Instruct the patient to lie on her right side.
    d. Stress the importance of adequate fluid intake.

34. The patient is in her first trimester of pregnancy. She has been started on a prenatal vitamin with iron. What teaching will the nurse provide for this patient? *(Select all that apply.)*
    a. Antacids can be taken with the iron tablet to help with epigastric discomfort.
    b. Ensure adequate fluid and fiber intake to assist with constipation.
    c. Iron can be taken with food if necessary to prevent nausea.
    d. Jaundice is a common side effect of iron supplements.
    e. Orange juice enhances iron absorption.

35. Which food(s) should the nurse recommend a pregnant woman eat to increase her iron intake? *(Select all that apply.)*
    a. Broccoli
    b. Cabbage
    c. Apples
    d. Potatoes
    e. Salmon

36. What is the recommended daily allowance of folic acid for a pregnant woman?
    a. 100–400 mcg
    b. 400–800 mcg
    c. 800–1200 mcg
    d. 1200–1600 mcg

37. Which is the most commonly ingested nonprescription drug for pain during pregnancy?
    a. Acetaminophen
    b. Aspirin
    c. Diphenhydramine
    d. Ibuprofen

38. Which priority intervention should the nurse implement for the patient receiving a beta-sympathomimetic drug?
    a. Auscultate breath sounds every 4 hours.
    b. Encourage patient to sleep on her back.
    c. Have atropine available as a reversal agent.
    d. Monitor maternal vital signs every 5 minutes when receiving IV dose.

39. Which nursing intervention(s) should a patient receiving magnesium sulfate for preeclampsia require? *(Select all that apply.)*
    a. Administer the loading dose as a bolus given IVP.
    b. Continuously monitor vital signs and fetal monitor.
    c. Encourage patient to ambulate in room to prevent blood clots.
    d. Have calcium gluconate available at the bedside.
    e. Monitor deep tendon reflexes (DTRs).

40. What clinical manifestation(s) would the nurse assess in someone experiencing magnesium toxicity? *(Select all that apply.)*
    a. Absent DTRs
    b. Fever
    c. Muscle pain
    d. Rapid decrease in respiratory rate
    e. Tachycardia
    f. Weight gain

41. The patient is in preterm labor and is receiving magnesium sulfate. She asks how long she will be on the drug. What is the nurse's best response?
    a. Until the time of delivery
    b. Until delivery or 4–8 hours after contractions have stopped
    c. Until delivery or 8–12 hours after contractions have stopped
    d. Until delivery or 12–24 hours after contractions have stopped

42. The patient is 38 weeks pregnant and is complaining of a sinus headache. Her blood pressure is 114/62 mm Hg, heart rate 88 beats/min, and respiratory rate 18 breaths/min. She has no edema and no protein in her urine. She tells the nurse that when she gets a headache she always takes a combination drug that contains aspirin, acetaminophen, and caffeine. What may occur with the use of aspirin late in pregnancy? *(Select all that apply.)*
   a. Decreased hemostasis in the newborn
   b. Increased maternal blood loss at delivery
   c. Increased risk of anemia
   d. Low–birth-weight infant
   e. Precipitous delivery

43. The patient is receiving magnesium sulfate for gestational hypertension. Which side effect(s) of this drug may be expected? *(Select all that apply.)*
   a. Dizziness
   b. Flushing
   c. Hyperreflexia
   d. Slurred speech
   e. Urinary incontinence

44. What is HELLP?
   a. A form of gestational diabetes
   b. Another acronym for premature rupture of membranes
   c. A disease process that occurs in mothers of multiples
   d. Severe sequelae of preeclampsia

45. Which drug(s) may be beneficial in the treatment of gestational hypertension? *(Select all that apply.)*
   a. Furosemide
   b. Hydralazine
   c. Lisinopril
   d. Methyldopa
   e. Nifedipine

CASE STUDY

Read the scenario and answer the following questions on a separate sheet of paper.

K.R., 40 years old, is pregnant with her fourth child. She is at 33 weeks' gestation. She has had one miscarriage and has two living children, ages 15 and 9 years. It is 2100 on Friday night, and her health care provider's office is closed, so she has left a message with the answering service. She contacts OB triage and states, "I think I may be having contractions, but I know I'm too early. My 15-year-old was born at 30 weeks, and I am so scared that this is happening again." She complains of lower abdominal tightening and back discomfort that comes and goes about every 8 minutes. K.R. was instructed to come to the hospital.

1. What are some priority questions for the nurse to ask while on the phone?

2. What puts K.R. at high risk for PTL?

3. What are some nonpharmacologic measures to treat PTL? What are some pharmacologic options to treat PTL?

4. What needs to be done for the fetus at 33 weeks' gestation?

50 Labor, Delivery, and Postpartum

STUDY QUESTIONS

Label the following areas for regional anesthesia.

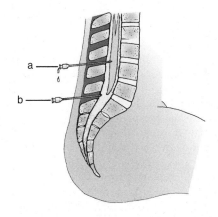

1.

Match the term in Column I to its definition in Column II.

Column I

_____ 2. Somatic

_____ 3. Visceral

_____ 4. Contraction

_____ 5. Regional

_____ 6. Ripening

Column II

a. Type of anesthesia for pain relief during labor and delivery without loss of consciousness

b. Type of pain caused by pressure of the presenting part and stretching of the perineum and vagina

c. Softening of the cervix

d. Type of pain carried by sympathetic fibers from the cervix and uterus

e. Tightening and shortening of uterine muscles

Match the stage in Column I with its definition in Column II.

Column I

_____ 7. Dilating stage

_____ 8. Pelvic stage

_____ 9. Placental separation and expulsion

_____ 10. Early postpartum

Column II

a. Placental separation from the uterine wall and its delivery

b. Cervical effacement and dilation occur

c. First 4 hours after delivery of the placenta

d. Complete cervical dilation and ends with delivery of the newborn

Complete the following.

11. The three *phases* of the dilating stage include _____, _____, and _____.

12. Sedative-hypnotics should be given at the onset of uterine contractions to decrease (maternal/neonatal) drug exposure. *(Circle the correct answer.)*

13. Adverse effects of opioids depend on the responses activated by the _____ and _____ receptors.

14. Barbiturates (should/should not) be given during active labor. *(Circle the correct answer.)*

217

15. Spinal anesthesia, also known as a _____ _____, is injected in the subarachnoid space.

16. A uterotropic drug, _____ stimulate(s) uterine contraction.

17. Progesterone on the smooth muscle _____ peristalsis, which can promote constipation during the postpartum period.

18. A mother with Rh-negative blood should receive _____ _____ to prevent fetal hemolysis in an Rh-positive fetus.

NCLEX REVIEW QUESTIONS

Select the best response.

19. The primary advantage of butorphanol tartrate and nalbuphine is their *dose ceiling effect*. What does this mean?
    a. Additional doses of the medication do not increase the degree of respiratory depression.
    b. Both of these drugs must be given together to get the dose ceiling effect.
    c. Only one dose is administered to obtain the desired effect.
    d. This means that there is no limit as to how much of the drug can be used to obtain the desired effect.

20. The patient has received spinal anesthesia for delivery. What should the nurse monitor in this patient?
    a. Hemoglobin and hematocrit
    b. Palpitations
    c. Pedal edema
    d. Postdural headache

21. What is/are treatment(s) for postdural headaches? *(Select all that apply.)*
    a. Analgesics
    b. Bed rest
    c. Blood patch
    d. Caffeine
    e. Decreased fluids

22. When should an IV drug for pain be administered to the laboring patient?
    a. At the beginning of the uterine contraction
    b. At the end of the uterine contraction
    c. Between uterine contractions
    d. In the middle of the uterine contraction

23. A baby was born within 15 minutes after his mother received opioids for pain and now has respiratory depression. Which drug is the best to provide reversal of neonatal respiratory depression?
    a. Calcium gluconate
    b. Calcium carbonate
    c. Flumazenil
    d. Naloxone

24. Before administration of general anesthesia, a laboring woman is given an antacid. What is the purpose of giving this drug?
    a. Decrease gastric acidity
    b. Enhance anesthesia induction
    c. Maintain a patent airway
    d. Prevent nausea and vomiting

25. What should be done before administration of an epidural?
    a. Bolus of crystalloids, 500–1000 mL IV
    b. Preprocedural echocardiogram
    c. The patient's verbal consent to the procedure
    d. Type and crossmatch for blood administration

26. A patient is receiving an epidural, and her blood pressure is beginning to drop. What is the first action the nurse should take?
    a. Administer oxygen.
    b. Expect an order to administer 5–15 mg of ephedrine IV.
    c. Expect an order to transfuse with 1 unit of packed red cells.
    d. Turn her on her left side.

27. Which value or greater on the Bishop score is associated with successful labor induction?
    a. 5
    b. 6
    c. 8
    d. 10

28. During which stage of labor do women commonly receive ergot alkaloids?
    a. First
    b. Second
    c. Third
    d. Fourth

29. Before administering methylergonovine, which baseline value should be measured?
    a. Blood pressure
    b. Fetal heart rate
    c. Maternal hourly urinary output
    d. Respiratory rate

30. If a patient has received meperidine and then receives a dose of naloxone, what will the woman in labor experience?
    a. Increased pain relief
    b. Increased pain
    c. Increased fetal heart rate decelerations
    d. Increased fetal heart rate variability

31. The nurse is aware that many factors influence the choice of pain control. What is the most important factor?
    a. Amount of time likely until delivery
    b. Frequency of contractions
    c. Intensity of contractions
    d. Patient preference

32. What should the nurse know about the use of barbiturates and narcotics in labor?
    a. Active labor is the most appropriate time for their use.
    b. Barbiturates make the delivery time unpredictable.
    c. The narcotic antagonists will counteract respiratory depression.
    d. Narcotics offer more complete pain relief.

33. Which priority information should be included in patient teaching about an analgesic during labor? *(Select all that apply.)*
    a. Effects on labor
    b. Effects on newborn
    c. Expected time delivery will occur
    d. Methods of administration
    e. Restrictions placed on mobility

34. Which statement about the patient who receives continuous lumbar epidural block anesthesia in repeated doses is accurate?
    a. Before 8-cm dilation, there is a risk of arresting the first stage of labor.
    b. Each repeated dose must have complete documentation.
    c. Following injection, ensure dispersion of the local anesthetic for effective pain relief.
    d. The method is suitable for vaginal delivery, but not for a cesarean delivery, because the density of the block cannot be manipulated.

35. In relation to uterine contractions, how should spinal anesthesia be administered?
    a. Before
    b. During
    c. Immediately after
    d. 1–2 minutes after

36. The nurse assesses a patient receiving a local anesthetic for side effects. What should the nurse monitor in this patient? *(Select all that apply.)*
    a. Dizziness
    b. Hypertension
    c. Metallic taste in mouth
    d. Nausea
    e. Palpitations

37. Which baseline data should the nurse collect on a patient having an IV oxytocin induction at 41+ weeks' gestation? *(Select all that apply.)*
    a. Deep tendon reflexes
    b. Fetal heart rate
    c. Pulse rate and blood pressure
    d. Type and crossmatch for blood
    e. Uterine activity

38. The nurse monitors a patient having an IV oxytocin induction at 41+ weeks' gestation for signs of uterine rupture. What would the nurse assess in a patient who has experienced uterine rupture? *(Select all that apply.)*
    a. Hemorrhage
    b. Hypertension
    c. Loss of fetal heart rate
    d. Projectile vomiting
    e. Sudden increased pain

39. Which type(s) of systemic drug group(s) is/are used during labor? *(Select all that apply.)*
    a. Antiepileptics
    b. Mixed narcotic agonists-antagonists
    c. NSAIDs
    d. Narcotic agonists
    e. Tranquilizers

40. The patient is complaining of labor pain. This somatic pain is caused by pressure of the presenting part and stretching of the perineum and vagina. This pain is experienced in which stage(s) of labor? *(Select all that apply.)*
    a. First
    b. Latent
    c. Second
    d. Transition
    e. Third

41. Which type(s) of anesthesia may be used for cesarean deliveries? *(Select all that apply.)*
    a. Caudal block
    b. Epidural anesthesia
    c. General anesthesia
    d. Pudendal anesthesia
    e. Spinal anesthesia

42. Which is/are the most commonly used drug(s) for the relief of perineal pain resulting from episiotomy or laceration? *(Select all that apply.)*
    a. Benzocaine
    b. Erythromycin
    c. Mineral oil
    d. Witch hazel compresses

43. The nurse is administering a stool softener to a postpartum patient. The patient asks what the purpose/action of this drug is. What is the nurse's best response?
    a. "To decrease perineal discomfort and facilitate stool passage postdelivery."
    b. "To decrease the incidence of gas, thus decreasing perineal pain."
    c. "To decrease the need for eating fiber while in the postpartum period."
    d. "To make sure you have a bowel movement before discharge."

44. A postpartum patient with a repaired fourth-degree laceration has benzocaine topical spray. She asks if she can also use a heat lamp on her perineum for additional comfort. What is the nurse's best answer?
    a. "No, the heat lamp will increase the incidence of bacteria growth."
    b. "No, use of a heat lamp with benzocaine may cause tissue burns."
    c. "What a good idea; it will decrease pain while improving healing."
    d. "Yes, you can use a heat lamp to augment the action of benzocaine."

45. When is the best time to administer the standard dose of $Rh_0(D)$ immune globulin?
    a. After chorionic villus sampling and at 38 weeks' gestation
    b. At 28 weeks' gestation and again within 72 hours after delivery
    c. Before amniocentesis and at 38 weeks' gestation
    d. Only at 28 weeks' gestation

46. After which procedure should the patient receive a microdose of $Rh_0(D)$ immune globulin?
    a. Abortion before 13 weeks
    b. Abortion after 16 weeks
    c. Amniocentesis
    d. Chorionic villus sampling

CASE STUDY

Read the scenario and answer the following questions on a separate sheet of paper.

K.E., 22 years old, is at 38 weeks' gestation and has intrauterine growth retardation (IUGR). She is scheduled for an induction.

1. What drugs are used to induce labor, and what other methods may be used to induce labor?

2. What priority teaching instructions will the nurse provide on arrival to the hospital?

3. What analgesic options are available to K.E.?

51 Neonatal and Newborn

STUDY QUESTIONS

Complete the following.

1. _____ _____ _____ can occur because of immature lung development and low _____ level, which is needed to decrease surface tension.

2. A patent _____ tube is required to administer surfactant.

3. _____ is excessive oxygenation and _____ is decreased carbon dioxide concentration.

4. Hepatitis B immunization should be initiated during the _____ period.

5. Erythromycin ophthalmic ointment is administered to newborns to prevent _____ _____, an eye infection among newborns.

NCLEX REVIEW QUESTIONS

Select the best response.

6. A baby is born at 30 weeks' gestation and is having respiratory distress. What type of drug will be given to help the baby's lungs?
   a. Antibiotics
   b. Benzodiazepines
   c. Calcium chloride
   d. Surfactant replacement

7. A nurse is preparing to assist in administering beractant intratracheally. What following action(s) is/are needed in preparing the drug?
   a. Warm for 5 seconds under hot running water.
   b. Shake the vial to mix the solution.
   c. Warm at room temperature for 20 minutes.
   d. Keep it refrigerated until immediately before administration.

8. Which of the following drugs could be administered to a newborn to mature lung development? *(Select all that apply.)*
   a. Erythromycin
   b. Beractant
   c. Vitamin K
   d. Poractant alfa
   e. Calfactant

9. A nurse is assisting with administering exogenous surfactant via endotracheal tube. Which of the following complications could occur with surfactant?
   a. Desaturation
   b. Bradycardia
   c. Pallor
   d. Hyperoxia

10. A preterm neonate becomes cyanotic and the oxygen level decreases during surfactant administration. What should the nurse do?
    a. Gently suction through the endotracheal tube immediately to raise the oxygen level.
    b. Reposition the neonate to disperse the drug throughout the lungs.
    c. Do nothing.
    d. Increase the amount of oxygen the neonate is receiving.

11. Which of the following would be administered to a neonate born to a hepatitis B carrier to provide passive protection against hepatitis B?
    a. Recombinant hepatitis B
    b. Varicella zoster
    c. Phytonadione
    d. Hepatitis B immune globulin

12. Which ophthalmic ointment is administered to the newborn immediately after birth?
    a. Bacitracin
    b. Erythromycin
    c. Gentamicin
    d. Penicillin

13. Which priority information should be included in patient teaching regarding ophthalmic and parenteral drugs administered to the neonate immediately after birth?
    a. Swelling of eyes usually disappears in the first 24–48 hours.
    b. All parenteral drugs can be administered in one injection.
    c. The injection is not painful for the baby.
    d. If the mother has had hepatitis immunizations, the newborn will not receive the hepatitis B immunization.

Read the scenario and answer the following questions on a separate sheet of paper.

J.G., 32 years old, is about to deliver her first baby and is anxious. Laboratory tests during one of her prenatal checkups revealed that J.G. was positive for HBs-Ag. Additional blood work was positive for active hepatitis B virus (HBV). J.G. is worried that her baby will also have hepatitis B.

1. How can HBV be transmitted to the neonate?

2. What is the nurse's best response to J.G.'s concerns?

3. What would the nurse administer to the neonate for hepatitis B? What are the rationales for the drugs?

4. What is the immunization schedule for recombinant hepatitis B?

52 Women's Reproductive Health

STUDY QUESTIONS

Match the medical disorder in Column I with its definition in Column II.

Column I

_____ 1. Endometriosis

_____ 2. Dysmenorrhea

_____ 3. Dysfunctional uterine bleeding

_____ 4. Polycystic ovarian syndrome

_____ 5. Premenstrual syndrome

Column II

a. Collection of cyclic physical and mood alterations

b. Abnormal location of endometrial tissue outside the uterus

c. A disorder in the metabolism of androgens and estrogens

d. A classification of irregular bleeding

e. Also called cyclic pelvic pain

Complete the following.

6. A women's reproductive life cycle begins with _____ and continues through _____.

7. Ethinyl estradiol is a synthetic _____ found in combined hormonal contraceptives.

8. Drospirenone is an analog of _____, a potassium-sparing _____.

9. If the minipill is delayed for more than 3 hours, a back-up contraceptive method should be used for _____ hours.

10. The inhibition of both FSH and LH secretion results in _____ and _____.

Match the term in Column I with its definition in Column II.

Column I

_____ 11. Amenorrhea

_____ 12. Dysmenorrhea

_____ 13. Mittelschmerz

_____ 14. Breakthrough bleeding

_____ 15. Chloasma

Column II

a. Episodes of bleeding during the active pill cycle of hormonal contraceptives

b. Absence of bleeding

c. Pain usually associated with ovulation

d. Painful periods

e. Hyperpigmentation of the skin

NCLEX REVIEW QUESTIONS

Select the best response.

16. Which of the following is/are the correct mode(s) of action when combined hormonal contraceptives are used as emergency contraception? *(Select all that apply.)*
    a. Causes an abortion
    b. Delays ovulation
    c. Interferes with hormones for implantation
    d. Interferes with tubal transport of embryo
    e. Menstruation starts immediately to remove any products of conception

17. Which individual should not take oral contraceptives?
    a. 20-year-old who is not sexually active
    b. 40-year-old with diabetes
    c. 38-year-old with breast cancer
    d. 48-year-old with emphysema

223

18. In which patient(s) should combined hormone contraceptives (CHCs) be used with caution? *(Select all that apply.)*
    a. 37-year-old who smokes
    b. 45-year-old who does not exercise
    c. 38-year-old with diabetes
    d. 28-year-old with epilepsy
    e. 18-year-old with depression

19. The patient works the night shift and realizes when she wakes up for work that she has missed a dose of her CHC. She calls the on-call nurse and asks what she should do. What is the nurse's best response?
    a. "It isn't a big deal. Just take one tomorrow."
    b. "Stop this pack and use alternative birth control for the next month."
    c. "Take your dose now, and then get back on schedule with the next one."
    d. "Take two now and use an alternative method of birth control."

20. A patient who has been taking conjugated estrogen for contraception reports a variety of side effects. Which clinical manifestation(s) is/are due primarily to an excess of estrogen? *(Select all that apply.)*
    a. Acne
    b. Breast tenderness
    c. Fluid retention
    d. Leg cramps
    e. Nausea

21. A patient who has been taking conjugated estrogen for contraception reports her current drug history. Which drug(s) will interact with her oral contraceptive? *(Select all that apply.)*
    a. Aspirin
    b. Fluoxetine
    c. Folic acid
    d. Phenobarbital
    e. Topiramate

22. Which laboratory value should be monitored closely in a patient who has been taking drospirenone for contraception?
    a. Blood glucose
    b. Hemoglobin
    c. Potassium
    d. Thyroid-stimulating hormone

23. A patient who has been using ethinyl estradiol and etonogestrel transvaginal for contraception calls and reports that the device fell out. What is the nurse's best advice?
    a. "Discard the current pill pack and start a new package of pills."
    b. "Do a home pregnancy test and report the results."
    c. "Rinse it off if it has been less than 3 hours and reinsert."
    d. "Throw it away and get a new one."

24. The family planning nurse would be correct to tell a patient to stop taking her combined oral contraceptive and notify her health care provider if she experiences which alteration?
    a. Increased vaginal discharge
    b. Severe headaches
    c. Lighter/shorter periods
    d. Menstrual cramping

25. What risk factor decreases with the use of progestin in hormone therapy (HT)?
    a. Breast cancer
    b. Cervical cancer
    c. Endometrial cancer
    d. Vaginal cancer

26. The patient is having complaints associated with menopause and presents to her health care provider to discuss HT. She states, "I just want to enjoy everything now and travel. I have too much to do to slow down with hot flashes and mood swings and taking a pill every day." The health care provider prescribes an estrogen patch. What is an advantage of this system?
    a. It is absorbed directly into the bloodstream.
    b. It is applied five times per week for 2 weeks using rotation of sites.
    c. It is less expensive than tablets.
    d. It results in fewer headaches.

27. Which drug(s) is/are used to treat osteoporosis? *(Select all that apply.)*
    a. Beta blockers
    b. Bisphosphonates
    c. Estrogen
    d. Progestins
    e. Selective estrogen receptor modulators (SERMs)

CASE STUDY

Read the scenario and answer the following questions on a separate sheet of paper.

During her gynecology intake interview with the nurse practitioner at her company's new health care clinic, C.W., age 55 years, states, "I seem to be having more discomfort when I have intercourse. I don't lubricate when I want and need to; if my husband hurries me, it is downright painful. This is probably my problem, but my husband thinks that after a 35-year marriage, I just don't really want to have sex anymore."

The nurse compiles a few more facts about C.W. for review and consideration. In addition to her dyspareunia, C.W. has urinary frequency and urgency, vaginal pruritus, thinning vaginal epithelium with a glazed-looking appearance, and minimal elasticity upon speculum examination.

C.W. is Caucasian, is very thin, and reports no periods for nearly 2 years. She has no history of vaginal infections, and her hygiene is excellent.

1. Given this history, what does the nurse suspect is occurring, and what other history would be important to obtain regarding symptoms?

2. What treatment options can be offered to this patient?

3. What other health concerns should be discussed?

53 Men's Reproductive Health

STUDY QUESTIONS

Match the terms in Column I with the definitions in Column II.

Column I

_____ 1. Anabolic steroids

_____ 2. Androgen

_____ 3. Hirsutism

_____ 4. Spermatogenesis

_____ 5. Virilization

_____ 6. Antiandrogens

_____ 7. Cryptorchidism

_____ 8. Gynecomastia

_____ 9. Oligospermia

_____ 10. Priapism

Column II

a. Low sperm count
b. Undescended testis
c. Breast swelling or soreness
d. Ongoing painful erection
e. Growth of facial hair and vocal huskiness in women
f. Formation of spermatozoa
g. Steroid hormones related to the hormone testosterone
h. Testosterone
i. Blocks the synthesis or action of androgens
j. Increased hair growth

NCLEX REVIEW QUESTIONS

Select the best response.

11. Of the following patients, which one should not receive sildenafil ?

   a. 56-year-old with hepatitis
   b. 58-year-old with seizure disorder
   c. 62-year-old with renal insufficiency
   d. 68-year-old with unstable angina

12. The 17-year-old patient is receiving androgen therapy for hypogonadism. He asks the nurse what androgen therapy does. What is the nurse's best response?
   a. "It ensures the ability to respond sexually."
   b. "It ensures adequate sperm production."
   c. "It promotes larger stature through protein deposition."
   d. "It stimulates the development of secondary sex characteristics."

13. A 16-year-old wrestler at a local high school tells the nurse during his annual sports physical that some of the athletes at his school use hormones to "bulk up" during the season. He wants to know if this is something he could do and if it is safe. What is the nurse's best response?
   a. "A safer way to bulk up is to eat an all-protein diet."
   b. "As long as they don't use other street drugs, this is probably safe."
   c. "This can cause serious, often irreversible, health problems even years later."
   d. "This is a safe practice as long as a health care provider adjusts the dose."

14. The patient is receiving androgen therapy. He has a history of cardiovascular disease, diabetes, and chronic obstructive pulmonary disease. What should the nurse be aware of with regard to the patient's drug and medical history?
   a. Androgens may decrease blood glucose levels, and insulin doses must be adjusted.
   b. Androgens decrease the effect of anticoagulants.
   c. Phenytoin potentiates the action of androgens.
   d. There are no interactions with steroids.

15. What is/are the indication(s) for androgen therapy in women? *(Select all that apply.)*
   a. Advanced carcinoma of the breast
   b. Delayed development of sexual characteristics
   c. Endometriosis
   d. Infertility
   e. Severe premenstrual syndrome

16. A teenage male patient is receiving androgen therapy for hypogonadism. What side effect(s) might this patient experience? *(Select all that apply.)*
   a. Gynecomastia
   b. Continuous erection
   c. A rise in voice pitch
   d. Urinary urgency
   e. Visual disturbances

17. What is/are the indication(s) for antiandrogen drugs? *(Select all that apply.)*
   a. Advanced prostatic cancer
   b. Erectile dysfunction
   c. Male pattern baldness
   d. Menopausal symptoms
   e. Benign prostatic hypertrophy (BPH)

CASE STUDY

Read the scenario and answer the following questions on a separate sheet of paper.

H.H., 60 years old, has a history of diabetes and hypertension and presents to his health care provider. He states, "I'm really kind of embarrassed about this, but I can't satisfy my partner anymore. Could I get some of that drug so I can keep an erection?"

1. What is erectile dysfunction, and how does it relate to the patient's history?

2. What class of drugs is the patient referring to, and how does it work?

3. What are common side effects associated with this class of drugs?

4. What health teaching should the nurse provide for the patient regarding erectile dysfunction?

54 Sexually Transmitted Infections

STUDY QUESTIONS

Match the infection in Column I to its description in Column II.

Column I

_____ 1. Gonorrhea

_____ 2. Primary syphilis

_____ 3. Secondary syphilis

_____ 4. Tertiary syphilis

_____ 5. Bacterial vaginosis

_____ 6. Chlamydia

Column II

a. Thin, white vaginal discharge with a strong fishy odor

b. Characterized by a skin rash that appears 2 to 8 weeks after the chancre

c. Second most common STI that is characterized by a greenish yellow or whitish discharge and dysuria in men

d. Most common STI in young adults and is often asymptomatic

e. A chancre at the site of original infection caused by *Treponema pallidum*

f. Occurs as early as 1 year after the initial infection, causing large sores inside the body along with systemic syphilis to the cardiovascular and neurologic systems

Match the STI in Column I with its appropriate drug in Column II.

Column I

_____ 7. Herpes simplex virus

_____ 8. Bacterial vaginosis

_____ 9. Chlamydia

_____ 10. Gonorrhea

_____ 11. Syphilis

_____ 12. Trichomoniasis

Column II

a. Benzathine penicillin G
b. Acyclovir
c. Ceftriaxone and azithromycin
d. Metronidazole
e. Nitroimidazole
f. Azithromycin

NCLEX REVIEW QUESTIONS

Select the best response.

13. The patient presents to the clinic complaining of dysuria and yellow-green discharge. Culture confirms *Neisseria gonorrhoeae*. Since this patient has presented with an STI, what other test should the patient be counseled to consider?
    a. Fasting blood sugar
    b. Fertility workup
    c. Human immunodeficiency virus (HIV) testing
    d. Liver panel

14. All recent sexual partners need to be informed of a patient's diagnosis of gonorrhea, and until reculturing demonstrates a cure, what will the nurse advise the patient to do to prevent further STI transmission?
    a. Abstain or use condoms during sex.
    b. Ask partners to take antibiotics.
    c. Douche before intercourse.
    d. Only engage in anal intercourse.

15. The patient, who has a history of repeated gonorrhea, chlamydia, and HPV, asks how long she has to abstain from sex. What is the nurse's best response?
    a. "For at least two months."
    b. "Until the drugs are finished."
    c. "Until your partner finishes his treatment."
    d. "You may have sex using condoms."

16. The patient asks if gonorrhea and syphilis are the same thing. What is the nurse's best response?
    a. "No, but if you have one, you should consider being tested for the other."
    b. "No, gonorrhea has no serious side effects."
    c. "No, only women get gonorrhea."
    d. "No, syphilis cannot be cured."

17. The patient would like to know how HIV is spread. What method(s) of transmission should be discussed with the patient? *(Select all that apply.)*
   a. Breast milk
   b. Contact with infected blood
   c. Vaginal secretions
   d. Sexual contact
   e. Mosquitoes

CASE STUDY

Read the scenario and answer the following questions on a separate sheet of paper.

K.E., 21 years old, presents to her health care provider complaining of abnormal vaginal discharge and pelvic pain that worsens during intercourse. She also complains of pharyngitis. On examination, the pharynx is erythematous with whitish patches. The pelvic examination revealed odiferous, whitish discharge with adnexal tenderness. She reports being sexually active, including oral sex, with multiple partners.

1. What is the presumptive diagnosis, and what are some of its clinical manifestations?

2. How should K.E. be treated pharmacologically? What are the dosages?

3. What information should be provided to K.E.?

55 Adult and Pediatric Emergency Drugs

STUDY QUESTIONS

Match the condition in Column I with the drug that treats it in Column II.

Column I

_____ 1. Anaphylactic shock

_____ 2. Angina pectoris

_____ 3. Opioid overdose

_____ 4. Extravasation of dopamine

_____ 5. Hypoxemia

_____ 6. Torsades de pointes

_____ 7. Frequent premature ventricular contractions (PVCs)

_____ 8. Atrial fibrillation

_____ 9. Increased intracranial pressure

_____ 10. Hemodynamically significant bradycardia

_____ 11. Paroxysmal supraventricular tachycardia (PSVT)

Column II

a. Magnesium sulfate
b. Diltiazem
c. Atropine sulfate
d. Mannitol
e. Phentolamine
f. Lidocaine
g. Nitroglycerin
h. Epinephrine
i. Oxygen
j. Adenosine
k. Naloxone

Match the drug in Column I with its classification in Column II. Answers may be used more than once.

Column I

_____ 12. Nitroprusside

_____ 13. Epinephrine

_____ 14. Lidocaine

_____ 15. Norepinephrine

_____ 16. Mannitol

_____ 17. Diltiazem

_____ 18. Albuterol

_____ 19. Furosemide

Column II

a. Antidysrhythmic, class IB
b. Osmotic diuretic
c. Calcium channel blocker
d. Catecholamine
e. Beta-adrenergic agonist
f. Vasodilator
g. Loop diuretic

Select the best response.

20. Sublingual nitroglycerin may be prescribed for chest pain. What is the most important vital sign to assess before giving this drug?
    a. Blood pressure
    b. Heart rate
    c. Respiratory rate
    d. Temperature

21. Following administration of IV morphine to treat chest pain associated with acute myocardial infarction, what is the most important aspect of patient monitoring?
    a. Assessment of respiratory status
    b. Documentation of neurologic function
    c. Measurement and strict recording of intake and output
    d. Measurement of central venous pressure

22. Which is the first-line emergency drug for the treatment of hemodynamically unstable bradycardia?
    a. Atropine
    b. Epinephrine
    c. Lidocaine
    d. Nitroglycerin

23. When monitoring a patient with a dobutamine infusion, the nurse must be alert to the development of adverse effects. Which one may require slowing or discontinuing drug administration?
    a. Bradycardia
    b. Confusion
    c. Diaphoresis
    d. Myocardial ischemia

24. Procainamide 1.4 mg/minute is infusing in a patient with supraventricular tachycardia. The nurse is closely monitoring the patient to determine if the procainamide should be discontinued. Which of the following is an end point of IV procainamide administration?
    a. Headache
    b. Hypotension
    c. Respiratory depression
    d. Vomiting

25. A 45-year-old post myocardial infarction complains of "heart racing" and is dyspneic. The cardiac monitor shows the patient to be in a tachyarrhythmia. Which dysrhythmia(s) is/are amiodarone IV used to treat? *(Select all that apply.)*
    a. Asystole
    b. Atrial fibrillation
    c. Bradycardia
    d. Second-degree heart block
    e. Ventricular fibrillation

26. What is the best indication for sodium bicarbonate?
    a. Metabolic acidosis
    b. Metabolic alkalosis
    c. Respiratory acidosis
    d. Respiratory alkalosis

27. The patient is admitted to the critical care unit after sustaining a severe closed head injury in a motorcycle collision. Mannitol is ordered to decrease intracranial pressure. Through which mechanism does mannitol exert its pharmacologic effects?
    a. Cerebral vasoconstriction
    b. Loop diuresis
    c. Osmotic diuresis
    d. Peripheral vasodilation

28. The patient presents to the emergency department after eating soup at a wedding reception. She is allergic to shellfish, and it is discovered that the soup was lobster bisque. She has hives and is anxious. Her tongue and lips are swollen. Which drug would be appropriate to administer to this patient in this situation?
    a. Atropine
    b. Diltiazem
    c. Diphenhydramine
    d. Lidocaine

29. An unresponsive patient presents to the emergency department in respiratory distress. Her friends say that she has been "using a lot of those pain pills for her back." Her pupils are pinpoint and her respiratory rate is 4 breaths/min. Which drug will the nurse be prepared to administer?
    a. Diltiazem 0.25 mg/kg IV piggyback
    b. Flumazenil 2.5 mg IV push
    c. Naloxone 0.4 mg IV push
    d. Magnesium 2 g IV piggyback

30. For which type(s) of shock should dopamine be administered? *(Select all that apply.)*
    a. Cardiogenic shock
    b. Hypovolemic shock
    c. Insulin shock
    d. Neurogenic shock
    e. Septic shock

31. Through which mechanism does dobutamine elevate blood pressure?
    a. Increasing cardiac output
    b. Positive alpha effects
    c. Vasoconstriction
    d. Vasodilation

32. The patient has a diagnosis of septic shock. A norepinephrine drip is infusing through a central IV line. The bag of norepinephrine is almost empty. The nurse prepares to hang another bag knowing that:
   a. hypertensive crisis can result if the infusion is interrupted.
   b. profound hypotension can occur if the infusion is abruptly discontinued.
   c. the patient is at high risk for bradycardia and heart block.
   d. the organisms responsible for septic shock will proliferate.

33. A 31-year-old unconscious male was brought to the emergency department with a blood glucose level of 15 mg/dL. The nurse will prepare to administer dextrose 50% (D50). Which of the following condition is D50 most commonly prescribed?
   a. As a maintenance infusion to keep a vein open
   b. To increase urine output
   c. To treat hyperglycemia
   d. To treat insulin-induced hypoglycemia

34. A patient was brought into the emergency department with supraventricular tachycardia. The nurse is preparing to administer adenosine. What is the proper method of administering adenosine?
   a. Slow IV push over 2 minutes
   b. Diluted in 50 mL as IVPB over 30 minutes
   c. Rapid IV push as a bolus followed by saline flush
   d. Via a nebulizer

35. What is a priority nursing action after administration of a total IV lidocaine dose of 3 mg/kg to an adult and the dysrhythmia has been suppressed?
   a. A continuous infusion of lidocaine must be initiated to maintain a therapeutic serum level.
   b. A therapeutic serum level will be achieved and maintained.
   c. Additional bolus doses must be administered to achieve a therapeutic serum level.
   d. 3 mg/kg is too much, and the patient has been overdosed.

36. The nurse is preparing to administer epinephrine IM to a patient with an allergic reaction. Which concentration should the nurse select?
   a. 1:10,000 concentration of epinephrine
   b. 1:1000 concentration of epinephrine
   c. 1:100 concentration of epinephrine
   d. 1:1 concentration of epinephrine

37. The patient is in cardiac arrest. To administer epinephrine IV, which concentration should the nurse select?
   a. 1:10,000 concentration of epinephrine
   b. 1:1000 concentration of epinephrine
   c. 1:100 concentration of epinephrine
   d. 1:1 concentration of epinephrine

38. The lowest adult dose of atropine for heart block or symptomatic bradycardia is 0.5 mg IV. What happens at lower dosages?
   a. Paradoxical bradycardia can occur.
   b. Miosis occurs.
   c. The patient is at high risk for tachycardia.
   d. Vagal activity is completely increased.

39. Flumazenil is used to reverse the effects of which drug type?
   a. Antipsychotics
   b. Benzodiazepines
   c. Opioids
   d. Paralytic agents

40. Magnesium sulfate is indicated for treatment of which alteration(s)? *(Select all that apply.)*
   a. Atrial dysrhythmias
   b. Hypokalemia
   c. Cardiac arrest with hypomagnesemia
   d. Refractory ventricular fibrillation
   e. Torsades de pointes

41. A 35-year-old female with heart failure has now developed pulmonary edema. Furosemide 60 mg IVP was ordered. Furosemide exerts its effects on pulmonary edema through which mechanisms?
   a. Bronchodilation and diuresis
   b. Bronchodilation and antiinflammatory actions
   c. Vasoconstriction and diuresis
   d. Vasodilation and diuresis

42. Which priority nursing intervention(s) should be implemented when caring for a patient with a nitroprusside infusion? *(Select all that apply.)*
   a. Always use nitroprusside with a blue or brown color to the solution.
   b. Monitor blood pressure continuously.
   c. Stop the nitroprusside abruptly if side effects are experienced.
   d. Protect the solution from light.
   e. Monitor thiocyanate levels.

43. Which side and/or adverse effect(s) is/are associated with atropine IV? *(Select all that apply.)*
   a. Dry mouth
   b. Miosis
   c. Mydriasis
   d. Urinary retention
   e. Vomiting

233

CASE STUDY

Read the scenario and answer the following questions on a separate sheet of paper.

M.E., 48 years old, calls emergency medical services (EMS) with complaints of chest pain and shortness of breath. He has a history of angina, asthma, and obesity. He states, "It just hit me hard. I think I'm going to die." He has taken three of his own nitroglycerin tablets, and he is given oxygen, an aspirin, and morphine en route to the hospital. On arrival at the hospital, an electrocardiogram is obtained. M.E. is not having a myocardial infarction but is diagnosed with unstable angina and is admitted to the coronary care unit. Vital signs on admission are temperature 97.3° F, heart rate 88 beats/min, respiratory rate 20 breaths/min, and blood pressure 214/118 mm Hg. A nitroglycerin drip is started.

1. How does nitroglycerin work to treat a patient with angina?

2. Why was the patient administered aspirin, oxygen, and morphine en route to the hospital? Why was the nitroglycerin drip started?

M.E. became unresponsive and developed widened QRS complex ventricular tachycardia with a ventricular rate of 190 beats/min. Code blue was called, and a crash cart was brought into the room. M.E. was shocked with 360 joules three times, without any change to the rhythm. A nurse prepares to administer emergency drugs.

3. What drug would a nurse prepare to first administer for pulseless ventricular tachycardia after unsuccessful defibrillation?

Answer Key

CHAPTER 1: DRUG DEVELOPMENT AND ETHICAL CONSIDERATIONS

1. b
2. e
3. d
4. a
5. c
6. trade
7. I
8. health information
9. FDA; health; innovative; safe; effective
10. nurse practice act
11. false
12. true
13. true
14. false
15. true
16. a
17. d
18. d
19. c
20. b
21. d
22. d
23. d
24. d
25. c
26. a, c, d, e. Differences in appearance, either in the drug or in the packaging, can be an indication of a counterfeit drug. However, it is important to remember that pharmacies may change their pharmaceutical supplier, so the drug may appear as a different color or shape to the patient. This is an opportunity for the nurse and the pharmacist to work together to provide patient education.

Case Study

1. The nurse will tell L.L. that his personal information will be shared with the pharmacist as it pertains to his care. The pharmacist will be able to discuss the drug and treatment with the patient in a separate counseling area, away from other patients.
2. HIPAA sets the standard for privacy of Individuals of their Identifiable health Information. The act allows patients more control on who has access to their health records.

CHAPTER 2: PHARMACOKINETICS, PHARMACODYNAMICS, AND PHARMACOGENETICS

1. absorption, distribution, metabolism, and excretion
2. half-life
3. Pharmacodynamics
4. bloodstream; administration
5. antagonists
6. receptors
7. f
8. e
9. c
10. a
11. b
12. d
13. g
14. a
15. d
16. c
17. b
18. c
19. c
20. b
21. d
22. b
23. b, c, e. The gastrointestinal tract is not considered vital to a patient in shock and hypotensive, so blood is shunted away and drug absorption is slowed. Blood flow is also slowed because of pain and stress, resulting in a prolonged emptying time of the stomach.
24. c. Both drugs are highly protein-bound. When two or more highly protein-bound drugs are taken at the same time, they compete for the protein-binding sites. The more highly bound drug could displace the weakly bound drug; ampicillin/sulbactam could displace diazepam, which results in increase activity of diazepam.
25. b
26. b
27. b
28. a. A drug that has a half-life of 24 to 30 hours will be taken once daily to maintain a steady state.
29. d
30. b. A decreased eGFR indicates renal dysfunction. Decreased eGFR is expected in older adults because of their decreased muscle mass. Many drugs,

235

including trimethoprim, are eliminated through the kidneys. To prevent toxicity, the dose would need to be decreased.

31. a
32. b
33. c
34. b
35. a. Measurements that check a drug's concentration include peak and trough levels; peak level measures the highest serum concentration and the trough level measures the lowest serum concentration of the drug.
36. a, b, d, e. The nurse must be completely familiar with any drug that he or she is administered. Information needs to be obtained not only on the drug but also on the specific patient's history. Drug reference books, drug pamphlets/inserts, or a pharmacist may be consulted with questions.
37. b
38. c
39. a, b, c. A time-response curve shows the dose-relationship of the drug's pharmacodynamics, which include onset, peak, and the duration of the drug's action.
40. a, b, d, e. The nurse should assess the patient for side effects (both desirable and undesirable) when administering drugs. This is especially important for drugs that have nonselective actions. The nurse must be familiar with the drug, including its dose range, desired effects, side effects, and adverse effects, before administration. This information can be obtained from a variety of sources including current reference books, drug inserts, and pharmacists. If the drug has a narrow therapeutic range or requires peak/trough levels, these should be evaluated before administration. Side effects may occur immediately or up to several days after a dose. There is no set time to wait and see if side effects disappear. The health care provider should be notified as soon as possible after the appearance of side effects, especially if they are undesirable.

Case Study

1. The receptor theory states that drugs bind to receptor sites to activate a receptor, produce a response, or inhibit (block) a response. Some receptor sites are specific to only one drug, whereas others may accommodate several different drugs. However, some "fit better" and are more active. The drug binding sites are located on cell membranes and are primarily protein, glycoprotein, proteolipids, and enzymes in nature. The four receptor families are cell membrane–embedded enzymes, ligand-gated ion channels, G protein–coupled receptor systems, and transcription factors.

   Verapamil is a calcium channel blocker. Ligand-gated ion channels stretch across the cell membrane. If the channel is open, ions (usually calcium and sodium) can flow across the membrane. A calcium channel *blocker* prevents the flow of calcium.

In the case of verapamil, this causes a decreased force of contraction, less spasm, and ultimately less anginal chest pain.

2. As with any new drug, the patient should be taught about how to take the drug (with or without food, timing during the day), what effects to expect and how soon to expect to see results, what undesirable side effects or adverse effects to expect, and what to report to the health care provider. It is important to stress that the drug must be taken "as prescribed" even if the patient is feeling better or not feeling any changes because some drugs work immediately and some medications may take several weeks to build up to a therapeutic level.

CHAPTER 3: CULTURAL CONSIDERATIONS

1. c
2. e
3. f
4. d
5. b
6. g
7. a
8. communication
9. deities; spirits
10. DNA variants; population
11. a
12. c
13. b
14. c. It is important for the nurse to recognize that people of African descent, which many Jamaicans are, use home remedies that have been passed down through generations. Clay is high in minerals such as calcium, iron, copper, and magnesium. Eating clay (geographia) or dirt is also considered a home remedy for nausea and vomiting associated with pregnancy.
15. d. Because the patient has consulted with a traditional healer, the patient may be more compliant with the drug regimen if he can continue to follow the guidance of the healer. Studies have not shown that sabila (aloe vera) will help control glucose levels.
16. a, b, d. Culturally competent care integrates pharmacogenetics with the social and cultural attributes of the patient, which includes their age, diet, and genetics.
17. a, c, d, e. When considering factors affecting adherence to a drug regimen, understanding the cultural phenomena of communication, social organization, time, environmental control, and biologic variations are important.

Case Study

1. The first concern for the nurse is the dose of erythromycin. A standard dose of erythromycin for this patient would be 570–950 mg per day every 6 hours. However, the instruction was to

give 1 teaspoon (tsp) every 6 hours. One teaspoon is equal to 5 mL. One tablespoon holds 3 tsp. An average porcelain soup spoon holds more than 3 tsp. The amount as originally instructed would be a potential overdose and puts the patient at risk for harm. The health care provider should be notified immediately.

2. The family and patient should be approached in a quiet and calm manner, using a quiet voice, and allowing periods of silence. Should a translator be required, a professional translator or language line should be utilized to obtain further history. Many non-native English speakers of Asian descent will simply nod when asked questions to avoid showing disrespect. The parents may not have understood the exact amount (teaspoon) of the drug required, and the spoon used in the home may have been what they used as a "teaspoon." To prevent any further misunderstandings regarding dosing, a syringe or measured spoon should be given at discharge.

CHAPTER 4: COMPLEMENTARY AND ALTERNATIVE THERAPIES

1. e
2. b
3. a
4. d
5. c
6. plants; infusion
7. tincture
8. Extract; liniment
9. decoction
10. volatile; herb-infused oils
11. d, h
12. g
13. h
14. j
15. a, h
16. f
17. b
18. c
19. e, h
20. i
21. a
22. c
23. a, b, c, d. Bilberry, garlic, ginseng, and licorice can interfere with anticoagulants, such as warfarin.
24. a, d, e. The nurse should intervene by discussing with the patient that ginseng can interfere with the anticoagulants and increase the chance of bleeding; therefore, the patient should report any signs or symptoms of bleeding, such as bleeding of gums, black and tarry stools, and blood in the urine. Although educating the patient about the potential food-drug interactions while taking an anticoagulant, it is not appropriate in this specific scenario.

25. b, d. Large quantities of any one herbal product can lead to an "overdosage" of that product. Because specific doses and quantities are not regulated in this country, it is difficult to determine the correct amount. More is not necessarily better. Infants and children should not receive herbal preparations because of the lack of standardization and testing in a pediatric population.
26. c, d
27. a, b, c, d. St. John's wort interacts with multiple drugs including anticoagulants and antiplatelets, anticonvulsants, antidepressants, and drugs for birth control. St. John's wort can increase bleeding time; it can cause decreased drug levels of anticonvulsants and oral contraceptives; it can increase serotonin levels, leading to serotonin syndrome.
28. a, b, d. The effects of antihypertensive medications may be decreased. Because licorice may have similar effects to aldosterone and corticosteroids, the effects of corticosteroid drugs may be increased. Taking licorice with digitalis may increase the effects of digitalis and lead to digitalis toxicity.

Case Study

1. The most commonly utilized herbal preparation for migraine headaches is feverfew. It is believed that this preparation may inhibit platelet aggregation and act as a serotonin antagonist, which may help in vascular and migraine headaches. Feverfew may also help with nausea and vomiting. Ginger is another herbal preparation that may help in the treatment of migraine headaches and the associated nausea. Although researched, the mechanism of action is unclear. St. John's wort may be taken for mild depression and anxiety, but it is not effective in treating headaches. St. John's wort has not been shown to be effective in moderate or severe depression; in fact, when combined with an SSRI, there is a higher risk for suicide. The mechanism of action is unknown.

2. Ginger interacts with antiplatelet and anticoagulant drugs. Feverfew also interacts with antiplatelet and anticoagulant drugs. St. John's wort has interactions with many drugs, including central nervous system (CNS) depressants, selective serotonin reuptake inhibitors (SSRIs), and oral contraceptives.

3. As with any herb or drug, the patient should be encouraged to keep a list of her drugs and dosages. Although many people believe herbs are automatically "safe" since they are natural, this is not always the case. Herbal preparations do not pass through an FDA approval process as drugs do, so strength, amount of filler, and impurities may vary. Herbal preparations may also vary from one company to another, so the patient should be encouraged to continue to obtain the preparation from the same reliable source or company.

CHAPTER 5: PEDIATRIC CONSIDERATIONS

1. fewer; increased
2. age; health status; weight; route of administration
3. 2; 3
4. body fluid composition; tissue composition; protein-binding capability
5. 2 years; higher
6. e
7. d
8. a
9. b
10. c
11. a, b. Absorption depends on the drug formulation (basic [alkalotic] or acidic). A low pH environment favors acidic drug absorption, whereas a high pH favors basic drug formulations.
12. c. The dosage for a water-soluble medication may need to be increased in this age group because their bodies are about 70% water up until age 2 years. Therefore, there is more water in which the drug will be distributed.
13. d
14. a
15. a, b, c, d. Pharmacokinetics include drug absorption, distribution, metabolism, and excretion.
16. a, b, c, e. In early adolescence, renal tubular function decreases, which may lead to impaired excretion and a higher risk for toxicity. Dehydration can also decrease renal function and may lead to toxicity. Because the patient is nauseated and vomiting, drugs should not be administered orally. When providing care to any patient, developmental levels should be considered.
17. b, c, d, f. If necessary, a child may be lightly restrained but should not be forcibly held down. The child should be praised for taking the drug. At no time should a child be threatened, forced, or made to view the medication as punishment. Depending on the developmental level of the child, explanations should be given to the child about what to expect, but the child should not be given the option of debating whether to take the drug. Herbal preparations are not usually given to children; however, cultural traditions should be respected as much as possible.

Case Study

1. Preschoolers may respond age-appropriate explanations. They may also benefit from a familiar toy or stuffed animal as support. Allow the child to verbalize being scared or upset. Whenever possible, allow the child options and control. Do not argue with the child or tell the child that she is being punished for falling from the tree. Tell the child what you are going to do before you do it. Do not just surprise the child.
2. A topical anesthetic like a eutectic mixture of local anesthetics (EMLA) or topical lidocaine may be utilized to lessen the pain of establishing an IV. The downside to using these topical anesthetics is that they must be in place 60 to 90 minutes before the IV can be started for them to be effective.
3. Answers can vary. Caregivers may be involved in patient care (if they choose to be) by helping to gently restrain the child. They can also provide distraction ("What color sling would you like?" or "What should we have to eat tomorrow morning when we get up?"). Reassuring the preschooler that she is doing a good job holding still can also be beneficial.

CHAPTER 6: GERIATRIC CONSIDERATIONS

1. absorption, distribution, metabolism
2. low; gradually; response
3. sensory; physical; aging
4. receptor; affinity
5. sotolol, all NSAIDs, meperidine, glyburide, metformin, exenatide, nitrofurantoin, potassium-sparing diuretics, thiazide diuretics, olmesartan, and new anticoagulants
6. c
7. b
8. d
9. a
10. ACE-I
11. Beta blockers
12. Psychotropics
13. ARBs
14. F
15. T
16. T
17. F
18. F
19. T
20. T
21. a.
22. b. Renal function is decreased in older adults, which can cause electrolyte imbalance. Also, decreased renal function can lead to prolonged half-life and elevated drug levels. Certain antihypertensives like ACE-I, potassium-sparing diuretics, and thiazide diuretics can worsen electrolyte imbalance.
23. a. There is no reason that the patient cannot work outside if he is taking digoxin, and the patient's symptoms are not related to the digoxin. Diphenhydramine can be very sedating in the geriatric population, and there are substitutes that are equally effective with fewer side effects. Fluoxetine, an SSRI, is prescribed for depression. Patients of all ages should be advised not to take each other's medications.
24. c. Drugs with a shorter half-life and less protein binding would have fewer side effects. There are fewer protein binding sites in older adults, resulting in more circulating drug. Because of less effective functioning of both hepatic and renal metabolism, drugs with a shorter half-life are safer.

25. a, b
26. d. Dizziness when going from a supine to a standing position is referred to as *orthostatic hypotension.* Although bradycardia may cause dizziness, this is not the most likely cause.
27. a. Changing positions slowly should assist in decreasing the dizziness associated with hypotension related to changes in position. Taking a deep breath and checking his heart rate will not affect his dizziness. Having a chair close to the bed may be beneficial if the patient feels dizzy but may also pose a safety risk. If the patient faints, he may strike the chair as he falls.
28. c. When a person has been hospitalized, a medicine reconciliation has been completed. Depending on the patient's response, drugs may be added to or subtracted from the regimen and dose adjustments may be made. The patient should take only those drugs that have been prescribed at discharge.
29. a. Although a family member could assist with the daily medication regimen, the patient will be able to maintain more independence using a non-childproof cap. Using a non-childproof cap should make the container easier for the patient to grasp and open.
30. b. Maintaining independence for as long as possible is crucial for a geriatric patient. A patient who has visual challenges can, with assistance, fill a medication-dispensing container for the upcoming week. The patient must have assistance in the setup to assure that the correct drugs are in each separate compartment. Leaving the drug bottles on the counter could lead to a mix-up if they are displaced. Writing down which drugs need to be taken is not beneficial if the patient has visual challenges. The patient does not forget what drugs need to be taken but is unable to clearly see which drug is to be taken at which time.
31. a, c, d, e. Of the listed factors, only height does not have a role in dosage adjustment. Older adults have more adipose tissue, so a greater amount of lipid-soluble drug would be absorbed. Protein is required for binding of some drugs, so if a patient is malnourished, there would be less protein available. Laboratory results, specifically those that assess renal and hepatic function, are important to trend, as well as those drug levels (digoxin, INR) needed to measure toxicity. As with any population, it is important to evaluate the patient for responsiveness to the drug.
32. a, b, d, e. Older patients have less protein available for binding, so it is important to know if a drug is highly protein bound. Drugs with a short half-life are less likely to cause problems for the patient. Certain drugs (some antibiotics, digoxin, warfarin) have very narrow therapeutic ranges, so they must be monitored closely. Vital signs may vary as a patient ages; therefore, it is important to obtain baseline vital signs to know the patient's norm.

Case Study

1. Because both renal function and hepatic function are important in drug metabolism and excretion, and both decrease with aging, the nurse would anticipate that measurement of liver enzymes, BUN, creatinine, and creatinine clearance would be ordered. Because this patient also has diabetes, the patient's blood glucose level will be evaluated.
2. There are a variety of sleep aids besides triazolam that could be utilized. Because this patient is also taking a diuretic, it would be important to suggest the patient take her diuretic in the morning to prevent frequent awakenings during the night to go to the bathroom. Some nonpharmacologic measures include taking warm baths, decreasing stimulation in the evening, and eliminating caffeine intake late in the day. The patient also states that she likes chamomile tea, which may help induce sleep. A light bedtime snack will help maintain blood sugar levels throughout the night.
3. The nurse should recognize and support the patient's desire to be compliant with her drug regimen; however, the patient does need further education about "doubling up" on medications. A variety of methods can be used to help the patient remember to take her drug. These can include using commercial pill dispensers, making a list, keeping a calendar, or setting an alarm.

CHAPTER 7: DRUGS FOR SUBSTANCE USE DISORDER

1. b
2. c
3. a
4. dopamine, neurotransmitters
5. reward circuit
6. epigenetics
7. inhibits
8. methadone or buprenorphine, or naltrexone
9. GHB (gamma-hydroxybutyrate)
10. euphoria, tranquility, blocks
11. CAGE
12. personality, behavior, job performance, job attendance
13. F. Electronic cigarettes are NOT safer than tobacco products.
14. F. DHEA is found in many dietary supplements, and there is NO evidence that DHEA slows aging, increases energy levels, or increases muscle strength.
15. T
16. b
17. a
18. d
19. c

20. a. Cocaine can cause dilated pupils (not pinpoint pupils) and restlessness. It can also cause hypertension (not hypotension), tachycardia, insomnia, erratic behaviors (not fine tremors), and tachypnea (not respiratory depression).

21. c. Methadone is a long-acting opioid that is effective in treating persons addicted to opioids by blocking the sensation of euphoria and tranquility produced by opioids, and it prevents opioid withdrawal and craving. Dronabinol is a synthetic cannabis, lorazepam is a benzodiazepine to decrease anxiety, and naloxone is a reversal agent for opioid-induced respiratory depression.

22. a, c, e. A patient must be ready and motivated to quit any addictive substance, or the likelihood of success is decreased. This is a difficult process that will require the patient's commitment. Certain triggers, like places where a person smokes or times that trigger the craving for a cigarette, should be identified and alternatives determined. There are a variety of aids, both pharmacologic and nonpharmacologic, that can be utilized to help a patient quit smoking. Ideally, a quit date of 1 to 2 weeks should be set so the patient stays motivated. Tobacco in any form is still addictive, so chewing tobacco or smoking tobacco in a pipe instead of a cigarette is still abusing tobacco. Although it is difficult, some patients prefer to quit smoking "cold turkey" or without the use of aids.

23. d. It is estimated that 10–15% of nurses have a substance use disorder, including cannabis, cocaine, narcotics, opiates, alcohol, and nicotine.

24. d. Bath salts are synthetic cathinones that have amphetamine-like stimulant effects.

Case Study

1. Even though the patient appears to be intoxicated, other causes of his unresponsiveness need to be evaluated. There is no antidote for alcohol intoxication other than supportive care. The patient's respiratory rate is insufficient and his respirations must be assisted. Treatment should be aimed toward airway management and supplemental oxygenation, supportive care, and IV hydration.

2. A person with alcohol toxicity can aspirate on vomitus and asphyxiate and develop severe dehydration, seizures, hypothermia, and eventually brain damage and death.

3. Disulfiram inhibits aldehyde dehydrogenase, the enzyme needed to metabolize alcohol. Disulfiram keeps patients from ingesting alcohol because of its side effects. It is slowly metabolized by the liver. The side effects can occur up to 2 weeks after cessation of drug therapy. Side effects can occur within 10 minutes of ingesting alcohol (including mouthwash, cough medicine, or foods containing or cooked in alcohol). Side effects include nausea,

headache, vomiting, chest pains, dyspnea (difficulty breathing), rash, drowsiness, impotence, acne, and a metallic aftertaste.

4. Metronidazole, an antimicrobial, and paraldehyde, a sedative, when taken concomitantly with disulfiram can produce the same side effects as if the person had been ingesting alcohol.

CHAPTER 8: THE NURSING PROCESS AND PATIENT-CENTERED CARE

1. safe, comprehensive
2. Evidence-based
3. Informatics
4. family-centered
5. quality
6. d, e, b, a, c
7. b
8. a
9. c
10. a
11. d
12. a
13. d or e
14. d
15. d
16. a
17. e
18. b
19. a
20. b
21. a
22. b
23. a
24. a
25. d
26. a
27. c
28. c
29. b
30. b
31. d
32. b
33. c
34. c

Case Study

1. The nurse will consider the nursing process: assessment, nursing diagnosis, planning, implementation, and evaluation.

   The assessment phase of the nursing process for this patient would include not only obtaining subjective and objective data, such as patient history and physical examination, but also reviewing current drugs and allergies. Physical examination should include physical reasons why the patient may not be able to administer the injection. Other items to assess include the home environment and, most importantly, the patient's readiness to learn and education level.

The next phase in the nursing process is the development of nursing diagnoses. These are based on actual concerns discovered in the assessment phase or potential problems attributable to risk factors that arise in the assessment. The patient's statements suggest several potential diagnoses, including those related to anxiety, knowledge deficit, and noncompliance.

In the planning phase, patient-centered, measurable goals are established in collaboration with the patient, family, and other members of the health care team. The goals must be realistic and measurable and occur in a certain time frame. A realistic goal for this patient could be *The patient will prepare the prescribed dose of insulin by the second day of instruction.*

During the implementation phase, the nurse provides the education necessary for the patient to be able to achieve the goal. In this situation, the teaching needs to address several areas, including the psychomotor skill of preparing and administering an insulin injection.

2. The nurse can determine the effectiveness of the teaching plan by a demo-return demo scenario could be utilized. Adequate time for questions must be provided, as well as contact information for the health care provider. The nurse must ensure that the patient is ready to learn, the material is presented in an appropriate manner for learning to occur, and the materials are culturally appropriate.

Continue to assess the attainment of the objectives and goals and revise the plan to ensure success. Evaluation is the final step in the nursing process. The goal must be evaluated and changes made if necessary. Was the patient able to correctly demonstrate insulin preparation? Did the patient have problems with anxiety surrounding the preparation? Was the patient able to verbalize concerns to the health care provider?

CHAPTER 9: SAFETY AND QUALITY

1. c
2. f
3. j
4. g
5. a
6. h
7. b
8. d
9. e
10. i
11. a
12. a
13. b
14. a
15. b
16. a

17. a. intradermal, yes; b. morphine sulfate or multiple sclerosis, no; c. every other day, no; d, drops, yes; e. kilograms, yes; f. 1 milligram, no; whole numbers should not contain trailing zeros; g. milligram, yes; h. every day or daily, no; i. keep vein open, yes; j. intravenous piggyback, yes; k. with, no; l. before, no; m. twice daily, yes

18.

Abbreviation	Meaning
CR	controlled release
ER	extended release
IM	immediate release
XR	extended release
XT	extended release

19. c. Antibiotics must be taken at regularly spaced intervals to maintain therapeutic blood levels.
20. b. ac is before meals and hs is at bedtime.
21. c
22. c. A nurse must never administer a dose that seems large or out of range without rechecking the calculations. If there continues to be a question, another nurse should double-check the dose as well.
23. a, b, d
24. a. The nurse's first action is to document the refusal immediately. It is important to remember that the refusal to take a medication is the patient's right. The nurse should determine the patient's reasoning behind refusing to take a medication and stress the importance of the medication regimen. The health care provider should be notified of the refusal.
25. b, c, d, e. The "Do Not Use List" of abbreviations include q.d., U, IU, and MS. q.d. should be written as "daily" or "every day"; U is to be written as "unit"; and IU as "International Unit." MS can be confused for morphine sulfate or magnesium sulfate; instead, write out the drugs.
26. b, d, e.

Case Study Answers

1. The "five rights" are 1) the right patient, 2) the right drug, 3) the right dose, 4) the right route, and 5) the right time.
2. Ask the patient to state his or her full name and birth date, and compare these with the patient's identification (ID) band and the medication administration record (MAR).

Many facilities have electronic health records (EHRs) that allow the nurse to directly scan the bar code from the patient's ID band. Once the band is scanned, the nurse can see the patient's medication record.

If the patient is an adult with a cognitive disorder or a child, verify the patient's name with a family member. In the event a family member is unavailable and the patient is unable to self-identify,

241

follow the facility's policy. Many facilities have policies that include a photo ID on the band with the patient's name and birth date affixed to the band.

Distinguish between two patients with the same first or last name by placing "name-alert" stickers as warnings on the medical records.

CHAPTER 10: DRUG ADMINISTRATION

1. Enteric-coated; timed-release
2. fine particle
3. semi-Fowler's or high Fowler's
4. 30
5. 5
6. c
7. a
8. b
9. ventrogluteal
10. vastus lateralis
11. deltoid
12. ventrogluteal
13. dorsogluteal
14.

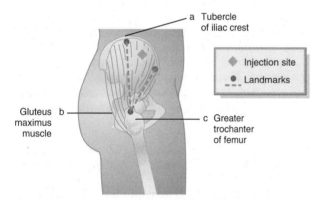

Ventrogluteal injection site

15. c
16. a
17. d
18. c is the preferred site because of easy access; however, ventrogluteal can also be used.
19. a. Over-the-counter drugs and herbal preparations may interact with prescription drugs. Patients must be encouraged to discuss the use of these preparations with their pharmacist or health care provider.
20. a, b, and e are correct. c is incorrect; not all drugs are stored in the refrigerator. d is incorrect; patients do not need to know how the drug was tested and developed.
21. b. The patient should rinse out the mouth after administering a dose from a metered-dose inhaler. This will help prevent secondary infection and irritation.

CHAPTER 11—DRUG CALCULATIONS

Section 11A: Systems of Measurement With Conversion Factors

1. b
2. f
3. g
4. c
5. i
6. j
7. o
8. e
9. n
10. m
11. d
12. l
13. a
14. k
15. h
16. A. 1000 mg; B. 1000 mL; C. 1000 mcg
17. 3000 mg
18. 1500 mL
19. 100 mg
20. 2.5 L
21. 0.25 L
22. 0.5 g
23. 4 pt
24. 32 fl oz
25. 48 fl oz
26. 2 pt
27. 3 mg
28. 5 mL
29. 1 fl oz
30. 3 tsp
31. 1000 mg
32. 0.5 g
33. 100 mg
34. 1 L; 1 qt
35. 8 fl oz
36. 1 fl oz; 2 T; 6 t
37. 1 t
38. 1½ fl oz; 9 t
39. 150 mL; 10 T

Section 11B: Calculation Methods: Enteral and Parenteral Drug Dosages

1. d
2. b, c, d, e. Parenteral routes are nonoral routes and generally bypass the hepatic system. These routes include subcutaneous, intramuscular, intradermal, and intravenous.
3. c, d. All insulins and heparinized products can be given subcutaneously. Regular insulin and fractionated heparin can be given intravenously.
4. self-sealing rubber tops; reusable if properly stored
5. a, b. Once a drug in a multi-dose vial has been reconstituted, the nurse should label the vial with the

date and time the drug was reconstituted or when to discard the vial and also with the nurse's initials.

6. c. The body's habitus must be considered when administering IM injection. 19, 20, and 21 gauges and 1, 1½, and 2 inches in length are appropriate.
7. b
8. b
9. c. Because the volume to be administered is less than 1 mL, a tuberculin (TB) syringe should be selected. A TB syringe is a 1-mL syringe. An insulin syringe is measured in units and not in mL. The 3-mL and 5-mL syringes can be used; however, they are too big and the amount drawn in these syringes may not be as accurate.
10. d
11. c. Since the drugs are compatible, use one syringe to draw up the correct amount of volume from each drug and attach the syringe to a syringe pump for infusion. Total volume of drug is 13 mL; one 20-mL syringe will suffice.

Interpreting Drug Labels

12. A. Viread;
    B. a generic name is not available;
    C. 300 mg/tab;
    D. tab
13. A. hydrocodone bitartrate and acetaminophen;
    B. 5 mg/300 mg per tab;
    C. yes;
    D.

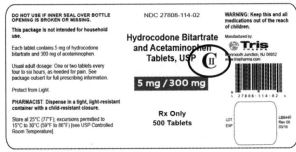

    E. Tab;
    F. controlled room temperature between 59° F and 86° F;
    G. Tris Pharma
14. A. phenytoin sodium;
    B. no;
    C. cap;
    D. 100 mg;
    E.

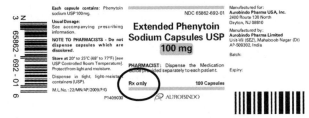

    F. in its original container at controlled room temperature and protect from light and moisture

15. A. dextromethorphan polistirex;
    B. Robitussin;
    C. no;
    D. liquid;
    E. 30 mg/5 mL;
    F. 89 mL;
    G. 10 mL q12h;
    H. approximately 9 doses
16. A. influenza A (H1N1)
    B. liquid;
    C. multi-dose;
    D. in an environment that is 35° to 46° F;
    E. IM
17. A. interferon gamma-1b;
    B. Actimmune;
    C. refrigerated

Drug Calculation

18. A. d;
    B. d; solution: ? = 1 tab/100 mg × 1000 mg/1 g × 0.5 g/x = 5 tab
19. A. a; B. b
20. A. d; B. b
21. d
22. b; concentration is 350 mg/mL after reconstitution. The amount 1 g does not need to be factored into the equation since the resulting concentration is given in mg.
23. A. b
24. A. losartan potassium;
    B. Cozaar;
    C. 30 tab;
    D. b
25. A. a; since both tab are scored, then 10 mg can be divided into ½ tab for the ordered dose;
    B. b
26. A. furosemide;
    B. Lasix;
    C. room temperature;
    D. c
27. A. Extended Release tablet; oral liquid is not extended release, and the bioavailability will be decreased;
    B. c;
    C. a; drugs in ER cannot be crushed; liquid solution can be given via NGT; b. 7.5 mL.
28. A. a; B. a
29. A. 1 tab; B. 2 tab
30. A. 5.7 mL; B. d
31. A. subcut;
    B. 40 mg/0.8 mL;
    C. 0.8 mL;
    D. a, c; tuberculin syringe is a 1-mL syringe. Insulin syringe is measured in units. Less accurate dosing can occur with 3-mL syringe.
32. A. c; B. c
33. A. a, b or just a or just b;
    B. 1 tab from 2.5 mg and 5 mg; 3 tab from 2.5 mg; or 1.5 tab from the 5-mg container.

243

34. d. This lithium level is too high, and adjustments need to be made. Withhold the dose and contact the health care provider.
35. A. b; B. a
36. A. d; B. d
37. b
38. d
39. c
40. c. The nurse should acknowledge the patient's concerns and provide an appropriate answer. The first two responses negate the patient's concerns, while the last response is incorrect.
41. a
42. d
43. A. No, Duramorph is morphine and is much weaker in strength than hydromorphone;
    B. d
44. d
45. c
46

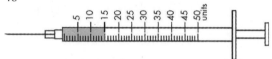

47. A. Topamax;
    B. topiramate;
    C. sprinkle capsules;
    D. 1 cap/dose

Body Weight and Body Surface Area
1. A. b;
   B. d; *solution:* ?
   $$mL = \frac{5\,mL}{400\,000\,\text{units}} \times \frac{200\,000\,\text{units}}{x}$$
   $$= \frac{1000\,mL}{400} = 2.5\,mL$$

2. A. b, *solution:*
   $$min = \frac{10\,mg}{1\,\text{kg}} \times \frac{1\,\text{kg}}{2.2\,\text{lbs}} \times \frac{75\,\text{lbs}}{24\,\text{h}} \times 12\,\text{h} = 170\,mg;$$
   $$max = \frac{15\,mg}{1\,\text{kg}} \times \frac{1\,\text{kg}}{2.2\,\text{lbs}} \times \frac{75\,\text{lbs}}{24\,\text{h}} \times 12\,\text{h} = 256\,mg;$$
   the dose of 200 mg is between the recommended dose;
   B. d
3. A. a; the dose is too low; child should receive 133–150 mg/dose;
   B. a; 225 mg/d
4. c
5. A. 2.1 mL;
   B. 350 mg/mL;
   C. b; *solution:* ?
   $$mL = \frac{1\,mL}{350\,\text{mg}} \times \frac{50\,\text{mg}}{\text{kg}} \times 8\,\text{kg} = 1.1\,mL$$
6. A. b; no, the dose is too low; B. d
7. A.

$$\frac{\left(20\,mg\,/\,1\,\text{kg} \times 1\,\text{kg}\,/\,2.2\,\text{lb} \times 22\,\text{lb}\right)}{3}$$
$$= 66.7\,mg \text{ and}$$
$$\frac{\left(50\,mg\,/\,1\,\text{kg} \times 1\,\text{kg}\,/\,2.2\,\text{lb} \times 22\,\text{lb}\right)}{3}$$
$$= 133.3\,mg;$$

B. Yes, the dose ordered is between the minimum and maximum dosage range;
C. b
8. A. b;
   B. b;
   C. a
9. A. 11 kg;
   B. 110 mg - 165 mg;
   C. Yes, it is within the recommended dose
10. 523 mg; *solution:* ?
    $$mg = \frac{50\,mg}{1\,\text{kg}} \times \frac{1\,\text{kg}}{2.2\,\text{lb}} \times 23\,\text{lb} = 522.7\,mg$$
11. A. 2954.5 mg; *solution:* ?
    $$mg = \frac{100\,mg}{1\,\text{kg}} \times \frac{1\,\text{kg}}{2.2\,\text{lb}} \times 65\,\text{lb} = 2954.5\,mg$$

    B. 1477.3 mg; *solution:* ?
    $$mg = \frac{2955\,mg}{2\,doses}$$
12. All answers are approximates.
    A. 0.17–0.18 m^2;
    B. 0.52 m^2;
    C. 0.9–0.95 m^2
13. All answers are approximates.
    A. 0.88 m^2;
    B. 0.9 m^2;
    C. 0.56 m^2
14. A. 0.51 m^2; *solution:*
    $$\sqrt{\frac{25 \times 32}{3131}} = \sqrt{0.256} = 0.51\,m^2$$
    B. 0.66 m^2; *solution:*
    $$\sqrt{\frac{58 \times 48}{3131}} = 0.94\,m^2$$
    C.
    $$\sqrt{\frac{40 \times 34}{3131}} = 0.66\,m^2$$
15. A. 0.25 m^2; *solution:*
    $$\sqrt{\frac{8 \times 28.2}{3600}} = 0.25\,m^2$$
    B. 1.02 m^2; *solution:*
    $$\sqrt{\frac{28.1 \times 133.4}{3600}} = 1.02\,m^2$$

244

C. 0.77 m²; *solution:*

$$\sqrt{\frac{85.5 \times 25}{3600}} = 0.77\,m^2$$

16. A. 1.06 m²;
    B. 1.01 m²; *solution:*

$$\sqrt{\frac{80 \times 40}{3131}} = 1.01\,m^2$$

    C. 101 mg; *solution:* 100 mg × 1.01 m² = 101 mg
17. A. 1.10 m²; B. 55 mg
18. A. 0.85 m²; B. 29.8 mg
19. A. 1.31 m²; B. 176 mg
20. A. 1.17 m²; B. 263.3 mg
21. A. 1.46 m²; B. 4.8 mg
22. A. 0.78 m²; B. 273 mg
23. A. 1.45 m²; B. 246.5 mg

Section 11C: Calculating Dosages: Drugs That Require Reconstitution

1. A. 5.4 mL; 250 mg/1.5 mL; B. c
2. A. 3.4; 250 mg/mL; B. b
3. b
4. c
5. d

Section 11D: Calculation Methods: Insulin Dosages

1. is not
2. units
3. a
4.

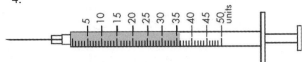

5. A.

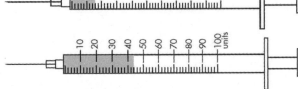

    B. c; first withdraw 8 units of regular insulin and then 44 units of NPH insulin.
    C.

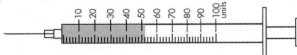

6. U-50; 8 units
7. U-30; 15 units
8. U-100; 52 units
9. U-30; 12 units
10. A.

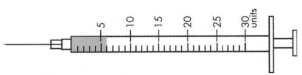

B.

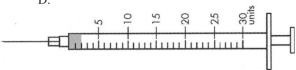

C. Notify the physician.
D.

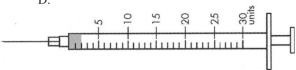

11E: Calculation Methods: Intravenous Flow Rates

1. c
2. d. Any method of drug calculation can be used, however dimensional analysis is the best method when conversion factors are needed.
3. d
4. a
5. c
6. a
7. b
8. d
9. 10–20 gtt/mL; 60 gtt/mL
10. keep vein open; 250-mL IV bag
11. calibrated cylinder with tubing
12. volumetric
13. uniform concentration of the drug, patient control and ownership of the pain
14. 28 gtt/min; *solution:* ?

$$\frac{gtt}{min} = \frac{10\,gtt}{1\,mL} \times \frac{1000\,mL}{6\,h} \times \frac{1\,h}{60\,min} = 28\,gtt/min$$

15. 31 gtt/min
16. 50 gtt/min; *solution:* ?

$$\frac{gtt}{min} = \frac{15\,gtt}{1\,mL} \times \frac{100\,mL}{30\,min} = \frac{50\,gtt}{min}$$

17. A. 1000 mL;
    B. 2500 mL;
    C. 104.2 mL/h; *solution:* ?

$$\frac{mL}{h} = \frac{2500\,mL}{24\,h} = 104.2\,mL/h$$

18. A. e;
    B. 28 gtt/min; *solution:* ?

$$\frac{gtt}{min} = \frac{10\,gtt}{1\,mL} \times \frac{500\,mL}{3\,h} \times \frac{1\,h}{60\,min} = \frac{28\,gtt}{min}$$

19. A. c;
    B. d
20. c

21. A. 3.4 mL;
    B. 250 mg/mL;
    C. b
22. 25 gtt/min
23. 67 gtt/min
24. A. 614 mcg;
    B. 204.7 mcg;
    C. 125 mL/h;
    D. 42 gtt/min; *solution:*

$$\frac{125\ mL}{1\ \cancel{h}} \times \frac{1\ \cancel{h}}{60\ \cancel{min}} \times 20\ \cancel{min} = 42\ mL\ infused;$$

therefore,

$$250\ mL - 42\ mL = 208\ mL\ left\ to\ be\ infused;$$

$$\frac{20\ gtt}{\cancel{mL}} \times \frac{208\ \cancel{mL}}{100\ min} = \frac{42\ gtt}{min}$$

25. 200 mL/h
26. A. 1.6 mL;
    B. 200 mL/h
27. 83.3. mL/h
28. 100 gtt/min
29. 50 gtt/min
30. A. 1250 units/h; *solution:* ?

$$\frac{units}{h} = \frac{30000\ units}{1\ \cancel{day}} \times \frac{1\ \cancel{day}}{24\ h} = 1250\ units\ /\ h$$

    B. 25 mL/h; *solution:* ?

$$\frac{mL}{h} = \frac{250\ mL}{12500\ \cancel{units}} \times \frac{1250\ \cancel{units}}{h}$$

31. A. 81.8 kg;
    B. 6544 units;
    C. 14.8 mL/h; *solution:* ?

$$\frac{mL}{h} = \frac{250\ mL}{25000\ \cancel{units}} \times \frac{18\ \cancel{units}}{1\ \cancel{kg}} \times \frac{81.8\ \cancel{kg}}{h}$$

$$= 14.7\ mL\ /\ h$$

32. A. 10.1 mL/h; *solution:* ?

$$\frac{mL}{h} = \frac{1\ mL}{100\ \cancel{unit}} \times \frac{18\ \cancel{unit}}{1\ \cancel{kg}} \times \frac{1\ \cancel{kg}}{2.2\ \cancel{lb}} \times \frac{123\ \cancel{lb}}{h}$$

$$= 10.1\ mL\ /\ h$$

    B. 2236.4 units; 11.2 mL/h
33. A. 11.3 mL/h;
    B. 2520 units; 12.6 mL/h
34. A. 25.2 mL/h;
    B. 21 mL/h
35. A. 39 mg; *solution:* (0.25 mg × 65 lb) + (0.35 mg × 65 lb) = 39 mg
    B. 10 mL/h
36. 7.6 mL/h (NOTE: both mcg and mg measurements are provided. Use the mcg measurement when calculating dosage.); *solution:*

$$\frac{mL}{h} = \frac{1\ mL}{1000\ \cancel{mcg}} \times \frac{2\ \cancel{mcg}}{1\ \cancel{kg}} \times \frac{63\ \cancel{kg}}{1\ \cancel{min}}$$

$$\times \frac{60\ \cancel{min}}{1\ h} = 7.6\ mL/h$$

37. A. 23.4 mL/h (NOTE: both mcg and mg measurements are provided. Use the mcg measurement when calculating dosage.)
    B. 32.8 mL/h
38. 16.7 mL/h (NOTE: no conversion factors are needed.)
39. 75 mL/h
40. 33 mL/h
41. 10.4 mL/h; *solution:* ?

$$\frac{mL}{h} = \frac{250\ mL}{500\ \cancel{mg}} \times \frac{1\ \cancel{mg}}{1000\ \cancel{mcg}} \times \frac{5\ \cancel{mcg}}{1\ \cancel{kg}} \times \frac{1\ \cancel{kg}}{2.2\ \cancel{lb}}$$

$$\times \frac{152\ \cancel{lb}}{1\ \cancel{min}} \times \frac{60\ \cancel{min}}{h} = 10.4\ mL\ /\ h$$

42. 14.3 mL/h
43. 11.1 mL/h
44. 11.3 mL/h
45. 8 mL/h
46. A. 4 mg/min; *solution:* ?

$$\frac{mg}{min} = \frac{1000\ mg}{1\ \cancel{g}} \times \frac{2\ \cancel{g}}{250\ \cancel{mL}} \times \frac{30\ \cancel{mL}}{1\ \cancel{h}} \times \frac{1\ \cancel{h}}{60\ min}$$

$$= \frac{4\ mg}{min}$$

    B. 30 mL/h. (NOTE: The flow rate is already provided in the question.)
47. A. 3 mcg/kg/min; *solution:* ?

$$\frac{mcg}{kg/min} = \frac{1000\ mcg}{1\ \cancel{mg}} \times \frac{100\ \cancel{mg}}{250\ \cancel{mL}} \times \frac{25\ \cancel{mL}}{1\ \cancel{h}}$$

$$\times \frac{1\ \cancel{h}}{60\ min} \times \frac{2.2\ \cancel{lb}}{1\ kg} \times \frac{1}{143\ \cancel{lb}}$$

    (NOTE: calculate for mcg/kg/min)
    B. 25 mL/h

CHAPTER 12: FLUID VOLUME AND ELECTROLYTES

1. d
2. f
3. b
4. e
5. a
6. c
7. b
8. a
9. c
10. d
11. a. Oral potassium supplements can be irritating to the stomach and should be taken with at least 6 ounces of fluid or with a meal.
12. d. IV potassium must be given using a rate-controlled device and cannot be allowed to run freely. In many hospitals, the nurse does not prepare this medication, and it is either mixed in the pharmacy or comes prepackaged from the manufacturer.

246

13.   d. Potassium is very irritating to the vein. If the site has become reddened and swollen, the IV should be discontinued immediately and the health care provider should be contacted to establish central venous access.

14.   b, c

15.   d. Administering sodium bicarbonate IV (50 mEq/L) as a one-time dose may help temporarily by driving potassium back into the cell.

16.   a, b, d, e. A patient who is taking a potassium supplement should be taught the signs and symptoms of both hypo- and hyperkalemia and when to notify the health care provider. Since there is a narrow range for potassium level, the patient should anticipate routine blood work to evaluate if the potassium level is in the expected range. Because potassium is irritating, the supplement should be taken with a meal or a full glass of liquid and the patient should remain upright for a minimum of 30 minutes to prevent esophagitis.

17.   b

18.   c

19.   b

20.   b

21.   a

22.   b

23.   b

24.   b

25.   b

26.   a

27.   a

28.   c, d. This patient is hypokalemic. Early signs of hypokalemia usually do not occur until serum K+ level falls below 3.0 mEq/L and may include muscle weakness, anorexia, nausea, and vomiting. Untreated hypokalemia can lead to cardiac arrest and death.

29.   a

30.   a. A potassium level of 3.2 mEq/L is considered hypokalemia and may require a supplement. Potassium supplements are taken over an extended period of time and not just a few days. Hypokalemia is rarely caused by inadequate intake. This response is also accusatory and is not therapeutic. GI losses attributable to vomiting and diarrhea may lead to hypokalemia; constipation will not.

31.   c. A sodium level of 150 mEq/L is considered hypernatremia. The normal range for serum sodium is 125–135 mEq/L. All other electrolytes are in normal range.

32.   a, d, e. GI disturbances; paresthesias of the face, hands, and feet; and arrhythmias are commonly seen with hyperkalemia.

33.   c, d, e

34.   a, b, e. This patient is hypocalcemic. Signs of hypocalcemia include anxiety, irritability, tetany, seizures, hyperactive deep tendon reflexes, and carpopedal spasms.

Case Study

1.   D.M. is in hemorrhagic shock from massive blood loss as indicated by his vital signs. Stab wounds to the chest and abdomen can penetrate vital organs, causing large blood loss and risk of death. The priority assessment for this patient is homeostasis, which includes circulation and airway. Circulation and airway are always a priority. After a systematic assessment of the patient, two large-bore IVs (14 or 16 gauge) should be established in large veins to replace fluids rapidly. Another option is to assist the health care provider in placing a central line for rapid fluid resuscitation with colloids and crystalloids.

2.   The patient needs to be resuscitated with blood and blood products.

3.   Whole blood may be more beneficial for this patient because it contains all of the components (plasma, platelets, and RBCs); however, uncrossmatched packed red blood cells (PRBCs) may be easier to obtain in the emergent setting of trauma. Volume can be expanded using volume expanders.

CHAPTER 13: VITAMIN AND MINERAL REPLACEMENT

1.   a
2.   b
3.   b
4.   a
5.   a
6.   a
7.   a
8.   a
9.   b
10.   b
11.   a
12.   d
13.   c
14.   e
15.   a
16.   b
17.

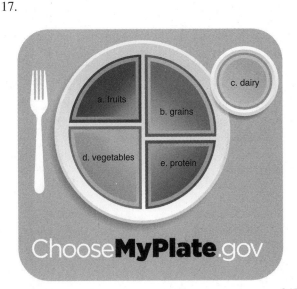

Answer Key

18. d

19. c. Newborns are vitamin K–deficient at birth, and it is a common practice in the United States to administer a one-time dose of vitamin K to prevent hemorrhagic disease of the newborn, which can present up to 6 months after birth.

20. c

21. a. Folic acid (folate) is very important during the first trimester of pregnancy to prevent neural tube defects such as anencephaly or spina bifida. All women who may become pregnant should be encouraged to take folate 400 mcg/day, since frequently a woman does not know she is pregnant until well into the first trimester.

22. c

23. b. Vitamin B_1 is also known as *thiamine*. Thiamine deficiency is evident in Wernicke encephalopathy, which, if left untreated, leads to Wernicke-Korsakoff syndrome and irreversible brain damage. Thiamine should be administered before dextrose. Vitamin B_6 deficiency can also be seen in alcohol abusers but does not necessarily create the above symptoms.

24. a

25. c

26. d

27. b. Vitamin A deficiency can be seen in patients with biliary and pancreatic disorders. Celiac disease damages the lining of the intestine and impairs absorption of vitamin A.

28. b

29. a, b, c, d. Any dose changes should be discussed with the health care provider before changes are made. Symptoms of hypervitaminosis A include nausea, vomiting, anorexia, lethargy, peeling skin, hair loss, and abdominal pain. Alcohol ingestion will decrease the absorption of vitamin A.

30. b. Pyridoxine or vitamin B_6 might be considered beneficial for a patient with neuritis from INH therapy. Signs and symptoms of neuritis include numbness, tingling, "pins and needles" feeling, and difficulty gripping an object.

31. d. Patients who are receiving parenteral nutrition are at risk for zinc deficiency. Zinc will also be crucial for this patient for wound repair and tissue healing. With continued PN, deficiencies of copper and iron can also occur.

32. c

33. d

34. d. Vitamin K is needed for synthesis of prothrombin and the clotting factors VII, IX, and X. Vitamin K_1 (phytonadione) is the only form that is available to treat an overdose of an oral anticoagulant.

Case Study

1. Vitamin A is a fat-soluble vitamin necessary for bone growth and for maintenance of epithelial tissues, eyes, and hair and has antioxidant properties. Excessive dosages can be toxic, causing alopecia, anorexia, abdominal pain, lethargy, nausea, and vomiting. Vitamin C is a water-soluble vitamin absorbed from the small intestine. Vitamin C helps absorb iron, assists in carbohydrate metabolism, and is involved in collagen, protein, and lipid syntheses. Toxicity from vitamin C is rare since excess dosages are excreted unchanged by the kidneys. Too much vitamin C can cause GI upset.

2. Vitamins C and D and certain foods can affect warfarin. Vitamin C has an antagonistic effect to oral anticoagulants; on the other hand, vitamin D has a synergistic effect. Vitamin K increases the synthesis of prothrombin, which is necessary for clotting. Vitamin K promotes clotting and is used as an antidote for warfarin. Foods high in vitamin K include dark green leafy vegetables, liver, cheese, egg yolk, and tomatoes.

3. Advise patient to consult with the health care provider if the patient wants to continue taking vitamins and eating fresh fruits and vegetables. The dose of anticoagulant may need adjustment. Explain the potential effects of the vitamins to the anticoagulant; complications of the atrial fibrillation can occur. Explain to the patient that a well-balanced diet usually negates the need for vitamin supplements. Educate on the signs and symptoms of hypervitaminosis.

CHAPTER 14: NUTRITIONAL SUPPORT

1. metabolic processes
2. 50%
3. hydration; electrolyte
4. multidisciplinary team approach
5. PEG; surgically; endoscopically; radiologically
6. True
7. True
8. False. Parenteral nutrition is delivered IV and enteral nutrition is delivered into the GI system.
9. True

10.

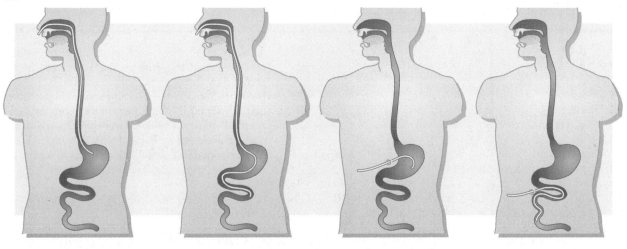

| Nasogastric | Nasoduodenal/nasojejunal | Gastrostomy | Jejunostomy |

11. d
12. a
13. b
14. c
15. a. The enteral nutrition of choice for a diabetic patient is Glucerna because it is low-carbohydrate, high-fat, and lactose-free.
16. d. Enteral tube feeding is best if the patient has a functioning GI system. However, a patient who is at risk for aspiration needs enteral feeding that will deliver the food below the pyloric sphincter or below the stomach; enteral via jejunostomy is the best answer.
17. c
18. d
19. b. Patients with burns have a higher calorie requirement than most other types of patients. In the acute phase, this is due to a hypermetabolic state. The patient requires nutritional support to assist in wound healing. Total parenteral nutrition (TPN) would be an option; however, there is an increased risk of infection. The best response is cyclic tube feeding in which the nutrition is administered over 8–16 hours, allowing the patient to be ambulatory and active during that time.
20. d. Because of the tonicity of the fluid from the high glucose levels, TPN must be administered through a central venous line.
21. d
22. b
23. b
24. c. If a patient is receiving continuous parenteral nutrition, residuals should be checked every 2–4 hours. A residual greater than 150 mL indicates potential delay in gastric emptying. If the residual is more than 150 mL, stop the infusion for 30 minutes to 1 hour and then recheck. If the residual continues to be high, stop the feeding and contact the health care provider.
25. a, c, d. Enteral nutrition is the preferred method if there is a functioning GI tract. It tends to be much less expensive than TPN and has a lower risk of infection, since TPN must be administered through central access. There is no risk of central line–associated bloodstream infection (CLABSI) from enteral feeding, because it is administered into the gastrointestinal tract.
26. a, c, d

Case Study

1. Transitioning a patient from TPN to enteral nutrition is common when a patient has a long-term need for nutritional support. Certain steps must be followed for a successful and safe transition. The first step is to see if a patient is ready for enteral feeding and how much he or she will tolerate. This is accomplished by giving small amounts of feeding at a slow rate while the TPN rate is gradually reduced. TPN can be discontinued when the patient is able to tolerate taking approximately 75% to 80% of his or her needs by the enteral method. It is important to remember that a critically ill patient may require between 3000 and 5000 calories/day.

2. A patient who will require long-term enteral nutrition will likely require a gastrostomy tube. Before that time, the patient may have received nutrition via a nasogastric or orogastric tube. Aspiration is a serious risk for those patients receiving tube feedings and may lead to aspiration pneumonia. Elevating the head of the bed between 30 and 45 degrees when possible may be beneficial. This is not an option if there is a question of spinal cord injury. The nurse should aspirate to check for residual before administering the next feeding and every 4 hours between feedings.

249

Answer Key

CHAPTER 15: ADRENERGIC AGONISTS AND ANTAGONISTS

1. c
2. d
3. b
4. e
5. a
6. effector
7. adrenergic
8. do
9. sympatholytics
10. phentolamine mesylate
11. propanolol
12. Beta blocker; many drugs can cause depression. Beta blockers should not be abruptly discontinued.
13. nonselective
14. asthma; COPD
15. Antagonism (The two drugs could counteract each other—as *antagonists*—thus negating a therapeutic action.)
16. d
17. a, c
18. a
19. a
20. b
21. d
22. c
23. d
24. b
25. b. Although albuterol will increase the patient's heart rate, this may cause a feeling of nervousness and not an ease of breathing. It has no effect on urinary output. Albuterol causes smooth muscle dilation, not constriction or contraction. Bronchodilation and relaxation of smooth muscles will improve air flow into the lungs.
26. a. Ensuring a patent airway is the first step in providing care to any patient. There is no indication at this time for an electrocardiogram. Although epinephrine is beneficial in allergic reactions, 1 mg of 1:1000 exceeds the subcutaneous dosage. Establishing an IV would not be the first action to take.
27. d. Although all pieces of information are important, the nurse should ask the patient how many puffs of the inhaler were taken to determine that the patient did not overdose on the drug. Other side effects of albuterol, besides shaking and trembling, include sweating, nausea, headaches, blurred vision, and flushing.
28. b, c, e. Albuterol is a beta agonist and amphetamine is a sympathomimetic.
29. c. Dopamine is a vasopressor (adrenergic agonist) that acts on alpha$_1$- and beta$_1$-receptor sites. Dopamine can cause tissue necrosis. Phentolamine mesylate is an adrenergic antagonist and is an antidote to stop further tissue necrosis. Dobutamine and epinephrine are also adrenergic agonists that can cause tissue necrosis. Although reserpine is an adrenergic neuron antagonist, it is used to treat hypertension.

30. a, b, c. Carvedilol is an adrenergic blocker. The other three drugs are adrenergic agonists. Adrenergic agonists are contraindicated in narrow-angle glaucoma.
31. b. Many OTC drugs, such as nasal decongestion, contain pseudoephedrine, which is a sympathomimetic; they can worsen hypertension.
32. b. Dopamine acts only on dopaminergic receptors and is located in renal, mesenteric, coronary, and cerebral arteries. These dopaminergic receptors can only be activated by dopamine. When these receptors are stimulated, vasodilation and increased blood flow occur, which can increase renal flow.
33. c, e
34. a. St John's wort can decrease the hypotensive effects of reserpine.
35. b. The proper dosage for timolol is initially 10 mg b.i.d., with a maximum dose of 60 mg/day. The above-ordered dose is 10 times the initial starting dose.
36. a

Case Study

1. An epinephrine auto-injector contains epinephrine, which is a naturally occurring catecholamine useful in the treatment of allergic reactions and anaphylaxis. It acts on both alpha and beta receptors and promotes CNS and cardiac stimulation and bronchodilation. It also decreases mucous congestion by inhibiting histamine release. Although epinephrine can be used for a variety of processes, including cardiac arrest and hypotension, an epinephrine auto-injector is used specifically for allergic and anaphylactic reactions and must be used at the first indication of difficulty breathing, hoarseness, hives, itching, or swelling of the lips and tongue.
2. The epinephrine auto-injector must be stored in a cool, dark place, and the solution must be clear and without particles. It is crucial that the patient appreciate and understand that the drug must be available at all times.
3. Proper use of an epinephrine auto-injector includes pressing the device firmly against the outer thigh and holding the device in place for 5–10 seconds. The injection must be delivered into the subcutaneous tissue. Massage the area for 10 seconds to promote absorption and decrease vasoconstriction.

CHAPTER 16: CHOLINERGIC AGONISTS AND ANTAGONISTS

1. c
2. e
3. g
4. d
5. h
6. a
7. b
8. f

250

9.

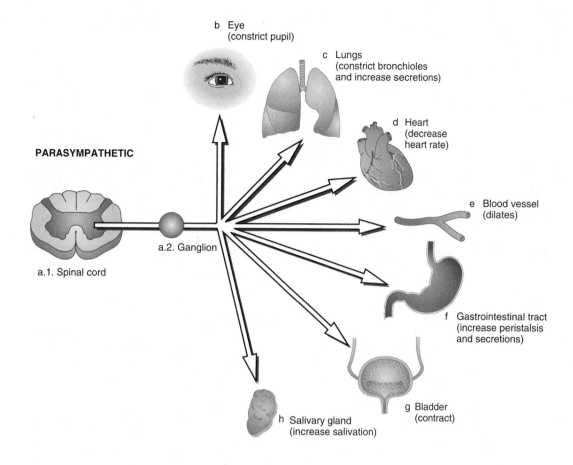

PARASYMPATHETIC

a.1. Spinal cord

a.2. Ganglion

b Eye
(constrict pupil)

c Lungs
(constrict bronchioles
and increase secretions)

d Heart
(decrease
heart rate)

e Blood vessel
(dilates)

f Gastrointestinal tract
(increase peristalsis
and secretions)

g Bladder
(contract)

h Salivary gland
(increase salivation)

10.   d. Pralidoxime chloride is an anticholinergics that inhibit the actions of acetycholine. It is given for cholinesterase inhibitor toxicity and oragnophosphate pesticide toxicity.

11.   a

12.   b

13.   c. Anticholinergic drugs are contraindicated in a patient with glaucoma because they increase the intraocular pressure.

14.   b

15.   c

16.   c

17.   a, c. Cholinergic drugs are parasympathomimetics in that they mimic the parasympathetic responses. One response is the dilation of blood vessels, which decreases blood pressure. Other responses include pupillary constriction (miosis), bronchoconstriction and increased bronchial secretions, decreased heart rate, increased gastrointestinal peristalsis and secretions, bladder contraction, and increased salivation.

18.   d. Bethanechol is used to treat urinary retention but will not be effective and should not be used in the case of a mechanical obstruction. If this patient was prescribed bethanechol for urinary retention and the urine output is decreasing, the health care provider should be notified to investigate another cause.

19.   d. Bethanechol is a cholinergic agonist. The patient is experiencing an adverse response, and the treatment of choice is atropine.

20.   c. Neostigmine bromide is used to *treat* myasthenia gravis (MG). Edrophonium chloride is used to *diagnose* MG.

21.   a, b. Atropine would be beneficial as a preoperative drug to help control oral secretions. It is also used for patients who are symptomatic with a heart rate less than 50 beats per minute.

22.   d. Atropine-like drugs should not be administered to patients with narrow-angle glaucoma because they will increase the intraocular pressure.

23.   c. Because of the decrease in gastrointestinal motility that can be associated with propantheline, the patient should be encouraged to eat foods that are high in fiber and drink adequate amounts of liquid to prevent constipation.

24.   a, b, c, e. Hyoscyamine is an anticholinergic drug that will have similar side effects to the prototype drug atropine. Adequate fluid intake will help prevent constipation. Vision may be blurry, and the patient should be advised not to drive until the effects of the drug on the vision are known. Sucking on hard candy or sugar-free ice pops, as well as increased fluid intake, may help with dry mouth. The patient should be educated as to baseline heart

251

rate and advised to report tachycardia (rates above 100 beats/minute) to the health care provider. Increased sweating is not a common side effect.

25. a, c, d. Anticholinergic drugs block the normal parasympathetic responses of the pupils, lungs, heart, blood vessels, gastrointestinal tract, bladder, and salivary glands.

26. d

27. b, c, d, e. Common side effects of anticholinergic drugs, like benztropine, may include dry mouth, constipation, and urinary retention. Dizziness and hallucinations should be reported to the health care provider because these may become dangerous to the patient. Because there is a decreased ability to perspire, life-threatening hyperthermia may develop. Palpitations may be due to tachycardia.

Case Study

1. Tolterodine tartrate blocks cholinergic receptors selectively in the bladder to decrease the incidence of incontinence.

2. The common side effects are those associated with other cholinergic drugs and may include dizziness, vertigo, dry mouth, nausea, vomiting, weight gain, and urinary retention.

3. Tolterodine is contraindicated in patients with glaucoma or gastric or urinary retention and in women who are breastfeeding.

4. Besides discussing side effects and adverse reactions with the patient, H.H. should be encouraged to take the drug on an empty stomach since absorption is delayed with food. Grapefruit juice should also be avoided because it decreases drug levels. Before taking any other drugs, the health care provider should be consulted because this drug interacts with several other classes of drugs such as phenothiazines, macrolides, and antifungals.

CHAPTER 17: STIMULANTS

1. brain; spinal cord
2. dysregulation
3. norepinephrine; dopamine
4. stimulant; suppress appetite
5. analeptics
6. a, c, d
7. c
8. a, b, c, d
9. b
10. a, b, c, d, f
11. b. An immediate-release drug can be taken in 2 or 3 divided doses. An extended-release drug should be taken once daily.
12. a. Phentermine hydrochloride should not be taken within 14 days of monoamine oxidase inhibitors (MAOIs) such as selegiline. Combinations of the two drugs intensify the stimulation and vasopressor

effects of phentermine that can cause severe cardiovascular and cerebrovascular responses.

13. d

14. b

15. a, b, e

16. c. Hemorrhagic stroke is the most likely diagnosis of those listed. There is a high risk for hemorrhagic stroke attributable to hypertensive crisis in those patients taking appetite suppressants or anorexiants. Pregnancy-induced hypertension is a possibility, but the patient has been trying to lose weight, not become pregnant. However, a pregnancy test should be obtained; anorexiants are contraindicated in pregnancy.

17. a, d, e. CNS stimulants are absolutely contraindicated in patients with coronary artery disease, hypertension, and liver failure. Cautious use is recommended for those patients with any degree of liver disease.

18. a

Case Study

1. Methylphenidate is absorbed from the GI tract and is before breakfast and lunch. It should be given at least 6 hours before sleep since it can cause insomnia. Methylphenidates decrease hyperactivity and improve attention span.

2. The drug is a CNS stimulant that is used in conjunction with appropriate counseling for treatment of ADHD. The best time to give the drug is 30–45 minutes before meals, so the nurse will need to review the lunch schedules of the students and plan accordingly on how best to administer the drugs.

   Baseline height, weight, and vital signs should be obtained and monitored throughout the course of treatment. A record of the students' complete blood count, including a white blood cell count with differential and platelet count, should be on file. Routine vital signs should be assessed since both of these drugs can cause an elevation in heart rate and blood pressure, especially if taken in conjunction with caffeine. Patients should also be monitored for an increase in hyperactivity.

   Health teaching is important not only for the student but also for the family and the teachers on staff. The goals of these drugs are to increase focus and attention and decrease impulsiveness and hyperactivity. The student and family should be encouraged to eat three nutritious meals per day along with healthy snacks because anorexia may be a side effect. Dry mouth may also occur, so, as possible within school policy, the student should be allowed to chew gum or suck on hard candy. The importance of avoidance of caffeinated beverages and foods, including chocolate, sodas, and energy drinks, must be stressed because high plasma levels of caffeine may be fatal.

   Drug administration at school must be handled with tact and ease. If possible, the school nurse's office should not be open and in the main hall where all other students can observe the comings and goings of the students requiring drug or care. Privacy is crucial.

CHAPTER 18: DEPRESSANTS

1. rapid
2. rapid
3. slow
4. rapid
5. rapid
6. rapid
7. sedative-hypnotics; general anesthetics; analgesics; opioid and nonopioid analgesics; anticonvulsants; antipsychotics; antidepressants
8. rapid eye movement; nonrapid eye movement
9. sedation
10. may
11. short
12. central nervous; pain; consciousness
13. surgical; analgesia; excitement or delirium; medullary paralysis
14. spinal
15. respiratory distress or failure
16. saddle block
17. are
18. short
19. zolpidem tartrate (also eszopiclone, zaleplon, and ramelteon)
20. flumazenil
21. esters; amides
22. d
23. f
24. e
25. a
26. b
27. c
28. c
29. b
30. c, d. Maintaining the patient flat in bed for 24 to 48 hours and encouraging adequate oral fluid intake as tolerated may help prevent a spinal headache. The patient may also require IV fluids to supplement intake.
31. c. By explaining the reason for positioning (either seated with an arched back or fetal position), the patient will feel as if she has more control. The nurse can reassure the patient that he or she will assist her in maintaining the proper position.
32. d
33. d, e
34. a, b
35. a, b, c, e. Older patients may have more problems with Stage 3 and Stage 4 nonrapid eye movement (NREM) sleep and awaken frequently. Establishing a bedtime routine, maintaining a schedule of going to bed and arising in the morning, and avoiding caffeine and alcohol at bedtime may

help. Although it sounds intuitive to take naps, they may actually hinder a patient getting a good night's sleep if they are longer than 20–30 minutes. Diuretics should be taken in the morning and fluids should be limited at bedtime to prevent frequent trips to the bathroom, which may interrupt sleep.
36. d, f

Case Study

1. Benzodiazepines are frequently prescribed before surgery. They increase the action of the inhibitory neurotransmitter gamma-aminobutyric acid (GABA) to the GABA receptors and reduce the excitability of the neurons. Drugs such as alprazolam or lorazepam might be prescribed for anxiety.

2. Balanced anesthesia includes many parts leading up to surgery. By using a variety of agents, less general anesthetic is needed, fewer cardiovascular side effects occur, less nausea and vomiting occur, pain is decreased, and a quicker recovery is promoted. This is also true of utilizing a laparoscopic approach instead of an "open" approach to this surgery.

   The night before the surgery, a medication such as zolpidem might be prescribed to ensure a good night's sleep. After the patient has arrived in the preoperative area and approximately 1 hour before surgery, a combination of an opioid or anxiolytic and an anticholinergic such as atropine might be given. The purpose of the anticholinergic is to decrease secretions, and therefore the risk of aspiration. Once the patient is transferred to the operating room, a short-acting sedative such as pentothal, propofol, or etomidate may be given and the patient will be given inhaled anesthetics. This procedure will require general anesthesia, so the patient will also receive a muscle relaxant to facilitate endotracheal intubation and maintain neuromuscular blockade.

CHAPTER 19: ANTISEIZURE DRUGS

1. d
2. a
3. e
4. b
5. c
6. electroencephalogram (EEG)
7. idiopathic
8. generalized; partial
9. preventing; do not
10. are not
11. phenytoin
12. over-the-counter
13. intramuscular
14. a, b
15. b. Although it is important to know the patient's medical history regarding seizures, the best response

253

is asking about the drugs that have been prescribed. Although no seizure medications for epilepsy are pregnancy category A or B, some category C medications may be utilized if the benefits outweigh the risks.

16. a, c, d
17. b
18. a, b, d. Valproic acid is taken in divided doses. Doses start at 10–15 mg/kg/day and increase to a maximum of 60/mg/kg/day until seizures are controlled. Increased fluid is not required with valproic acid. There are no food restrictions with valproic acid, as may be seen with other anticonvulsants.
19. b, c, d. An absolute contraindication is heart block and bradycardia. Cautious use is recommended for patients with hypoglycemia and hypotension. Dilantin is excreted in small amounts in the urine. Urine output should be monitored afterward.
20. d. Intravenous phenytoin is irritating to the tissue, and it is recommended that a central line or peripherally inserted central catheter (PICC) line be utilized when possible. The health care provider does not need to be notified immediately to change the medication to oral form. Continuing the infusion, even with a saline flush, may cause sloughing of the tissue.
21. a. Although a variety of anticonvulsants may be utilized over a patient's lifetime, at this time, there is no cure for seizure disorders. The patient will need to take a medication for the duration of his life.
22. b
23. a, b, d, e. Documenting the types of movements (tonic/clonic), the duration of seizure activity, and the locations where the movements started and progressed are important pieces of gathering the history of the seizure event. It is important to know, if possible, what the patient had been doing before the event and if the patient reported any warning before the seizure. The patient is unable to stop true seizure activity voluntarily.
24. c. Nosebleeds and sore throats may be a sign of blood dyscrasias and should be reported to the health care provider. A reddish pink discoloration of the urine may be expected. To prevent injury to the gums, a soft toothbrush should be utilized. Orthostatic hypotension is not associated with phenytoin use.
25. a
26. a. The first-line drug of choice for status epilepticus is either diazepam or lorazepam. Midazolam, propofol, and high-dose phenobarbital are administered for continued seizures.
27. a, b, c
28. c

Case Study

1. Oxcarbazepine is taken by mouth with an initial dose of 300 mg twice daily. One of the benefits of this medication is that there are fewer adverse effects than with carbamazepine and drug level monitoring is usually not necessary, which may be more convenient in the patient's role of elementary school teacher. Patient teaching is required for safe handling of the drug. As with other antiseizure medications in the iminostilbene family, dizziness, drowsiness, and ataxia can occur.

2. The nurse should tell the patient that many antiseizure medications have teratogenic properties that increase the risk for fetal malformations. Carbazepines have been known to cause fetal anomalies; whereas there is a decreased risk with oxcarbazepine. However, as with any drug, caution is advised in taking drugs while pregnant. If the patient is contemplating pregnancy, then she should consult her health care provider to determine risk versus benefit.

CHAPTER 20: DRUGS FOR PARKINSONISM AND ALZHEIMER DISEASE

1. c
2. a
3. d
4. e
5. b
6. dopamine; acetylcholine
7. dopamine
8. levodopa
9. carbidopa
10. donepezil or rivastigmine
11. enhance
12. selegiline
13. carbidopa, levodopa, entacapone
14. trihexyphenidyl (also benztropine)
15. a, c, d. Carbidopa/levodopa combination drug is available in 10/100 mg and 25/250 mg tablets or capsules and can be taken tid or qid.
16. a
17. b, c, d, e. Carbidopa-levodopa may make the patient's movements smoother, although at high doses, dyskinesia may be noted. Jaundice will not result from missing doses. Extended release drugs should not be crushed or cut; if the patient is unable to swallow tablets, then other preparations, such as liquid or oral disintegrating tablets, are available. Nausea and vomiting are side effects, so taking the drug with meals may be beneficial. There is no indication that carbidopa-levodopa affects glucose levels.
18. a, b, e. Aged cheeses, chocolate, and yogurt are all foods that are high in tyramine. These foods should be avoided when taking selegiline to prevent a hypertensive crisis from occurring.
19. d. Tricyclic antidepressants decrease the effect of rivastigmine.
20. c. When taken with levodopa, COMT inhibitors like entacapone will increase the levodopa combination in the brain.

21. a, e. Glaucoma and angina are contraindications for the use of anticholinergic drugs. Shingles and diabetes are not contraindications. A patient with a history of urinary retention, not frequency, should not take anticholinergic drugs.

22. a, c. Even though most drugs for alzheimer's disease can cause hallucinations, they are more common with bromocriptine and pramipexole.

23. c. Memantine is prescribed for the treatment of mild to severe Alzheimer disease. Increased wandering and hostility can indicate that the disease is progressing and an increase in the dose may be beneficial. The maximum dose for memantine is 20 mg per day.

24. a. Sucking on hard candy or chewing sugarless gum may help with dry mouth associated with anticholinergic drugs such as benztropine mesylate. This drug is initially taken at bedtime and twice per day in divided doses as a maintenance dose. The nurse should remind the patient that all drug adjustments need to be made by the health care provider. Urinary retention is a side effect of anticholinergic medications; however, the nurse should encourage the patient to urinate when he or she feels the urge and not on a set schedule.

Case Study

1. Alzheimer disease a progressive disease of cognitive decline, and the progression may occur over many years or decades. During the early stages of Alzheimer disease, symptoms are usually considered mild, and the patient may start to show some signs of decreased ability to function in work or social settings and have problems with recall and memory. Anxiety may also be a component. As the disease progress, patient may require to have more assistance with performing complex tasks, leading to the need for a higher level of assistance as the patient needs reminders to bathe, lock doors, and turn off stoves, for example. Disorientation becomes more noticeable and the patient may become tearful; this marks the beginning of early dementia. Later in the disease, the patient needs assistance with activities of daily living and may have incontinence of urine and feces. Psychological disturbances such as paranoia, agitation, delusions, and violent behavior become more prominent. In late dementia, the patient is unable to care for him- or herself and may make only sounds or speak a few words. Patients will eventually become comatose.

2. Rivastigmine is an acetylcholinesterase inhibitor (AChE) that is used in the treatment of mild to moderate Alzheimer disease. Rivastigmine increases cognitive function by preventing the breakdown of acetylcholinesterase, which allows for more acetylcholine to be available as a transmitter.

3. Safety is a primary concern for the grandmother as she moves into a new home with her family. As Alzheimer disease progresses, the patient may begin to wander more and is at higher risk for falling. Removing obstacles from the patient's path may help prevent falls, as will eliminating loose rugs and quickly cleaning up spills. Assuring adequate locks on outside doors may prevent the patient from wandering outside unattended; however, the patient should be able to have an escape route from the house as needed. Door alarms are also available. Covers may be placed over dials for the burners on a stove. These are similar to those utilized for preventing young children from adjusting the burners. The family will need additional resources and support, as caring for a patient with Alzheimer disease is a full-time job. Organizations such as the Alzheimer's Association can provide direction.

CHAPTER 21: DRUGS FOR NEUROMUSCULAR DISORDERS AND MUSCLE SPASMS

1. b
2. d
3. a
4. c
5. traumatic; debilitating disorders
6. hyperactive; antiinflammatory
7. decrease; increase
8. Myasthenia gravis is an autoimmune disorder that involves an antibody response against AChR sites, eventually destroying the receptor sites for ACh. Drugs used to treat MG are the AChE inhibitors (cholinesterase inhibitors and anticholinesterase), such as neostigmine or pyridostigmine. They inhibit the action of AChE, which allows more activation of the cholinergic receptors.
9. Multiple sclerosis is an autoimmune disorder that attacks the myelin sheath of the nerve fibers of the central nervous system, resulting in plaques. Drugs used to treat MS include the immunomodulators teriflunomide, alemtuzumab, and glatiramer acetate and corticosteroids.
10. b
11. b. Drooling, excessive tearing, sweating, and miosis are signs of a cholinergic crisis.
12. a
13. c
14. d. There is an increased toxicity when taken with tetracycline.
15. c. Azathioprine and interferon-β are biologic response modifiers and immunosuppressants. They are used to decrease the inflammatory process of the nerve fibers.
16. b
17. a, c. Centrally acting muscle relaxants, such as methocarbamol, can cause drowsiness and change

the color of the urine green, brown, or black. Other side effects inlude dizziness, lightheadedness, headaches, and altered taste.

18. b. Diazepam can increase intraocular pressure and is contraindicated in narrow-angle glaucoma.

Case Study

1. Patients with spinal cord injuries may have spasticity attributable to hyperexcitability of neurons caused by increased stimulation from the cerebral neurons or lack of inhibition in the spinal cord or at the skeletal muscles.

2. Carisoprodol is a centrally acting muscle relaxant and is utilized for muscle spasms. Baclofen is used specifically for muscle spasticity, either caused by trauma or resulting from multiple sclerosis.

3. Side effects of these drugs include drowsiness, dizziness, nausea, and hypotension. They should not be taken with other central nervous system depressants or alcohol. Baclofen can be used for an extended period of time without developing tolerance. It does not have abuse potential. Carisoprodol is now a Schedule IV drug and has the potential for abuse.

CHAPTER 22: ANTIPSYCHOTICS AND ANXIOLYTICS

1. e
2. d
3. f
4. g
5. a
6. h
7. b
8. c
9. thought processes; behaviors; dopamine
10. dihydroindolones; thioxanthenes; butyrophenones; dibenzoxazepines
11. drowsiness
12. pruritus; photosensitivity
13. decrease
14. are not
15. tolerance
16. sedative-hypnotics
17. c
18. a
19. a
20. b
21. b
22. c
23. c
24. b
25. b. Orthostatic hypotension may occur with phenothiazines and nonphenothiazine medications within this class. The patient should be encouraged to change positions slowly to prevent orthostatic hypotension.

26. d
27. a
28. b
29. c, d, e. Either hypo- or hypertension may be an indication of an adverse reaction. Although it may be safe to take some herbal medications while taking fluphenazine, taking kava kava may increase dystonic reactions. There are numerous side effects associated with fluphenazine, including dizziness, headache, and nausea.

30. c. Because of less effective hepatic and renal function, doses of antipsychotics should be decreased by 25% to 50% in older patients.

31. d. The correct answer is always maintaining the airway. It does not matter what the suspected overdose or illness may be. Airway is always the top priority.

32. a
33. c
34. c
35. d
36. b. Hyperglycemia is a side effect of taking risperidone. Blood glucose levels should be obtained at baseline and monitored carefully.

37. b
38. b, c, d. Patients with liver damage, subcortical brain damage, and any continued blood dyscrasia should not take fluphenazine.

39. a, b, d, e

Case Study

1. Clonazepam is a benzodiazepine that is in the same family as diazepam and alprazolam. It is used for anxiety associated with depression and seizures.

2. Benzodiazepines enhance the action of gamma-aminobutyric acid (GABA), an inhibitory neurotransmitter. It has a fairly rapid action and is readily absorbed from the gastrointestinal tract.

3. Side effects include drowsiness, dizziness, and coma if taken in large doses. The action of benzodiazepines is potentiated when taken with alcohol.

4. H.K. may have taken an overdose. A respiratory rate of 8 breaths/minute and an O_2 saturation of 78% require immediate action by the nurse. Maintaining an airway is the priority intervention. Oxygen should be administered, and an airway adjunct should be inserted. Her ventilations should be assisted with a bag-mask and high-flow oxygen until her airway can be secured. An IV will need to be established and flumazenil administered. Flumazenil acts very quickly but is only effective for benzodiazepine overdoses. An emetic is not an option for this patient because she is unresponsive. Gastric lavage is the intervention of choice. Blood pressure may need to be supported with IV vasopressors.

CHAPTER 23: ANTIDEPRESSANTS AND MOOD STABILIZERS

1. False
2. True
3. False
4. False
5. True
6. 2 to 4 weeks
7. increase; increase; decrease
8. St. John's wort
9. second-generation antidepressants; dopamine, norepinephrine, serotonin
10. stimulate; central nervous system
11. Lithium; bipolar affective
12. narrow; 1 to 1.5 mEq/L
13. increase; caffeine; loop; decrease
14. major depression, generalized anxiety disorder, and social anxiety disorder
15. grapefruit juice; toxicity
16. b, c
17. c
18. b, c
19. b, c
20. c
21. b, c
22. a, b, c
23. a
24. a
25. b
26. d
27. c
28. b
29. c
30. d
31. b. Orthostatic hypotension is a frequent side effect of tricyclic antidepressants (TCAs). The patient should be encouraged to change positions slowly to avoid this side effect.
32. a, b, e. Bananas, chocolate, and wine are contraindicated in a patient who is taking a monoamine oxidase inhibitor (MAOI). Any food that is high in tyramine such as aged cheeses, processed meats, and soybeans or soy products should also be avoided.
33. d. St. John's wort is a common herbal remedy for depression. St. John's wort, when taken in combination with selective serotonin reuptake inhibitor (SSRI) drugs, can precipitate serotonin syndrome, which presents as headache, sweating, and agitation.
34. c
35. c. Monitoring the patient is one of the most important roles of the nurse. Trending vital signs, weight, and lab work will be important to the patient's ongoing care. The patient needs to maintain a fluid intake of 2–3 L of fluid/day initially and must be especially vigilant to maintain an adequate intake in hot weather. Manic patients frequently stop taking their drug when they feel better. They must be advised to continue taking the drug even if they feel better.

36. a. Monitoring hepatic and renal function in a patient taking lithium should be completed with weekly blood work, which includes BUN and creatinine level measurements.
37. b. The patient's lithium level is still subtherapeutic, and he remains in a manic phase. Therapeutic range is usually reached in 1–2 weeks.
38. a. The patient needs further education requiring the purpose of the drug. Lithium may be used in bipolar disorder as a mood stabilizer, but its effect is on the manic phase.
39. d. Venlafaxine is a serotonin-norepinephrine reuptake inhibitor. Side effects of this venlafaxine may include drowsiness, insomnia, photosensitivity, and ejaculatory dysfunction, among others. Taking St. John's wort while taking venlafaxine increases the risk of serotonin syndrome or neuroleptic malignant syndrome.
40. a, d. Some studies have linked lithium to a congenital anomaly involving the tricuspid valve of the heart if taken during the first trimester of pregnancy. Lithium is a pregnancy category D drug.

Case Study

1. SSRIs block the reuptake of the neurotransmitter serotonin at the nerve terminal. One of the possible causes of depression is a lack of circulating serotonin. By preventing the reuptake, more serotonin is available and depression is lessened. SSRIs may be effective in the treatment of depression in cases where the patient was nonresponsive to a TCA.
2. In the initial interview, the nurse should inquire about medical history, prescription and OTC drugs, allergies, and past coping behavior. The nurse should directly ask the patient about suicidal thoughts. The use of herbal agents should also be investigated. A thorough psychiatric history should be obtained with a specific focus on past episodes of depression and treatments. Vital signs should be obtained as well as weight. Baseline laboratory work should be reviewed, since fluoxetine should be used with caution in patients with a history of renal or liver problems.
3. Discharge teaching should include recommendations for counseling, since studies have shown that medication and counseling together are more successful than either modality alone. Support groups have also shown benefit. The nurse should teach the patient to take fluoxetine as prescribed and inform the patient that it may take 2–4 weeks for the onset of action. Alcohol should be avoided while taking SSRIs. Fluoxetine should be taken with food. Dry mouth may be a side effect that can be relieved somewhat with sucking on hard candy or chewing gum. If the patient feels suicidal at any

257

time, she should contact the health care provider or suicide hotline or go to the emergency department immediately.

CHAPTER 24: ANTIINFLAMMATORIES

1. d
2. c
3. e
4. h
5. b
6. a
7. f
8. g
9. i
10. injury; infection
11. redness (erythema); swelling (edema); heat; pain; loss of function
12. delayed
13. does
14. higher (or increased)
15. 24
16. d
17. a, c, d, e. Heartburn can be a side effect of NSAIDs. Taking NSAIDs with food may help decrease heartburn. Dark, tarry, or bloody bowel movements are an indication of GI bleeding, which is an adverse effect of NSAID use. The dosage range for NSAIDs varies from drug to drug, but large doses may cause erosive esophagitis, which would cause indigestion-type pain. There are many types of heartburn, including those associated with acute myocardial infarction. Not all heartburn is of GI origin attributable to a drug effect.
18. b
19. a. Warfarin is an anticoagulant that may be taken by patients with atrial fibrillation. Aspirin displaces warfarin from its protein-binding site. This increases the anticoagulant effect and may lead to excessive bleeding, which may initially be indicated by bruising. Although the other drugs may have drug-drug interactions, they do not cause increased anticoagulant effects, as evidenced by the bruising.
20. d
21. c. Ibuprofen can cause bronchospasms in a patient with asthma; therefore, its use is contraindicated to those with known sensitivity.
22. a
23. b. Since ibuprofen is excreted in the urine, adequate fluid intake and urine output should be maintained. Ibuprofen is category C in early pregnancy and category D in the third trimester.
24. c
25. a
26. b
27. a
28. c
29. a, c, d. Corticosteroids may be used for a variety of disease processes including flare-ups of arthritic

conditions. They have a long half-life and are usually taken once a day in a large prescribed dose and then the dose is tapered for 5–10 days. Lengthy corticosteroid therapy is never stopped abruptly. They may be given in combination with other drugs including prostaglandin inhibitors.

30. b, c, d, e. Fluid intake should be increased to promote uric acid excretion. Avoiding alcohol is important because alcohol causes an overproduction, as well as an underexcretion, of uric acid. Purine is required to synthesize uric acid. Taking the drug with food will help avoid GI upset. Some studies have shown that vitamin C may help increase uric acid elimination; however, large doses of supplemental vitamin C are not recommended, and since vitamin C is an acid, there is a higher risk of kidney stone formation.

31. d. Although side effects of infliximab may include headache, dizziness, cough, nausea, and vomiting, an adverse reaction to the drug is severe infection attributable to immunosuppression. A fever of 38.8° C in an adult who is taking infliximab needs to be evaluated.

Case Study

1. The normal therapeutic dosage is 325–650 mg q4h as needed, up to a maximum of 4 g/day. If the patient takes 975 mg every 4 hours as stated, this patient will be taking 5850 mg/day, which exceeds the maximum daily dose.
2. Side effects may include anorexia, nausea, vomiting, dizziness, abdominal pain, and heartburn.
3. Signs of overdose or adverse reactions include tinnitus, GI bleeding, blood dyscrasias including thrombocytopenia and leukopenia, and liver failure.
4. The patient appears to be hypotensive, tachycardic, and tachypneic. These vital signs could be indicative of a hypovolemic state, potentially attributable to a GI bleed. Interpretation of the vital signs is compounded because of the use of caffeine with the aspirin. Metabolic acidosis, as can be seen in aspirin overdose, can also cause tachypnea.

CHAPTER 25: ANALGESICS

1. gate, nociceptors
2. endorphins
3. peripheral, prostaglandins
4. increased
5. c
6. f
7. e
8. a
9. b
10. d
11. central nervous system; peripheral nervous system
12. respiration; coughing
13. antitussive; antidiarrheal

14. head injury; respiratory depression (shock and hypotension are also acceptable answers)
15. side effect; health care provider
16. IV
17. c
18. b
19. e
20. a
21. f
22. g
23. d
24. a. All opioids have the potential to decrease pulse rate and urine output, but a major side effect of meperidine is decreased blood pressure (hypotension).
25. c. Opioid toxicity will cause pinpoint pupils, not dilation. Respiratory depression, nausea, vomiting, constipation, and urinary retention can also occur with opioid overdose.
26. b. Monitoring fluid intake is the least important. The nurse should monitor bowel sounds to identify constipation, a common side effect of opioids. The patient's pain should be frequently assessed. The nurse should assess vital signs, noting rate and depth of respirations for future comparisons; opioids commonly decrease respirations and systolic blood pressure.
27. b, c, d, e. There are no dietary restrictions associated with the use of opioids. The patient should not exceed the recommended dosage. Adequate fluid intake and inclusion of fiber in the diet will assist with constipation. Patients should always be taught the side effects to report.
28. d. Drugs with long duration of action (long half-life) are more beneficial to patients dealing with chronic pain.
29. b. An opioid antagonist is naloxone. Flumazenil is an antagonist to benzodiazepines. Butorphanol and pentazocine are opioid agonist-antagonists.
30. b. Opioid agonist-antagonists may be used to decrease opioid abuse, but there is still a potential to cause dependence.
31. b. Withdrawal symptoms attributable to physical dependence can result 24 to 48 hours after the last opioid dose and include irritability, diaphoresis, restlessness, muscle twitching, tachycardia, and hypertension.
32. c
33. b, d, e. The best people to assess how a child is acting are those who are with the child the most. Ask the parents or other caregivers how the child usually acts when he is in pain or upset. Utilizing developmentally appropriate communication skills and pain scales should yield the best result for the nurse treating this patient's pain. Opioids are appropriate to utilize if nonopioid methods are ineffective.
34. b. Cholestyramine will decrease the effectiveness of acetaminophen. An alternative nonopioid would

be an option for the patient instead of stopping the cholestyramine.
35. a, b, e. Constipation, urinary retention, and respiratory depression are priority assessments for patients taking opioid agonist-antagonists. Nausea and vomiting is usually mild and is not a priority. Hypotension can occur with opioids, not hypertension.
36. b. It does not appear that the patient's pain is well controlled with the current medication or scheduling. The health care provider should be notified so adjustments can be made or other options can be explored. Unrelieved pain can lead to a variety of health issues, such as tachycardia, hypertension, increased stress response, and glucose intolerance, among others.
37. c. The dose may be too high for the patient. Older adults should use a lower dose fentanyl transdermal patch to avoid severe side effects. Side effects from the use of opioids are more pronounced in older adults. The rates of metabolism and excretion of drugs are decreased; thereby, drug accumulation may occur.
38. c. Alcohol must be avoided while taking opioid pain medications. Alcohol can intensify the CNS effect of the opioid.
39. c
40. a, b, d. Nonopioid pain medications, such as acetaminophen, ibuprofen, and aspirin, are appropriate for minor injuries such as abrasions and minor aches and pains. Some nonopioids, such as aspirin and ibuprofen, have antiinflammatory effects that can further lessen pain and swelling. Aspirin also has an antiplatelet effect and should not be taken concomitantly with other antiplatelets or anticoagulants.

Case Study

1. Migraines are caused by neurovascular events in the brain causing neuronal hyperexcitability in the cerebral cortex. The exact cause is unknown, but specific factors that trigger a migraine headache include foods with monosodium glutamate and aspartame, fatigue, stress, missed meals, odors, light, and hormone changes, among others.
2. Two types of migraines include migraine with an aura and migraine without an aura. Migraine headaches, with or without an aura, are characterized by a unilateral throbbing headache accompanied with nausea, vomiting, and photophobia. Migraines are more common in women. Cluster headaches are also unilateral, but nonthrobbing pain behind the eyes and they are not associated with an aura. Cluster headaches are more common in men.
3. Treatment may include analgesics, beta-adrenergic blockers, anticonvulsants, and tricyclic antidepressants. Other treatments include ergot alkaloids and selective serotonin$_1$ receptor agonists (triptans). The triptans, 5-HT receptor agonists (i.e., sumatriptan, naratriptan, zolmitriptan), should be taken as early as possible during a migraine to be effective. All triptans are contraindicated if the patient has coronary artery

259

disease, uncontrolled hypertension, cerebrovascular disease, and peripheral vascular disease.

CHAPTER 26 —ANTIBACTERIALS

Section 26A—Penicillins and Cephalosporins

1. f
2. h
3. g
4. i
5. a
6. b
7. c
8. d
9. e
10. d. Superinfection is a secondary infection caused by the disturbance of the normal microbial flora during antibiotic therapy. Fungal infections frequently result in superinfections.
11. a
12. d. Cefprozil monohydrate is given for skin infections. The usual dosage range for adults is 250 to 500 mg/d, with a maximum dose of 1 g/d.
13. c. The appropriate dose would be 1500 mg q8h. The range for an adult dose is 1 to 2 g q8h to q12h, with a maximum dose of 8 g/d.
14. c
15. a. Anorexia and also nausea and vomiting are common side effects of ceftriaxone. It is possible the patient will begin to eat more and regain weight as her illness is cured; however, this is not the best answer.
16. b. Acidic fruits or juices may make dicloxacillin less effective. Abdominal pain is a possible side effect. The entire course of antibiotics must be completed to prevent the development of resistance. Rashes can be associated with dicloxacillin but may also be an indication of an allergic reaction. The patient would need to be evaluated for other indications of an allergic reaction, such as difficulty breathing or hives.
17. d
18. b. Penicillin's beta-lactam ring structure inhibits bacterial cell-wall synthesis. Penicillins, including penicillin V, can be both bacteriostatic and bactericidal.
19. c. Antibiotics, especially penicillins, may make oral contraceptives less effective, so an alternate method of birth control should be utilized.
20. a, c, d. Ideally, culture and sensitivity should be obtained before starting antibiotics. Allergic reactions are a possibility with any antibiotic. Because cephalosporins are eliminated in the urine, monitoring for adequate urine output is important. Ceftazidime is administered q8-12h, not daily.
21. c. Amoxicillin is contraindicated in a patient with asthma. Use in pediatric patients and diabetic patients is not contraindicated. Amoxicillin is pregnancy category B.
22. c. A dose of 750 mg every 8 hours would not provide the correct blood levels. The standard dose for adults is 250–500 mg q6h or 500 mg to 1 g q12h. The maximum dose is 4 g/day.

Section 26B—Macrolides, Oxazolidinones, Lincosamides, Glycopeptides, Ketolides, Tetracyclines, and Glycylcyclines

1. b
2. f
3. a
4. c
5. a
6. e
7. a
8. d
9. c, d, e. Doxycycline should be taken with meals or milk for improved absorption. There are no restrictions regarding eggs.
10. a, b, c, e. Outdated drugs of any kind should be discarded; however, tetracycline will break down into toxic by-products so it must be assured it is discarded. Superinfections, which occur when normal bacteria are destroyed, are common with the use of antibiotics. Tetracycline should not be taken during the first and third trimesters of pregnancy because of possible teratogenic effects. Tetracycline does not cause urinary urgency.
11. a, b, c, e. Iron, which is found in prenatal vitamins, and antacids prevent absorption of doxycycline. Studies have shown that the effects of warfarin may be increased by taking doxycycline, placing the patient at higher risk for bleeding. Cautious use should be exercised in a patient taking doxycycline and a proton pump inhibitor like omeprazole.
12. b, c, d, e. Drugs in the tetracycline family should be stored away from light to prevent breakdown. Cautious use is recommended in patients with renal and/or liver disease. Baseline levels should be assessed and reevaluated as needed. Because of mutations within the strains of various sexually transmitted infections, a culture and sensitivity should be obtained before starting treatment. It is also possible that various sexually transmitted infections could be present at the same time, and it would be beneficial to the patient if the most effective antibiotic is prescribed for each. Tetracyclines may make oral contraceptives less effective, so additional contraceptive use is recommended.
13. c
14. c. Contact the health care provider. Vancomycin may be nephrotoxic, and a decrease in urine output may be an early indication of renal damage.

Decreasing renal function is also a part of normal aging, putting this 70-year-old patient at higher risk for renal failure.

15. c. Conjunctivitis is a possible side effect of azithromycin. If this occurs, the patient should not wear contact lenses. Photosensitivity is not a side effect of this medication. Taking azithromycin with food may help prevent nausea. If a headache occurs as a side effect, drugs such as ibuprofen or acetaminophen are not contraindicated.

16. a

Section 26C—Aminoglycosides, Fluoroquinolones, and Lipopeptides

1. aminoglycoside
2. children
3. loop diuretics or methoxyflurane
4. DNA gyrase; DNA
5. increase
6. a
7. b
8. a
9. b
10. c
11. a
12. a
13. b, e. Ototoxicity is a serious adverse effect of gentamicin. Elevated renal function tests may indicate a decrease in renal function, which increases the risk of nephrotoxicity. Nausea, headache, and photosensitivity may be side effects; however, they are usually not considered serious.
14. b. Peak blood levels are drawn 30–60 minutes after a drug has been administered.
15. b. The correct trough level for gentamicin is less than 1 to 2 mcg/mL. The health care provider should be contacted before administering the dose because it is elevated, which can cause an adverse reaction such as nephrotoxicity.
16. c. Superinfection or secondary infection, such as vaginitis, can occur resulting from antibacterial therapy.
17. a, b, c. Because gentamicin can cause hepatotoxicity, liver enzymes (AST and ALT) need to be monitored for signs of liver failure. Gentamicin can also be nephrotoxic; therefore measurement of the characteristics of urine is necessary. Ototoxicity can occur with gentamicin, causing hearing loss.
18. b. A trough of 5.9 mcg/mL is usually achieved by the third dose. The units are in mcg/mL, not mg/mL.

Section 26D—Sulfonamides and Nitroimidazoles

1. folic acid
2. penicillin
3. trimethoprim

4. are not
5. is not
6. liver; kidneys
7. bacteriostatic
8. increases
9. b
10. b
11. a
12. d
13. b, c, d, e. TMP-SMZ is contraindicated in a nursing mother. It is possible that there is cross-sensitivity between sulfonamides, so it is important to determine if the patient is allergic to any other antibiotics. There are a variety of etiologies for kidney stones; however, crystallization of the urine may occur with sulfonamides, which can lead to kidney stone formation. Some patients are more prone to kidney stones than others. TMP-SMZ has a variety of interactions with several drugs, including warfarin, oral hypoglycemic agents, ACE inhibitors, digoxin, phenytoin, and potassium-sparing diuretics.
14. a, b, c, d. To prevent crystallization in the urine, fluids should be encouraged. Urine output should be carefully monitored since this medication is excreted in the urine. Adverse reactions are possible and include abdominal pain, nausea, vomiting, diarrhea, and anorexia. A desired effect of TMP-SMZ will be resolution of the bronchitis as evidenced by decreased coughing and clear lung sounds.
15. b
16. c
17. d
18. a

Case Study

1. TMP-SMZ is a sulfonamide that is bacteriostatic. Trimethoprim and sulfamethoxazole inhibit the bacterial synthesis of folic acid, which is required for bacterial growth. The standard oral dosage is 160 mg of TMP/800 mg of SMZ q12h.
2. Patient and family teaching will include the need for adequate fluid intake to maintain a urine output of more than 600 mL/d to prevent crystalluria. The drug should be taken on an empty stomach. The nurse will advise the patient of the potential side effects of anorexia, nausea, vomiting, diarrhea, and abdominal pain. Other side effects include headache, fatigue, vertigo, and insomnia. The patient should be advised to ask for help when getting out of bed or ambulating because of the potential for vertigo and risk of falling. Other plan of care instructions include teaching the patient and family to monitor for any rash or bruises, and if observed to notify the provider. TMP-SMZ can increase the effects of warfarin. The blood glucose level should be monitored more closely because of increased risk for hypoglycemia.

3. The nurse will need to be aware of the potential for increased effects of anticoagulation, such as bruising and bleeding, because of the interaction between warfarin and TMP-SMZ. There is also a potential for increased hypoglycemic effects of glyburide. The nurse will need to carefully monitor lab work, including BUN and creatinine levels for renal function as well as liver panel (AST, ALT, ALP). The nurse will also need to monitor for life-threatening adverse effects, including electrolyte imbalances (hyperkalemia, hyponatremia, hypoglycemia), seizures, angioedema, anemias, leukopenia, pseudomembranous colitis, and Stevens-Johnson syndrome (erythema multiforme major). Stevens-Johnson syndrome is characterized by fever, malaise, joint pain, and skin lesions. Severe cases can be life-threatening and may require intensive care hospitalization and the use of immunoglobulins.

CHAPTER 27: ANTITUBERCULARS, ANTIFUNGALS, AND ANTIVIRALS

1. acid-fast, tuberculosis
2. do not
3. speak, sneeze, cough; inhale
4. latent tuberculosis infection
5. kidney, liver; renal or hepatic disorders, alcoholism, diabetic retinopathy, severe hypersensitivity to pyrazinamide or ethionamide, concurrent MAOI therapy
6. is not (Psychotic behavior is an adverse effect and isoniazid should be discontinued should it occur.)
7. Combination
8. vitamin B_6 (pyridoxine)
9. isoniazid (INH), 9
10. a
11. a
12. a
13. b
14. a
15. b
16. b
17. b
18. a
19. opportunistic
20. histamine-mediated
21. cold sores, genital herpes
22. shingles, dermatome
23. A, B
24. does not
25. B, C
26. b. Other life-threatening effects include blood dyscrasias, seizures, and exfoliative dermatitis.
27. b. Alcoholism is a contraindication for treating tuberculosis with isoniazid. Alcohol ingestion with this drug can increase the incidence of peripheral neuropathy and hepatotoxicity.
28. c

29. a, b, d. Side effects can occur 1 to 3 hours after starting amphotericin B infusion. Side effects include chills, flushing, fever, nausea, vomiting, headache, dyspnea, and tachypnea. To alleviate side effects, diphenhydramine, acetaminophen, and hydrocortisone can be administered 30 to 60 minutes before administering amphotericin B.
30. d. Ribavirin is labeled to treat hepatitis C virus. Acyclovir is given for herpes virus, amphotericin B is an antifungal, and zanamivir is for influenza.
31. b, c, e. It will be important to obtain a history of medications taken and drug allergies before starting treatment. A history of tuberculosis (TB) exposure and the results and dates of most recent purified protein derivative (PPD) and chest x-rays will also be important information. A history of IV drug use, although important overall, is not necessary at this time. Blood glucose level is not pertinent in this patient; important baseline laboratory values include monitoring liver and renal functions.
32. b
33. c
34. c. Antacids should not be taken at the same time as INH. Antacids decrease the absorption of INH.
35. a, b. Vitamin B_6 supplements or increased intake may be necessary to prevent peripheral neuropathy. Alcohol should be avoided since INH can be hepatotoxic. Rifampin, not INH, may turn body fluids brownish-orange.
36. b. Combination therapy is more effective in eradicating TB infection than any single drug.
37. b
38. b. The standard dose range is 0.25–1.5 mg/kg/day. The drug should be further diluted and infused slowly via an in-line filter while monitoring for side effects, such as fever, chills, flushing, nausea, and vomiting. The drug must be protected from light.
39. c. Amphotericin B is only given intravenously, and side effects include flushing, nausea, vomiting, hypotension, and chills. The patient does not need to be NPO before receiving a dose of amphotericin B, and it may in fact be beneficial to have a light, nongreasy meal or even some crackers to help decrease the nausea. Amphotericin B is nephrotoxic, so any changes in urination should be reported immediately to the health care provider.
40. a, c, d, e. The patient should abstain from sexual intercourse or use a barrier method, such as condoms, correctly and consistently.
41. a, b, c. Peginterferon can cause mild to serious side effects. Mild side effects such as flulike symptoms and myalgia can be treated with antiinflammatories. Other side effects are more serious; peginterferon can cause papilledema (which can lead to vision changes), pancytopenia (placing the patient at risk

for infection, so fever should be reported), and mood changes (which may indicate depression).

42. b
43. a, b, c, e. Laboratory values that assess hepatic and renal function should be obtained at baseline and trended. Fluconazole can cause hypokalemia. Prothrombin time (PT) may be altered if the patient is taking warfarin.

Case Study

1. The nurse must complete a thorough assessment including questions regarding medications currently taken, allergies, and vital signs. Specific questions regarding vaginal or anal itching should also be asked because nystatin can cause pruritus, urticaria, and rash.
2. Frequent use of antibiotics can destroy the normal flora in the body and cause an opportunistic infection to occur. This infection is likely thrush, which is caused by *Candida* species.
3. To correctly take nystatin, the patient should put 4 to 6 mL in her mouth and swish for several minutes to coat the mucous membranes and the tongue. Nystatin should then be swallowed to treat the throat. If ordered, the patient can spit out the nystatin.

CHAPTER 28: PEPTIDES, ANTIMALARIALS, AND ANTHELMINTICS

1. c
2. e
3. a
4. b
5. d
6. g
7. f
8. b
9. c. Malaria is caused by multiple species of protozoan parasites that are carried by mosquitos.
10. b. Chloroquine is a commonly prescribed drug for malaria. If drug resistance to chloroquine occurs, then other treatments can be used.
11. c, d, e, f. With the use of chloroquine, red blood cell count, hemoglobin, and hematocrit levels may be lowered. Liver enzymes such as AST may be elevated. Baseline laboratory values should be obtained and monitored.
12. b. Chloroquine is taken for 2 weeks before and 8 weeks after exposure to potentially infected mosquitoes to prevent growth of the parasites. Abdominal cramping, nausea, and vomiting are among the expected side effects. Ringing in the ears may be an indication of ototoxicity and needs to be reported immediately. Taking either antacids or laxatives may decrease the effectiveness of chloroquine.
13. b. Artemether/lumefantrine is a combination drug that has a high success rate and may be used if

other drugs have failed because of resistance. It is especially useful in patients with high fevers.

14. b, d, e. Proper hygiene for a patient who has worms includes frequent handwashing, especially after using the toilet and before eating. Because the worms may live on a variety of materials, all clothing, towels, and bedding should be changed on a daily basis and washed in hot water. The patient should shower instead of sitting in a bathtub and should not swim in pools or use hot tubs while infected. To prevent trichinosis, caused by *Trichinella spiralis,* all pork and pork-containing products must be thoroughly cooked to destroy the larvae.
15. c, d, e
16. a, c, d. Antibiotics should be taken as prescribed and the full course should be completed, even if the person feels better.

Case Study

1. Helminths are parasitic worms that have been transmitted from infected soil to the person. Helminths feed on the person's tissue.
2. Groups of helminths that infest humans include tapeworms, flukes, and roundworms. They enter humans when the person eats contaminated food, the person is bitten by carrier insects, or the helminth directly penetrates the skin.
3. Helminths are treated with anthelmintics taken orally. The type of helminth infestation will determine the type(s) of anthelmintic(s) prescribed.

CHAPTER 29: HIV- AND AIDS-RELATED DRUGS

1. a
2. d
3. c
4. f
5. b
6. b
7. e
8. a
9. e
10. a
11. binding, fusion, replication, assembly
12. should
13. 95
14. CYP450
15. Efavirenz
16. dosing frequency, food requirement, fluid requirement, pill burden, drug interaction potential, side effect profile
17. IRIS (immune reconstitution inflammatory syndrome)
18. a, d. HIV is transmitted via contact with blood and body fluids, such as semen, vaginal fluids, and breast milk; this also includes donated sperm from an HIV-infected person. Increased risk occurs in those who have unprotected sex; those who have sex with multiple partners; and IV drug users who

263

share contaminated personal care items, such as razors.

19. b. CD4+ T-cell count can be used to determine when to initiate drug therapy and to monitor the efficacy of therapy. Other laboratory tests include plasma HIV RNA quantitative assay (or viral load) and HIV resistance testing.

20. c. Two laboratory tests used to determine the efficacy of treatment include CD4+ count and HIV viral load. CD4+ count reflects the immune status and should increase in response to ART. HIV viral load is indicative of the virus circulating in the blood, which should decrease in response to ART.

21. a, c, e. It is recommended that all who are HIV positive be treated. Tools to promote medication adherence should be provided, which include using a pill planner and setting alarms.

22. b, c. Adherence improved because newer drug formulations decreased dosing frequency or pill burden. Also, some ARTs have been combined into one pill, to further reduce pill burden. Newer ARTs have increased potency and/or have fewer side effects.

23. b

24. b

25. a, b, c. Zidovudine can cause hepatotoxicity, lactic acidosis, pancytopenia, and myelosuppression. Therefore, CBC with differentials will be monitored for indications of pancytopenia and myelosuppression. A metabolic panel will be checked for signs of hepatotoxicity (elevated ALT/AST) and lactic acidosis (creatinine).

26. a, b, c, d. Seizures would be an adverse reaction, not a side effect.

27. c. Efavirenz is the only NNRTI that crosses the blood-brain barrier (cerebrospinal fluid); neural tube defects to fetuses can occur. Neuropsychiatric symptoms can also occur, such as dizziness, sedation, nightmares, euphoria, and loss of concentration.

28. d

29. d. All NNRTIs can cause hepatotoxicity, including hepatic failure; therefore, liver panels should be monitored.

30. a, c, d. Most of the side effects associated with efavirenz are CNS side effects such as dizziness, insomnia, agitation, and hallucinations. Gastrointestinal side effects include nausea and diarrhea. Other side effects include rash. Seizures are adverse reactions, not side effects.

31. a, c, d. Efavirenz has effects on the liver and increases the potential for liver failure. Efavirenz crosses the cerebrospinal fluid. Alcohol can increase the risk of hepatotoxicity and neuropsychiatric symptoms and should not be consumed while taking efavirenz. The patient should discuss the use of any herbal preparations with the health care provider. St. John's wort should not be taken with efavirenz. Vomiting is one of the common side effects, not an adverse reaction.

32. b, c, d. Monitoring of liver enzymes and lipid panels (cholesterol and triglycerides) are important while taking tenofovir.

33. a, b, d. St. John's wort should not be taken with any antiretrovirals, as it may change the levels in the blood. A benefit of tenofovir is that it may be taken with or without food. This is important because nausea, vomiting, diarrhea, and flatulence are potential GI side effects.

34. a. Combination therapy is the standard of care for both treatment of maternal HIV infection and prophylaxis to reduce the risk of transmitting HIV to the fetus. During intrapartum, zidovudine IV should be given if the viral load is greater than or equal to 400 copies/mL, regardless of current ART.

35. a, b, c, e. Atazanavir has few side effects. They include rash, cough, diarrhea, vomiting, and nausea.

36. a, b, d, e. Anything that will help the patient keep track of timing on drug and increase adherence will be of benefit. This can be in the form of pill organizers, timers to remind the patient of medication schedule, and wall calendars or charts where the drug can be crossed off after it has been taken. Also, taking the drug at the same time each day can increase adherence.

Case Study

1. Although occurring less frequently than in years past, exposure to HIV still occurs to health care workers. The first step the nurse should take is to completely wash the exposed area with soap and water and report the incident.

2. Postexposure prophylaxis (PEP) should start within 72 hours of exposure and continue for 4 weeks.

3. The common side effects mostly reported include nausea, malaise, and fatigue.

CHAPTER 30: TRANSPLANT DRUGS

1. cadaveric transplantation
2. interleukin 2–mediated
3. lovastatin or simvastatin, or pravastatin or atorvastatin, or statin drugs
4. posttransplant lymphoproliferative disorder, Epstein-Barr virus
5. mTOR, T-cell and B-cell
6. hypokalemia
7. skin, sun
8. Induction therapy includes transplant drugs that provide *immunosuppression.*
9. An example of a living-donor transplantation is when *one kidney* is donated by a living person is transplanted into the body with *end-stage kidney* disease. Another example of a living-donor transplantation is when a *portion of a liver* by a living person is transplanted into the body with *severe liver disease.*
10. Transplant recipients receiving immunosuppressive drugs *cannot* receive live vaccines.

11. Sirolimus is primarily excreted in the *feces.*
12. Antithymocyte globulin alters *T-cell* function and prolongs T-cell *deletion.*
13. c
14. e
15. g
16. c
17. f
18. e
19. a
20. d
21. b
22. a, c, e. Cytokine release syndrome is a complex event associated with cytokine release because of an infusion reaction. When cytokines are released into the circulation, systemic symptoms can occur, such as hypotension, tachycardia, dyspnea, and fever (hyperthermia). Other symptoms include chills, nausea, headache, rash, scratchy throat, and asthenia.
23. a. Before receiving immunosuppressive drugs, antipyretics, antihistamines, and/or corticosteroids are administered to reduce the severity of the symptoms associated with cytokine release syndrome.
24. d. Grapefruit and grapefruit juice affect the metabolism of cyclosporine; they increase the blood concentration of cyclosporine.
25. c. Many drugs can interact with cyclosporine, including antibiotics, histamine$_2$-receptor blockers (e.g., cimetidine), antiinflammatories (e.g., ibuprofen), and herbal preparations. Fever can indicate an infection, and the patient should call the health care provider.
26. a. The dose ordered is incorrect. The maintenance dose for belatacept is 5 mg/kg starting week 17 post renal transplant. The nurse should not give the drug; instead, the nurse should notify the physician for the correct dose. Giving belatacept without an order is not within the scope of nursing practice.
27. d. Mammalian target rapamycin inhibitor (mTOR) is appropriate for persons who had a kidney transplant. Individuals who had other organ transplants are at risk for lymphoma and other malignances.
28. a, c, d
29. c. The adrenal cortex produces and secretes natural glucocorticoids that are necessary for the immune system. High doses of corticosteroids, such as prednisone, suppress adrenal function, more specifically the adrenal cortex. If corticosteroids are discontinued abruptly, the adrenal cortex does not have time to adjust and starts producing and secreting its hormones.
30. d. To decrease the incidence and severity of adverse reactions while receiving antithymocyte globulin, a corticosteroid and an antihistamine should be administered. A prophylactic antibiotic is not necessary.
31. a. Infection is a major risk factor for patients on immunosuppressive therapy. Patients and their family and/or caregiver should be taught to wash hands frequently, especially after toileting, and to avoid sick people or crowds. Taking daily blood pressure and temperature is not necessary. Exercise and proper nutrition are encouraged, but cooking all fruits and vegetables is not necessary.

Case Study

1. Cyclosporine modified is a calcineurin inhibitor that inhibits T-lymphocyte proliferation and reduces the synthesis of cytokines. Methylprednisolone sodium succinate is a corticosteroid that decreases the inflammatory response; suppresses neutrophils, the immune system, and adrenal function; and alters vascular permeability.
2. Common side effects for cyclosporine and methylprednisolone sodium succinate include hypertension, edema, acne, hirsutism, nausea and vomiting, headache, and hyperglycemia. Adverse effects include diabetes mellitus, malignancy, infections, and seizures.
3. Immunosuppressive drugs such as cyclosporine and methylprednisolone sodium succinate suppress the immune response and place the patient at risk for disseminated infection resulting from the live virus.

CHAPTER 31: VACCINES

1. d
2. f
3. e
4. c
5. b
6. a
7. g
8. 20
9. vaccinations, ages, dosage, route
10. mosquitoes
11. VAERS (Vaccine Adverse Events Reporting System)
12. Herpes, varicella
13. d
14. b, c, e. Acquired passive immunity is provided through administration of antibodies pooled from another source. Fetuses are protected by the maternal immune system. Pregnant women should not receive immunizations, with a few exceptions such as the seasonal flu vaccine.
15. c. Passive immunity involves antibodies that are preformed and short lived. On the other hand, active immunity is when the body's own immune response recognizes a pathogen and produces antibodies.
16. d
17. d. All vaccines stimulate an immune response against a specific pathogen.
18. a. A patient actively infected stimulates his or her own immune response and acquires natural immunity.
19. a. Immunization recommended at birth is hepatitis B.

265

20. a
21. a. Adolescents should receive the two doses of VZV 4–8 weeks apart.
22. c
23. a. Td is a vaccine that contains inactivated tetanus and diphtheria toxins that stimulate the formation of antitoxins to produce active immunity.
24. c
25. c. Fever, myalgia, and cough are typical signs and symptoms of influenza. Other manifestations include headaches, malaise, and nasal congestion.
26. d
27. a. Redness and tenderness are common side effects.
28. a, b, c, e. Parents should be given a copy of the immunization record as well as an appointment card with a contact phone number for the clinic at the time of discharge. A Vaccine Information Statement should be given to any patient, not just children, before he or she receives any immunizations.
29. a
30. c. Although diphenhydramine is used for allergic reactions, in the case of an anaphylactic reaction, epinephrine should be readily available.

Case Study

1. A concern for a patient who has sustained a puncture wound is the potential for tetanus.
2. Signs and symptoms of tetanus include stiffness in the neck ("lockjaw") and abdominal muscles, difficulty swallowing, muscle spasms, and fever. If not treated, tetanus can cause broken bones and difficulty breathing, and can be fatal.
3. The patient should receive a Td vaccine. If there are no contraindications, zoster, pneumonia, and, if in contact with infants or young children, pertussis vaccines could also be given.

CHAPTER 32: ANTICANCER DRUGS

1. h
2. j
3. a
4. d
5. i
6. c
7. g
8. b
9. f
10. e
11. Benzene
12. Skin cancer
13. Non-Hodgkin lymphoma or Hodgkin disease, or nasopharyngeal cancers
14. Cancer of the colon, rectum, breast, uterus, prostate, and ovary
15. Cancer of mouth, throat, esophagus, liver, and breast

16. a. Combination chemotherapy is used as a treatment across all (or most) phases of cell life; therefore, it tends to be more effective.
17. d
18. c
19. a. The goal of palliative chemotherapy is not to cure but to help improve the patient's quality of life by treating symptoms such as pain or shortness of breath that may be associated with advanced disease.
20. a. White blood cells are used to fight infection. If the white blood cell count is decreased (leukopenia), the patient is at higher risk for an infection. Temperature changes, even if slight, may be an indication of a developing illness.
21. a. Chemotherapy causes myelosuppression, involving red cells, white cells, and platelets. Platelets are involved with clotting and healing injured tissue. If the platelet count is low (thrombocytopenia), the patient is more prone to occult bleeding (from the GI tract, for example) and may be unable to effectively develop clots to prevent bleeding.
22. d. Caffeine may have a laxative effect, so it should be limited in patients with diarrhea.
23. b. When both drugs are given orally, cyclophosphamide decreases digoxin levels by impairing GI absorption.
24. d. Metronidazole may increase the toxicity of 5-FU by inhibiting elimination.
25. a. Adriamycin has serious cardiac side effects. Cardiac function should be assessed before and during treatment with adriamycin. Measurement of cardiac ejection fraction should be obtained before commencing treatment. Depending on studies, a drop in the ejection fraction between 5% and 10% can be an early indication of cardiotoxicity.
26. c. Doxorubicin may cause cardiac toxicity, including congestive heart failure. Shortness of breath and crackles could be an indication of early heart failure. Methotrexate can cause hematologic and GI toxicities. Although cyclophosphamide can cause hematologic, pulmonary, and cardiac toxicity, CHF is more prevalent in patients taking doxorubicin.
27. c
28. c. When the blood count is at its lowest, the patient is at the highest risk for infection.
29. c. Hemorrhagic cystitis is a result of severe bladder inflammation, which may occur with cyclophosphamide. Adequate hydration while giving this drug is important to potentially prevent this complication.
30. a. Hydration should be started before treatment and maintained throughout. Antiemetics should be given 30–60 minutes before beginning treatment prophylactically.
31. d. Pregnancy should be prevented during chemotherapy treatment, including use of cyclophosphamide, because of the effects on the fetus.

32. a. Signs of IV infiltration include pain, swelling, and erythema at the IV site. Infusion should be stopped until another IV has been established. Oral hygiene is very important, and the mouth should be rinsed every 2 hours.

33. c. Nausea, vomiting, and diarrhea associated with chemotherapy can place the patient at risk for altered nutrition. Adequate nutrition is required for healing. Small, frequent meals and snacks may be better tolerated than three large meals per day.

34. d. Doxorubicin may change the urine to a pink or reddish color. This is due to bladder irritation.

35. c. Adriamycin has both cardiac and pulmonary side effects. These should be reported to the health care provider.

36. a

37. b. Chemotherapeutic drugs suppress the bone marrow. Laboratory work should be monitored for abnormalities. The nadir for many chemotherapeutic drugs occurs between 7 and 10 days.

38. d. Two pairs of disposable gloves, preferably powder-free gloves (nitrile, polyurethane, Neoprene), should be worn when preparing chemotherapy and changed every 30 minutes or if they become punctured or contaminated.

39. b. The patient and his family will need to be alert for signs of infection attributable to the effects of chemotherapy. Assessing the temperature will need to become a part of his routine.

40. a. Antiemetics should be administered prophylactically before chemotherapy is initiated.

41. c. Petechiae, ecchymoses, and bleeding gums are an indication of bleeding.

42. a

43. d. Vincristine lowers the effects of phenytoin, so the patient must be carefully observed for an increase in seizure activity.

44. a, c, d. Each of these herbals has shown some effect when taken with vincristine. A daily multivitamin may be beneficial in patients undergoing chemotherapy. There is no contraindication for taking valerian.

45. c. An alcohol-based mouthwash will be very uncomfortable for a patient with stomatitis. Also, if the skin barrier is broken, using an alcohol-based mouthwash will potentially cause further irritation.

46. c. Neutropenia, or a lowered white blood cell count, puts the patient at risk for infection.

Case Study

1. Cyclophosphamide (Cytoxan) is an alkylating agent. It works by causing the DNA strand to cross-link, strands to break, and abnormal base pairing to occur. This prevents the cancer cells from dividing. Cyclophosphamide is also a CCNS (cell cycle–nonspecific) drug that kills cells across the life span.

2. Some major side effects of cyclophosphamide include nausea and vomiting, anemia, risk for infection, and bleeding. Some side effects specific to this medication include the potential for hemorrhagic cystitis, discoloration of the nails, cardiomyopathy, and syndrome of inappropriate antidiuretic hormone (SIADH) secretion.

3. A thorough nursing history and physical assessment are crucial for this patient throughout the course of therapy. A baseline assessment of laboratory values, x-rays, and vital signs is very important. A psychosocial assessment should also be completed. Careful monitoring of the patient's temperature on a daily basis is crucial to watch for early signs of infection.

4. The patient should be taught that adequate fluid intake (both oral and IV) will be very important to prevent hemorrhagic cystitis. Even if the patient is nauseated, small sips of water at frequent intervals may be beneficial. The goal for fluid intake is 2–3 L/day. The patient should be advised not to become pregnant while undergoing treatment. Cyclophosphamide is pregnancy category D. Also, before using any OTC drugs or herbal preparations, the patient should confer with her health care provider since there are several herbs (ginseng, garlic, kava kava, echinacea, ginkgo, St. John's wort) that may have interactions with chemotherapy. If the patient has a desire for complementary therapy, it should be respected as much as possible.

CHAPTER 33: TARGETED THERAPIES TO TREAT CANCER

1.   growth factor
2.   Cellular communication, signal transduction
3.   phosphorylation
4.   Transcription factors
5.   Cyclins
6.   Proteasomes
7.   autophagy, lysosomal, recycling
8.   block, growth, spread
9.   EGFR (epidermal growth factor receptor)
10. Kinases
11. d
12. b
13. a
14. e
15. c
16. d. Shortness of breath could be an indication of an anaphylactic reaction. The infusion must be stopped immediately and the reaction treated.
17. c
18. b. Diarrhea is a common side effect for gefitinib. Other side effects include skin reactions, anorexia, vomiting, and elevated liver enzymes.
19. a. Gefitinib is extensively metabolized by the liver, and it can increase the levels of other drugs, such as warfarin, which can increase the international normalized ratio (INR).
20. b. Other drugs, such as ketoconazole, that are CYP3A4 enzyme inhibitors can increase the plasma concentration of sunitinib, leading to toxicity.

21. c. Erlotinib can cause interstitial lung disease. Assessing lung sounds for adventitious sounds is the most important action by the nurse in a patient beginning to receive erlotinib. Patients who have preexisting respiratory problems are cautioned in receiving erlotinib because pulmonary fibrosis may occur.

22. a. Imatinib may cause thrombocytopenia and increase the risk for bleeding. This may be initially apparent with bleeding gums, bruising, and petechiae.

23. c. Ziv-aflibercept is an angiogenesis inhibitor. Its primary action is to prevent the development of new blood vessels.

24. a, b, e. MAbs are antibodies that are specific to tumor cells that express the target antigen. MAbs include fully human antibodies, murine antibodies, chimeric antibodies, and humanized antibodies.

25. b. Notify the health care provider. Rituximab can worsen hypotension when given with antihypertensive drugs. The dose may need to be decreased or the nurse may need to give a bolus of IV fluids; but the nurse must first notify the provider for the order.

Case Study

1. For metastatic ovarian cancer, bevacizumab 10 mg/kg is administered intravenously every 2 weeks in combination with paclitaxel.

2. Bevacizumab binds to vascular endothelial growth factor (VEGF) and prevents the binding of VEGF with its receptors. It blocks angiogenesis, and the goal is to slow the disease progression.

3. Side effects include hypertension, headache, rhinitis, asthenia, dry skin, and back pain. Adverse effects of bevacizumab are GI perforations, encephalopathy, renal toxicity, thromboembolic events, and congestive heart failure. Although there are many side effects and/or adverse effects, bevacizumab is used for those patients with metastatic disease where the benefits outweigh the risks.

4. Because of the many potential side and adverse effects, the patient should be informed of when to notify the health care provider. S.M. should notify her provider if she develops any GI symptoms, such as nausea, vomiting, or diarrhea, because of the risk for GI perforation or formation of fistulas. Chest pain, abdominal pain, or swelling with redness or pain in the legs should be reported immediately. She should also report any blood in the stools. The patient should not take NSAIDs because of the risk for bleeding. The patient should avoid dehydration and should wear loose clothing to prevent thrombosis.

CHAPTER 34: BIOLOGIC RESPONSE MODIFIERS

Complete the following.
1. biologic response modifiers; restore
2. recombinant DNA; hybridoma technology

3. immunomodulation; metastasizing
4. monocytes
5. red blood cells
6. endothelium; neutrophils
7. capillary leak syndrome
8. b
9. c
10. a
11. d
12. a, b, d
13. d. Granulocytes may become sequestered in the pulmonary system and cause dyspnea. This will cause an additional stress on the already compromised patient. Special attention should be paid to complaints of difficulty breathing.
14. b. It is important to assess the hemoglobin level. Risk for complications is higher when EPO is administered to patients with a hemoglobin level >11 g/dL.
15. a, b, c. Interferons should be stopped if patients develop severe depression, hematologic toxicity (severe neutropenia and thrombocytopenia), and hepatic decompensation. Dosages are adjusted for hematologic toxicity other than neutropenia or thrombocytopenia.
16. a
17. a, c, d,
18. a, b, d. The patient should be educated regarding side effects, adverse effects, and how to administer interferon alpha. The side effects from BRM administration usually disappear 72–96 hours after discontinuation of therapy.
19. b, c. GM-CSF should be administered to both allogeneic and autologous BMT recipients. It is not recommended for Kaposi sarcoma. GM-CSF is used for an ANC <1500/mm³, and it should not be used within 24 hours of chemotherapy.
20. a, c, e

Case Study

1. G-CSF is not a chemotherapeutic drug, but is used in conjunction with myelosuppressive chemotherapy to increase production of neutrophils and enhance phagocytosis to help fight infection. It is an adjunct to chemotherapy.

2. Side effects of G-CSF are similar to those of other BRMs (nausea, vomiting, fatigue, etc.); however, bone pain is consistently reported with G-CSF because of the action on the bone marrow. Bone pain occurs more frequently in patients receiving higher doses.

3. Priority teaching instructions include the use of nonopioids to help relieve bone pain. Should the patient become pregnant, she should notify her health care provider immediately, as caution should be used in administering this G-CSF to pregnant patients. The patient should also report any abdominal pain, including pain referred to the left shoulder, as well as chest pain or unusual bleeding, such as hematuria or bloody stool.

CHAPTER 35: UPPER RESPIRATORY DISORDERS

1. c
2. a
3. d
4. b
5. H_1, smooth
6. first-generation; dry mouth; drowsiness
7. nonsedating; anticholinergic
8. tolerance; rebound nasal congestion; 3 days
9. alpha-adrenergic; vasoconstriction; hypertension
10. a
11. b
12. b
13. a
14. b
15. a
16. b
17. a
18. d
19. a
20. d
21. a
22. c
23. a, b, d, e
24. d
25. c
26. a, b, c, d
27. a, b, c, d. Decongestants are not contraindicated in obesity unless the patient also has any of the other diagnoses.
28. c, d. Antihistamines may cause drowsiness. Diphenhydramine is a common ingredient in OTC sleeping preparations. Should the patient choose to take any OTC drugs, he or she should be instructed to read the label carefully to check for interactions. The best option, however, is to check with the health care provider or pharmacist. Decongestants taken at bedtime may cause insomnia or jitteriness. Antibiotics are ineffective against a virus.

Case Study

1. Oxymetazoline is a decongestant nasal spray that is used to help constrict the vessels within the nasal cavity. The nasal mucous membranes shrink, and it is easier for the patient to exchange air through the nose.
2. The correct dose for this patient would be 2 or 3 sprays in each nostril, morning and night. It should not be used for longer than 3–5 days because of the potential for rebound congestion.
3. Rebound congestion occurs because of irritation of the nasal mucosa leading to vasodilation instead of vasoconstriction. Use of nasal decongestants can also lead to nasal dryness and, if overused, epistaxis. Some brands of oxymetazoline are listed as moisturizing. Another option is to use saline nasal drops, although this will only moisturize and not serve as a decongestant. Oral decongestants such as phenylephrine or pseudoephedrine may also be used. Also important with this patient

is to determine the cause of the nasal congestion. Allergies may be treated with intranasal glucocorticoids and first- or second-generation antihistamines. A common cold will not be treated with glucocorticoids.

CHAPTER 36: LOWER RESPIRATORY DISORDERS

1. d
2. e
3. b
4. f
5. c
6. a, b
7. b
8. f
9. cyclic adenosine monophosphate (cAMP)
10. epinephrine
11. beta$_2$-adrenergic agonists
12. cAMP
13. increases
14. synergistic
15. shorter
16. methylxanthine (xanthine); asthma
17. glucocorticoids
18. prophylactic; histamine
19. rebound bronchospasm
20. beta$_2$
21. is
22. evening
23. 10 mg/day; 5 mg/day
24. mucolytics
25. antibiotic
26. c. The inhaler should be shaken well before each use. Inhalers do not require refrigeration. By testing the inhaler each time to see if the spray works, the patient is losing a dose of the medication.
27. a, b, d, e. Inhaled doses of drugs for asthma have a more rapid onset and fewer side effects than oral preparations. They are shorter-acting. Some inhaled and oral drugs can be taken together.
28. b
29. a
30. a, c
31. b
32. c, d
33. d. Taking theophylline and ephedra together may increase the risk of theophylline toxicity. Hyperglycemia is a sign of theophylline toxicity.
34. a, b, c, d. It is not necessary to wait 5 minutes between inhalations.
35. d, e
36. a, b, c, e. Beta blockers increase the half-life of theophylline. Theophylline increases the risk of digitalis toxicity and decreases the effects of lithium. Phenytoin decreases theophylline levels.
37. a, c, d, e
38. b. Cromolyn sodium is used as a prophylactic medication to prevent asthma attacks by preventing

269

the release of histamine and suppressing inflammation in the bronchioles. It will not stop an attack once it has started and is not a bronchodilator.

39. c. The therapeutic range for theophylline is 10–20 mcg/mL.

Case Study

1. Albuterol is a selective beta$_2$ agonist. It is considered a "rescue inhaler" and can be used on an as-needed basis during an acute asthma attack because it is fast-acting and provides bronchodilation. Since it is a selective beta$_2$ agonist, there are fewer side effects than with nonselective beta agonists. Montelukast sodium is a leukotriene modifier. Leukotrienes are chemical mediators that cause airway edema and increased mucous production. Leukotriene modifiers decrease inflammation. They must be taken daily and are not effective to treat an acute asthma attack. Fluticasone propionate/salmeterol 100/50 is a glucocorticoid combination drug that contains fluticasone propionate 100 mcg and salmeterol 50 mcg. Glucocorticoids have antiinflammatory properties, and they work synergistically with beta$_2$ agonists.

2. H.K. should be encouraged to keep all appointments as scheduled and to contact the health care provider before taking any over-the-counter drugs. If H.K. smokes, information on smoking cessation programs should be given, and she should be advised to notify the health care provider if she is contemplating pregnancy. Patients with asthma should be encouraged to stay hydrated and report any increased use of "rescue inhalers" like albuterol. A patient with asthma should also be encouraged to wear a medical identification bracelet or necklace to indicate the drugs being taken.

CHAPTER 37: CARDIAC GLYCOSIDES, ANTIANGINALS, AND ANTIDYSRHYTHMICS

1. b
2. e
3. c
4. d
5. a
6. weakens; enlarges
7. increase
8. digitalis glycosides; inhibit
9. increase; decrease
10. positive inotropic action (increases heart contraction); negative chronotropic action (decreases heart rate); negative dromotropic action (decreases conduction of the heart cells); and increased stroke volume
11. decrease
12. warfarin (or other anticoagulants)
13. hypokalemia, hypomagnesemia, hypercalcemia
14. dilating; arterioles; renal; decreases
15. first-pass metabolism by the liver
16. smooth muscle of blood vessels
17. 1–3; 3
18. headache
19. beta blockers and calcium channel blockers
20. verapamil; diltiazem
21. reflex tachycardia; pain
22. stressed (or exerted)
23. occurs frequently, is unpredictable, and manifests with progressive severity
24. is at rest
25. spasm
26. reduction of venous tone or coronary vasodilation
27. hypoxia; hypercapnia
28. fast sodium channel blockers; beta blockers; calcium channel blockers; also drugs that prolong repolarization
29. alcohol; cigarettes
30. b
31. a
32. a
33. c
34. d
35. b
36. c. Phosphodiesterase inhibitors promote positive inotropic response and vasodilation, not vasoconstriction.
37. c
38. d. Quinidine is a fast sodium channel blocker that decreases sodium influx into cardiac cells. The response is slowed conduction speed, suppressed automaticity, and increased repolarization time.
39. d
40. a. Amiodarone prolongs repolarization and is given intravenously in emergency treatment for ventricular dysrhythmias when other antidysrhythmics are not effective. Atropine is for symptomatic bradycardia; acebutolol is for premature ventricular contractions and is given orally.
41. a, b
42. d. Lidocaine is used to treat ventricular dysrhythmias. Atrial fibrillation, bradycardia, and complete heart block are atrial dysrhythmias.
43. a, c. Constipation is a side effect of verapamil, which is taken three times per day. Verapamil may cause hypotension, not hypertension.
44. c
45. d. Calcium channel blockers may have an effect on kidney and liver function, so baseline liver enzymes should be obtained and trended.
46. c. ANP and BNP are elevated in persons with HF. Both are secreted from the atrial cells of the heart.
47. d. Normal values are less than 100 pg/mL. Greater than 100 pg/mL is considered elevated. Older women tend to have higher normal BNP levels than older men; however, a level of 420 pg/mL is markedly elevated and is of concern for heart failure.

48. a. Digitalis drugs, such as digoxin, can be used for heart failure or atrial fibrillation. Atrial fibrillation is a cardiac dysrhythmia of the atria.

49. a. The usual maintenance dose of digoxin is 3.4 to 5.1 mcg/kg/d. Answers b and c are too low and answer d is too high of a dose. The therapeutic serum level for digoxin is 0.8 to 2 ng/mL.

50. b

51. d. Vision changes, fatigue or malaise, headache, and bradycardia are signs of digitalis toxicity. The patient cannot wait until his next appointment to be seen. Digoxin levels will need to be evaluated and an antidote may need to be given.

52. b

53. a, b, c. Cortisone, furosemide, and hydrochlorothiazide all promote loss of potassium, which increases the effect of digitalis and can lead to digitalis toxicity. A person taking a potassium-wasting diuretic or cortisol should avoid hypokalemia by eating potassium-rich foods or taking potassium supplements.

54. a. Pulse rate should be checked before taking digoxin, and the health care provider should be notified if it is less than 60 beats/min or irregular.

55. c a. There are no specific drug-food contraindications for digoxin. The patient should be encouraged to eat foods high in potassium such as fruits and vegetables (including potatoes). A patient with heart failure should avoid hot dogs because of their high sodium content.

56. a, b, c, e, f. All but sodium channel blockers can be used to treat heart failure. Sodium channel blockers prolong repolarization of cardiac cells and are used to treat dysrhythmias.

57. a, b, d. Headache is a very common side effect of NTG. Other side effects include dizziness and weakness because of vasodilation and hypotension.

58. a, b. Nitroglycerin tablets should not be chewed but should be placed under the tongue. There are no dietary restrictions when taking nitroglycerin. Tablets must be stored in their original amber glass container and away from light to prevent decomposition. A very dry mouth will hinder absorption, so sips of water may be taken. If chest pain persists or worsens after three tablets, 911 should be called.

59. c

60. b

61. a, c. The initial dose for acebutolol is 200 mg q12h. The maintenance dose is 600 to 1200 mg/d in 2 divided doses.

62. c

63. a. Acebutolol is a beta blocker and should not be abruptly stopped because abrupt discontinuation can lead to reflex tachycardia or dysrhythmias.

64. a, b, d, e. Acebutolol can cause diarrhea, edema, vomiting, erectile dysfunction, and hypotension.

65. a, d, e. Aloe, Ma-huang, and ginseng should be avoided while taking digoxin. Aloe and Ma-huang can increase the risk of digoxin toxicity; ginseng can falsely elevate digoxin levels.

66. a, b, e. Electrolyte imbalances, especially potassium, calcium, and magnesium, can lead to cardiac dysrhythmias. Excessive catecholamines may lead to rapid atrial or ventricular rates as well as ectopy. Hypoxia and *hyper*capnia may also cause dysrhythmias.

Case Study

1. The three different types of angina are classic, unstable, and variant. Classic angina is fairly predictable and occurs with stress or exertion. Unstable angina is also known as *preinfarction angina.* It is unpredictable and increases in frequency and severity. Unstable angina may or may not be related to stress. Variant angina is also known as *vasospastic* or *Prinzmetal angina.* It occurs at rest. Patients frequently have a combination of both classic and variant angina. Classic angina is caused by an actual narrowing of the coronary arteries, whereas variant angina is caused by vessel spasms. Unstable angina often indicates an impending myocardial infarction (MI).

2. Vasospastic angina or variant angina occurs at rest. But since stress plays a part in anginal attacks, avoiding strenuous activities, heavy meals, and emotional upset may be beneficial nonpharmacologic methods to treat vasospastic angina. Smoking cessation is very important to overall cardiac health. Preventive measures include adequate rest and relaxation techniques.
Pharmacologic treatments for angina include nitrates, beta blockers, and calcium channel blockers. Antianginal drugs either increase oxygen supply or decrease oxygen demand by the myocardium. Nitrates reduce venous tone, promote vasodilation, and decrease cardiac workload. Beta and calcium channel blockers decrease oxygen demand by decreasing the workload of the heart. Nitrates and calcium channel blockers are effective for treating vasospastic angina.

3. Beta blockers and calcium channel blockers can be used to treat angina. Beta blockers include atenolol, metoprolol, and nadolol. Calcium channel blockers include amlodipine, diltiazem, and verapamil hydrochloride. Beta blockers should be used in persons with stable angina. Nitrates and calcium channel blockers can be used for variant angina. Nitrates are also used for unstable angina.

4. Nitrates cause relaxation and dilation of blood vessels, including coronary vasculature, which decreases resistance; hence, blood pressure drops. Nitrates also decrease preload and afterload, reducing myocardial oxygen demand.

1.

Thiazides (e.g., hydrochlorothiazide)
Distal tubule c
Bowman capsule
Osmotics (mannitol) and carbonic anhydrase inhibitors
Glomerulus
Proximal tubule a
H_2O
Na^+
ADH
ADH
Na^+
H_2O
d Collecting tubule
Potassium-sparing diuretics (e.g., triamterene)
H_2O
K^+
H_2O
Ascending loop
Descending loop
Na^+
b
Loop of Henle
Loop diuretics (e.g., furosemide)

a. Proximal tubule; osmotic and carbonic anhydrase inhibitors; Na^+
b. Loop of Henle; loop diuretics; Na^+ and K^+
c. Distal tubule; thiazides; Na^+
d. Collecting tubule; potassium sparing; retains K^+

Laboratory Test	Normal Levels	Abnormal Results
2. Potassium	3.5–5 mEq/L	hypokalemia
3. Magnesium	1.8–3 mg/dL	hypomagnesemia
4. Ionized calcium	4.5–5.5 mEq/L	hypercalcemia
5. Chloride	95–105 mEq/L	hypochloremia
6. Bicarbonate	24–28 mEq/L	minimal bicarbonate loss
7. Uric acid	2.8–8 mg/dL	hyperuricemia
8. Blood sugar	70–110 mg/dL	hyperglycemia
9. Blood lipids	Total chol: <200 mg/dL LDL: <100 mg/dL Trig: <190 mg/dL	hyperlipidemia

10. The two main purposes for diuretics are to decrease fluid and decrease hypertension.
11. Most diuretics promote sodium and water loss by blocking sodium and chloride reabsorption from the renal tubules. This causes a decrease in fluid volume in the tissues and circulation, which lowers blood pressure.
12. b, d, e
13. d
14. b
15. b
16. a
17. c. Spironolactone blocks the action of aldosterone and inhibits the sodium-potassium pump, so potassium is retained. This is important in maintaining a regular cardiac rhythm. It is frequently prescribed by cardiologists and is not contraindicated in patients who have had a myocardial infarction. Sodium is excreted with this drug. Patients should be advised not to overindulge in foods rich in potassium such as bananas, because this could cause above-normal levels of potassium (hyperkalemia).
18. d. To prevent hearing loss, furosemide must be administered slow IV push over at least 1–2 minutes. It does not need to be diluted and does not require a central line for administration. Cardiac monitoring is not essential, because furosemide does not cause arrhythmias.
19. a, b, d. Hypokalemia, or low serum potassium level, is a risk for patients taking thiazides. This could be a life-threatening condition. Sodium is also lost, causing hyponatremia. Calcium level is elevated because thiazides block calcium excretion. There is minimal effect on bicarbonate levels. Cautious use in hepatic failure patients is recommended, but trending of AST/ALT levels is not always indicated. Baseline values may be beneficial.
20. a. The normal range for serum potassium level is 3.5–5 mEq/L. A level of 5.8 mEq/L is considered hyperkalemia. The dose of spironolactone may be held or decreased, and the patient should decrease intake of potassium-rich foods such as bananas, apricots, leafy greens, and salmon.
21. a. Acetazolamide is recommended for patients with open-angle glaucoma.
22. a. Acetazolamide is a carbonic anhydrase inhibitor. It blocks the action of carbonic anhydrase, which is an enzyme that affects hydrogen ion balance. If the action is blocked, more bicarbonate will be excreted, leading to metabolic acidosis.
23. d. Because the onset of action is 2 hours, it may be best to take the drug when the patient will be awake for several hours so sleep is not disturbed. Hydrochlorothiazide can be taken with food to prevent GI upset. The drug needs to be taken consistently, even if the patient is not having symptoms.

24.   a. Furosemide will cause an increased loss of potassium (hypokalemia) when given with amiodarone, which may predispose the patient to ventricular arrhythmias.

25.   c. Muscle weakness, abdominal distention, severe leg cramping, and cardiac arrhythmias are indications of hypokalemia (low potassium levels). Low potassium levels may occur with the use of loop diuretics.

26.   b

27.   a, b

28.   b

29.   c. The combination of furosemide and alcohol can increase orthostatic hypotension.

30.   a. Loop diuretics are contraindicated in patients with anuria. Giving diuretics to a patient without any urine output will not force urine production.

31.   d. Daily weights and vital signs need to be trended at home on a daily basis. The patient and family should be educated on how to take these measurements or arrangements should be made for assessment by home health services, at least initially. The onset of action for hydrochlorothiazide is 2 hours. Hyperglycemia is a side effect of hydrochlorothiazide, so blood sugar level should be monitored. This medication can be taken with food to prevent nausea.

Case Study

1.   Mannitol is an osmotic diuretic that is used for patients with increased intracranial pressure and increased intraocular pressure. Osmotic diuretics increase osmolality and sodium reabsorption. Sodium, chloride, potassium, and water are excreted. This shift in fluid will cause, at least temporarily, a decrease in intracranial pressure.

2.   The standard dosage range in adults for mannitol is 1–2 g/kg, followed by 0.25 mg/kg to 1 g/kg infused over 30–60 minutes. Mannitol crystallizes easily, so it must be warmed before administration. It is suggested that it be given through an IV administration set with a filter.

3.   For this patient, the correct dose would be 80–160 g, followed by 20–80 g over 30–60 minutes.

CHAPTER 39: ANTIHYPERTENSIVES

1.   beta-adrenergic blockers; centrally acting alpha$_2$ agonists; alpha-adrenergic blockers; also adrenergic neuron blockers, alpha$_1$- and beta$_1$-adrenergic blockers

2.   diuretics, direct-acting arteriolar vasodilators; also ACE inhibitors, angiotensin II-receptor blockers, and calcium channel blockers

3.   prehypertension; stage 1; stage 2

4.   beta blockers; ACE inhibitors; also angiotensin II–receptor blockers, potassium-sparing diuretics, centrally acting alpha$_2$ agonist

5.   diuretics

6.   Stage 2

7.   diminished; lowered

8.   cardioselective

9.   decrease very-low-density lipoprotein (VLDL) and LDL; increase HDL

10.   c

11.   d

12.   b

13.   a

14.   e

15.   f

16.   g

17.   h

18.   b. According to the guidelines, the patient falls in the category of prehypertension with a reading of 136/82 mm Hg, since prehypertension is defined as systolic blood pressure of 120–139 mm Hg or diastolic blood pressure of 80–89 mm Hg.

19.   d

20.   b. Nonselective alpha-adrenergic blockers are used for severe hypertension associated with pheochromocytomas (catecholamine-secreting tumors of the adrenal medulla).

21.   d

22.   d. Diuretics are frequently given with a variety of antihypertensive agents to decrease fluid retention and peripheral edema.

23.   a, b, c. ARBs inhibit the binding of angiotensin II to angiotensin I receptors, cause vasodilation, and decrease peripheral resistance. ARBs do not increase sodium retention or decrease heart rate.

24.   b

25.   a. The primary side effect of ACE inhibitors is a constant, irritated cough and may be relieved upon discontinuation of the drug. ARBs do not have the side effect of coughing.

26.   d. African Americans are not as responsive to ACE inhibitors given as monotherapy but may respond better if an ACE inhibitor is combined with a thiazide diuretic.

27.   c. Calcium channel blockers and alpha$_1$ blockers may be more effective in the African American patient population for treating hypertension. They do not respond well to direct renin inhibitors, beta blockers, and ACE inhibitors. ARBs are similar to ACE inhibitors, affecting the RAAS.

28.   a. Ma-huang decreases or counteracts the effects of antihypertensives and can even increase the hypertensive state.

29.   a

30.   c

31.   d. Captopril has low protein-binding power (25%), so there will be no or minimal drug displacement.

32.   b. ACE inhibitors, such as captopril, when taken with nitrates, diuretics, or adrenergic blockers can increase the risk of hypotension. Nitrates cause vasodilation, diuretics cause sodium and water loss, and adrenergic blockers decrease sympathetic tone.

33. b. Aldosterone, a hormone secreted by the adrenal cortex, promotes sodium retention and potassium excretion. Captopril is an ACE inhibitor that inhibits the release of aldosterone. This action can increase serum potassium level, and if captopril is taken with a potassium-sparing diuretic, such as spironolactone, hyperkalemia is more likely.

34. b. Adherence with the medication regimen can be very frustrating to a patient who "feels better." Stopping an antihypertensive abruptly can lead to rebound hypertension.

35. c. Nifedipine is a potent calcium channel blocker, and the immediate-release form has been associated with profound hypotension, MI, and death.

36. a. Amlodipine, a calcium channel blocker, is highly protein-bound (93%).

37. a, b, d. Metoprolol is a cardioselective beta blocker that lowers blood pressure, which can cause dizziness, nausea, vomiting, and headache.

38. d

39. d

40. b. Ankle edema may occur with calcium channel blockers such as amlodipine because of its vasodilator effect. There are other options that may be utilized to treat the patient's hypertension.

41. b

42. b

43. d, e. Cardioselective beta blockers will help maintain renal blood flow and have fewer hypoglycemic effects than those associated with noncardioselective beta blockers. Rebound symptoms are a possibility if the medication is stopped abruptly. Cardioselectivity does not confer absolute protection from bronchoconstriction.

44. a, b, c

45. b. Aliskiren can be used for mild to moderate hypertension, either as a monotherapy or with combination of other antihypertensives or diuretics. Aliskiren is not effective in reducing blood pressure among African Americans. Because aldosterone concentration is decreased, aliskiren can cause hyperkalemia, not hypokalemia.

Case Study

1. Chlorthalidone with clonidine combines a thiazide diuretic with a centrally acting alpha$_2$ agonist. Centrally acting alpha$_2$ agonists decrease the sympathetic response from the brainstem to the peripheral vessels. The result is decreased peripheral vascular resistance and increased vasodilation, thereby reducing blood pressure. Because clonidine can cause fluid retention, a diuretic is frequently prescribed, which accounts for the combination of clonidine with chlorthalidone.

2. *Hypertensive emergencies* are episodes of uncontrolled blood pressure that can cause acute impairment of one or more systems (cardiovascular, renal, neurologic). If left untreated, permanent damage may occur. The blood pressure needs to be lowered, but in a controlled setting, such as with sodium nitroprusside. Sodium nitroprusside is a potent vasodilator and is administered intravenously in a critical care unit; it is the drug of choice for hypertensive emergencies. The patient must be monitored closely in a critical care unit during administration.

3. Priority teaching instructions at discharge for this patient include the importance of taking the medication as prescribed. Determining why the patient skips doses is important. Missing doses can cause rebound hypertension, tachycardia, and headache. Priority teaching instructions may need to be directed toward the cause of missing doses. If the patient remains on a similar drug that is combined with a diuretic, the nurse should suggest the patient take the drug during waking hours so sleep is not interrupted. Decreasing stress, increasing exercise, and evaluating the diet are important pieces of the entire care plan for a patient with hypertension.

CHAPTER 40: ANTICOAGULANTS, ANTIPLATELETS, AND THROMBOLYTICS

1. artery; vein
2. clot formation; do not
3. do not have
4. venous thrombus that may lead to pulmonary embolism
5. subcutaneously; intravenously
6. standard heparin; lower the risk of bleeding
7. warfarin
8. decrease
9. 4
10. plasminogen; plasmin
11. bleeding/hemorrhage
12. fondaparinux
13. Order of heparin activity: d, b, a, c
14. c
15. d
16. a
17. a
18. e
19. d
20. f
21. b
22. f
23. c
24. a, b, c. Most patients on warfarin therapy are maintained at an International Normalized Ratio (INR) of 2–3. Patients with mechanical heart valves or recurrent systemic embolism should have an INR of 2.5–4.5.
25. c
26. b, d. Clopidogrel is an antiplatelet and apixaban is a selective factor Xa inhibitor.
27. a. Abciximab is an antiplatelet medication in the glycoprotein (GP) IIb/IIIa receptor antagonist

family. It is used primarily for acute coronary syndromes and for preventing reocclusion of coronary arteries following PTCA. Aminocaproic acid is an antagonist to thrombolytics (antithrombolytic) to stop bleeding by inhibiting thrombolysis. Protamine sulfate is an antidote to stop bleeding attributable to heparin or LMWH. Warfarin is an oral anticoagulant.

28. a. The correct dose for continuous infusion is 0.125 mcg/kg/min. This patient weighs 76 kg (168 pounds ÷ 2.2 = 76 kg). 76 kg × 0.125 mcg/kg/min = 9.5 mcg/min.

29. d

30. a. Various laboratory values will be monitored while a patient is taking warfarin. The most important levels to trend will be PT, aPTT, and INR. The INR and PT are closely related, and the patient will have the aPTT evaluated before changing to warfarin completely.

31. b

32. d. Vitamin K is the antidote for warfarin poisoning or overdose. Protamine sulfate is the antidote for heparin poisoning.

33. a. Warfarin is 97% protein-bound.

34. b. In drugs that are highly protein-bound, such as fluoxetine, there is the potential for drug displacement of warfarin, leading to higher free drug levels in the blood. This can result in bleeding.

35. a. Bleeding is considered an adverse reaction to fondaparinux.

36. a

37. a, b, c, d

38. b. Used after bleeding during cardiovascular surgery, aminocaproic acid may also be used to help with bleeding from thrombolytics.

39. a, c, e. Vital signs should be continually assessed while a patient is receiving thrombolytics. Cardiac monitoring should be performed to observe for reperfusion arrhythmias. The nurse should also monitor for signs and symptoms of bleeding.

40. a, b, d. Anticoagulants would be beneficial for patients with a history of deep vein thrombosis and for those who have received an artificial heart valve. They are also beneficial in patients who have had major orthopedic surgeries, such as hip or knee replacements, to prevent pulmonary emboli.

Case Study

1. Heparin combines with antithrombin III, which accelerates the anticoagulant cascade of reactions that prevents thrombus formation. By inhibiting the action of thrombin, conversion of fibrinogen to fibrin does not occur and the formation of a fibrin clot is prevented. Heparin will not dissolve a clot like a thrombolytic, but it prevents the formation of further clots. Before discharge home, a patient must be transitioned to either a low–molecular-weight heparin (LMWH) like enoxaparin sodium, which is administered subcutaneously, or an oral medication such as warfarin.

2. Warfarin inhibits hepatic synthesis of vitamin K, thus affecting clotting factors II, VII, IX, and X. If the blood cannot clot as well, the likelihood of another pulmonary embolus forming is lower.

3. Priority teaching for this patient before discharge includes information regarding compliance with lab testing (INR) and communication with the health care provider before taking any medications, herbals, or OTC preparations. Dietary restrictions include limiting the amount of vitamin K–rich foods, such as green leafy vegetables, in the diet, as well as careful consumption of vitamin C. Herbals such as St. John's wort, ginkgo, kava, and ginseng also decrease the effectiveness of warfarin. The nurse should also advise the patient that aspirin and NSAIDs should be avoided; acetaminophen may be used as a substitute for pain relief as needed.

Safety precautions should also be taken to prevent anything that would lead to a risk of bleeding. The patient should be advised to use a toothbrush with soft bristles and only shave with an electric razor. If the patient does sustain an injury, bleeding should be able to be controlled with direct pressure for 5–10 minutes with a sterile dressing. If this is not effective, the patient should notify the health care provider or go to the nearest emergency department. Any indications of bleeding such as epistaxis, hematemesis, or blood in the stool should be reported to the health care provider as well.

CHAPTER 41: ANTIHYPERLIPIDEMICS AND PERIPHERAL VASODILATORS

1. LDL, VLDL, HDL, chylomicrons
2. protein; fat
3. atherosclerotic plaques; heart disease
4. apolipoprotein
5. HMG-CoA reductase; HMG-CoA reductase inhibitors (statins)
6. homocysteine
7. arteriosclerosis; hyperlipidemia
8. b
9. c
10. a
11. a
12. b
13. e
14. d
15. c. There are two forms of apolipoproteins, apoB-48 and apoB-100. Of the two, apoB-100 is a better indicator for CAD.
16. d. Rhabdomyolysis is a severe side effect associated with statin drugs, such as atorvastatin. This occurs when muscle tissue breaks down.
17. b. High levels of homocysteine have been linked to loss of flexibility (elasticity) to the vessel walls.

Other effects associated with homocysteine include cardiovascular disease, stroke, blood clotting, damage to the vascular endothelial lining, and thickening of the vasculature.

18. c. Intermittent vascular claudications cause vasospasms, and vasodilators improve blood flow to the extremities. Gingko has been taken to treat intermittent claudication.

19. c

20. d. LDL contains 50–60% of cholesterol in circulation and with an elevated level increases the risk for atherosclerotic plaques and heart disease.

21. d

22. a. An HDL level of 22 mg/dL is low. The normal value should be greater than 60 mg/dL. Low levels of HDL put the patient in the high-risk category for cardiovascular disease. A value less than 35 mg/dL is considered high risk.

23. b. Lifestyle changes, such as eating a low-fat, low-cholesterol diet, generally lower the cholesterol level by only 10–30%. Other activities should be instituted, such as implementation of routine exercises to increase HDL level and cessation of smoking.

24. c. Diet, exercise, weight loss, and medication all play a vital role in decreasing cholesterol level. Diet continues to play a vital role, in spite of the antihyperlipidemic medication that is taken.

25. a. Cilostazol doses are in the range of 50–100 mg q12h with a maximum dose of 200 mg/d.

26. b, d, e. Cilostazol should be taken 30 minutes before or 2 hours after meals. Grapefruit juice will increase the levels of cilostazol, so it should be avoided. There is no contraindication for the use of acetaminophen. Headache and abdominal pain are both side effects of cilostazol. Blood pressure should be monitored frequently, and the patient should be encouraged to change positions slowly to prevent a precipitous drop in blood pressure.

27. a, d, f

28. a

Case Study

1. Atorvastatin is an HMG-CoA reductase inhibitor, or a "statin" drug. By inhibiting cholesterol synthesis in the liver, atorvastatin decreases LDL ("bad") cholesterol, slightly increases HDL ("good") cholesterol, and decreases triglycerides.

2. Atorvastatin is pregnancy category X. Atorvastatin is contraindicated to be used during pregnancy and breastfeeding. S.S. should use a reliable birth control to prevent pregnancy while on atorvastatin.

3. Monitoring the patient for the desired effect is an obvious priority, although it is important for the nurse to advise the patient that changes in lipid profiles may take several weeks for lipid levels to decline. Liver enzymes should also be drawn at baseline and monitored throughout therapy. Many statin drugs are contraindicated in acute hepatic disease.

Vision should be tested at least yearly, because there have been some studies that indicate an increased risk of cataracts in patients taking statins. This risk is higher in patients with diabetes.

4. The nurse should emphasize that treatment of hyperlipidemia is a lifelong commitment. Making dietary changes, exercising, and using pharmacologic therapy will help decrease LDL levels, and therefore potentially decrease the risk of heart disease. Other important points in the health teaching plan for S.S. include the importance of keeping follow-up appointments with health care providers, taking the medication as scheduled even if she does not feel she is making any progress, and reporting any muscle pain or tenderness immediately, because this can be an indication of the life-threatening adverse effect of rhabdomyolysis. She should report any vision changes. The nurse should also emphasize to not abruptly stop taking atorvastatin because of a serious rebound effect that could lead to a heart attack.

CHAPTER 42—GASTROINTESTINAL TRACT DISORDERS

1. f
2. d
3. e
4. b
5. g
6. c
7. a
8. chemoreceptor trigger zone (CTZ), medulla
9. antihistamines, bismuth subsalicylate, phosphorated carbohydrate
10. anticholinergics
11. glaucoma
12. dopamine antagonists
13. nausea, vomiting, serotonin or 5HT₃
14. cannabinoid
15. Laxatives, cathartics
16. sodium, magnesium
17. deficit, electrolyte
18. antihistamines, anticholinergics, dopamine antagonists, benzodiazepines, serotonin antagonists, glucocorticoids, cannabinoids, miscellaneous
19. fecal impaction, chronic laxative use, neurologic disorders, bowel obstruction, immobility, delayed defecation, insufficient fluid intake, poor dietary habits, certain drugs such as opioids and anticholinergics
20. Mix psyllium in 8–10 oz of water, stir, and drink immediately, followed by another glass of water.
21. False. Antiemetics are not recommended for pregnant women to consume because of the risk to the fetus. Instead nonpharmacologic treatment should be tried, such as flat soda or weak tea and crackers.
22. False. A "normal" bowel movement varies from one person to another. A "normal" number of

bowel movements can range from one per day to three per week.

23. True. Chronic use of laxatives can cause a person to become dependent on the laxative for a bowel movement, especially in older adults.

24. False. Castor oil should not be used during pregnancy because it can stimulate uterine contractions.

25. a, e. The CTZ lies near the medulla, and the vomiting center is in the medulla. These two areas, when stimulated, can cause vomiting. The medulla is an organ that contains the two areas.

26. a, b, c, e. All but the opioids can be used as antiemetics. Opioids can cause constipation that can decrease intestinal motility, thereby decreasing peristalsis; opioids can be used as antidiarrheals.

27. b. Promethazine is a phenothiazine that blocks H_1-receptor sites on effector cells, impedes histamine-mediated responses, and inhibits the CTZ.

28. a, b, c, d. Drinking weak tea and sodas that have gone flat may help with nausea. Open a can or bottle of soda and let it sit for several hours to remove its carbonation. Unsweetened gelatin may also be helpful. Crackers and dry toast may provide something to stay in the stomach. Relaxed breathing may help with the feeling of nausea, but it is usually more beneficial to breathe in through the nose and out through the mouth as is used in relaxation techniques.

29. c

30. c, d. Nonpharmacologic measures are now recommended for morning sickness. Some prescription antiemetics can be taken during pregnancy, but they are classified as pregnancy category C. Hydroxyzine is classified as pregnancy category X. OTC antiemetics are no longer considered safe. Some herbals are used during pregnancy, but they are not FDA approved. Telling the patient it will just go away in a few months, while this may or may not be true, negates the patient's feelings.

31. b. Antihistamines, such as diphenhydramine, are frequently used to treat motion sickness. They are available OTC. Anticholinergics and cannabinoids, while they can be used as antiemetics, are not generally used for motion sickness. Osmotics are considered laxatives.

32. a. When poison is ingested, vomiting should not be induced because regurgitating these substances can cause esophageal injury. Instead, activated charcoal is administered to absorb the poison.

33. a, b, c. Adsorbents, anticholinergics, and opioids can be used for diarrhea. Proton pump inhibitors inhibit the production of gastric acid. Selective serotonin reuptake inhibitors, such as ondansetron HCl, can be used as antiemetics.

34. a, b, e. Diphenoxylate with atropine is an antidiarrheal. Usual side effects are caused by atropine, an anticholinergic; these include headache, drowsiness,

and urinary retention. It also causes hypotension (not hypertension), nausea, and vomiting. It does not cause hypoglycemia.

35. c. Laxatives stimulate peristalsis, allowing for passage of soft stools.

36. b, d, e. Laxatives and/or cathartics include bulk-forming, emollients, and stimulants. Adsorbents are considered antidiarrheal, and emetics are used to induce vomiting.

37. a. Bisacodyl is a stimulant laxative used for bowel preparation and for prevention and short-term treatment of constipation. Its action increases peristalsis by directly affecting the smooth muscle of the intestine.

38. b. Stool softeners, such as docusate sodium, soften stools to allow easier passage of stool without straining. They are not used to treat diarrhea, vomiting, or nausea.

39. d. Patients with heart failure are not candidates for the use of saline cathartics. Saline cathartics pull fluid into the system, potentially making the heart failure worse.

40. b. Mineral oil absorbs the fat-soluble vitamins so the body cannot absorb them. This can lead to vitamin deficiency.

41. d. Patients with any kind of bowel obstruction or severe abdominal pain should not take laxatives.

42. a, c, d, e. Promethazine is an antihistamine given for nausea and/or vomiting. Antihistamines inhibit histamine-mediated responses and have anticholinergic effects, which include blurred vision, drowsiness, dry mouth, and hypotension.

43. a. Dronabinol, a cannabinoid, should be given 1–3 h before chemotherapy, then q2-4h with a maximum dose of 15 mg/m^2/dose or 6 doses/day.

44. d. Certain antidiarrheals, including those containing diphenoxylate, difenoxin, or loperamide, are contraindicated in patients with severe hepatic disease.

45. c, d. A patient with diarrhea should avoid "heavy" fried foods and milk products. Promoting fluid intake and replacing electrolytes are priority interventions when the patient is experiencing diarrhea.

Case Study

1. Constipation has a variety of causes, including decreased fluid intake, poor diet, lack of exercise, and current drugs. Lack of appetite is a frequent complaint among the older adult. Poor dentition may lead to inability to eat raw fruits and vegetables. The opioid L.B. is taking for her postoperative hip pain, as well as the potential for decreased mobility and lack of exercise, may also lead to constipation.

2. Bisacodyl is a stimulant laxative that promotes defecation by irritating the smooth muscle of the intestine.

3. Omeprazole and other proton pump inhibitors will decrease the effect of bisacodyl, so dosage

adjustments may need to be made. Calcium supplements can decrease the dissolving of bisacodyl. There are no serious interactions with either digoxin or hydrocodone.

4. It will be important for the nurse to encourage L.B. to eat well and exercise as much as possible. Including bran and whole grain in the diet may be beneficial. Bulk-forming laxatives can provide the fiber that she may not be getting in a regular diet. When possible, the patient should discontinue use of the opioid pain reliever. The nurse should also advise L.B. that the drug should be taken whole, with a glass of water. Milk should be avoided around the time of administration, because milk also reduces the effectiveness of the laxative. L.B. should be instructed on the side effects of bisacodyl, such as abdominal cramps.

CHAPTER 43: ANTIULCER

1. g
2. a, h
3. e
4. b
5. f
6. c
7. i
8. a
9. e
10. d
11. c
12. d
13. a
14. d
15. c
16. e
17. b
18. d
19. b
20. b. Antacids neutralize hydrochloric acid and should be taken 1–3 hours before meals and at bedtime. They should not be taken with meals because of the delayed gastric emptying time, which can increase acid production.
21. a. Taking a liquid antacid with water increases gastric emptying time.
22. b, c, d, f. Antiulcer drugs include anticholinergics, antacids, H_2 blockers, and PPIs. Other antiulcer drugs include tranquilizers, pepsin inhibitors, and prostaglandin E_1 analogues.
23. c, e. Commonly used drugs to treat GERD include H_2 blockers and PPIs. Anticholinergics and pepsin inhibitors are commonly used to treat ulcers. Antacids are used to prevent ulcers.
24. a, b, d, e. There are various nonpharmacologic methods to help prevent the discomfort associated with gastroesophageal reflux disease (GERD). Nicotine relaxes the lower esophageal sphincter so acid can reflux back into the esophagus. Elevating

the head of the bed will allow the body to work with gravity instead of against it to keep acid in the stomach. NSAIDs can cause gastric ulcers. Spicy foods are irritating to the lining of the esophagus.

25. d. Propantheline is an anticholinergic that inhibits gastric secretions and is used to treat peptic ulcers. Anticholinergics should be taken before meals to decrease acid secretion and at bedtime. It should not be used as a monotherapy.
26. a, b, e
27. a, b, c. Nizatidine should not be taken with meals, because it will delay absorption. The abdominal pain should have improved within 1–2 weeks, depending on the cause. Healing of the ulcer may take 4–8 weeks.
28. a. All the drugs are PPIs that are effective in treating GERD and ulcers; however, esomeprazole has the highest success rate for *erosive* GERD.
29. a, b, d, e. Side effects of ranitidine and other H_2 blockers include confusion, headache, decreased libido, and nausea. Other side effects include dizziness, constipation, abdominal pain, diarrhea, vomiting, blurred vision, malaise, and weakness.
30. a, b, c. There are no documented interactions between esomeprazole and either lisinopril or propranolol. Esomeprazole interferes with the absorption of ampicillin, digoxin, and ketoconazole.
31. c. Hyperglycemia is an adverse reaction to sucralfate. Although the normal range for blood glucose may vary, a blood glucose level of 185 mg/dL is considered elevated. Another adverse reaction includes hypophosphatemia.

Case Study

1. There are seven groups of antiulcer drugs: tranquilizers, anticholinergics, histamine$_2$ blockers, proton pump inhibitors, pepsin inhibitors, prostaglandin E_1 analogues, and antacids.
2. Aluminum hydroxide is a nonsystemic antacid composed of alkaline salts and aluminum. Antacids, as their name implies, neutralize acids that destroy the gastric mucosal barrier. They may be taken alone or in combination with other medications for ulcers.
3. The usual dose for aluminum hydroxide is 10 mL, 1 to 3 hour after meals and at bedtime, however the dosage is variable and may be more depending on the reason for taking antacids.
4. The priority teaching right now for this patient is in regard to the proper dose. The patient should be advised to drink 2–4 ounces of water with the aluminum hydroxide and to decrease or eliminate consumption of alcohol and caffeinated beverages. Aluminum hydroxide should not be taken with milk or foods high in vitamin D because of the risk for hypophosphatemia and hypercalcemia. S.S. should also avoid spicy or high-fat foods and caffeinated beverages, which can further irritate the gastric mucosa. There are many

predisposing factors for ulcers, including environmental factors such as a high-stress job. Learning to utilize relaxation techniques and decrease stress may help the patient's discomfort. The patient should also be advised of the potential side effects, including anorexia and constipation.

CHAPTER 44—EYE AND EAR DISORDERS

1. locally
2. artificial eyes
3. NSAIDs; corticosteroids
4. tear
5. intraocular; trabecular
6. angle-closure glaucoma
7. diuretics; glaucoma
8. cycloplegics
9. increase
10. conjunctivitis
11. carbonic anhydrase inhibitors
12. parasympathomimetic
13. h
14. f
15. i
16. a
17. b
18. d
19. c
20. j
21. g
22. e
23. c. Mydriatics dilate pupils for better visualization during a diagnostic procedure.
24. c. Acetazolamide is a systemic carbonic anhydrase inhibitor used to decrease IOP. Acetazolamide is also a diuretic and can cause fluid and electrolyte imbalances.
25. a, b, c, d. Small pupils or miosis is not a side effect of this medication.
26. d. Before ear irrigation, direct visualization of the tympanic membrane is necessary to avoid damaging the TM. A perforated TM is a contraindication for ear irrigation.
27. b. Carbamide peroxide is an OTC medication that helps break up cerumen so it can be washed away.
28. a, c, d, e. Pilocarpine is a cholinergic agonist with minimal systemic effects, but they do occur. Most common side effects include blurred vision, eye pain, and headache. Cardiac dysrhythmias and respiratory depression are adverse reactions and are deemed an emergency.
29. a, d
30. e. There are two types of age-related macular degeneration, wet and dry. Dry AMD is more common, with vision being gradually lost. There is no known treatment or drug for dry AMD.
31. a, b, c, d. Tetracaine is a topical anesthetic. The other medications listed are decongestants to help

with the eye irritation attributable to allergies. Ophthalmic allergy drugs contain antihistamines and/or mast cell stabilizers.
32. c. *S. pneumoniae* is the most common, followed by *H. influenzae* and *M. catarrhalis*.
33. b. A cotton wick is placed inside the EAC for medication to reach the length of the EAC. When the swelling subsides, the wick will fall out or it can be manually removed.

Case Study

1. Open-angle glaucoma occurs when there is too much aqueous humor that causes pressure and damages the optic nerve, which leads to decreased vision. As aqueous humor is formed, excess fluid drains through the trabecular meshwork structure of the eye. In open-angle glaucoma, the trabecular network is clogged and the excess fluid cannot drain. Open-angle glaucoma occurs gradually, and the cause is unknown.
2. There are several different classes of medications that are used to treat glaucoma. Timolol is a nonselective beta-adrenergic blocker. Beta blockers are usually the first-line drugs in glaucoma treatment. Beta blockers work by decreasing the production of aqueous humor.
3. The patient should wash her hands before administration of the drug and be very careful not to touch the tip of the bottle to the eye. The head should be tipped back and one drop instilled in the conjunctival sac of the lower lid. The patient should not rub her eyes after the drug is instilled. A tissue can be used to dab at the extra drug. Eyedrops should be instilled before any eye ointment.
4. No. This dose is too high. The standard dose is 1 gtt of 0.25–0.5% solution bid initially; then it can be decreased to 1 gtt/day as the condition stabilizes. The patient must be carefully observed for bradycardia, bronchospasm, and indications of developing or worsening heart failure, since this drug may cause systemic effects.

CHAPTER 45: DERMATOLOGIC DISORDERS

1. c
2. d
3. b
4. a
5. f, i
6. h
7. b, c, d, e
8. a
9. athlete's foot, ringworm
10. Comedones, whiteheads, blackheads
11. teratogen, iPLEDGE
12. multisystem, skin, joints
13. rebound
14. T-cell

15. desquamation
16. thinning, atrophy
17. a, c, d. Acne vulgaris is a common skin disorder treated nonpharmacologically or with pharmacotherapy. Drugs used to treat acne include antibiotics, corticosteroids, and keratolytics. Antifungals can be used for skin disorders caused by tineas. Nonsteroidal antiinflammatories are not effective for skin inflammation. A T-cell antagonist, such as methotrexate, is a folate antimetabolite for systemic treatment of psoriasis.
18. b
19. a. Calcipotriene is a synthetic vitamin D analogue that enhances keratinocyte differentiation while inhibiting their proliferation. There is no cure for psoriasis, but there are periods of remissions and exacerbations.
20. b. Infliximab is a biologic response modifier; specifically it inhibits tumor necrosis factor and is given in a controlled environment via IV injection at prescribed intervals.
21. b, c, e. Contact dermatitis, a common form of eczema, can cause local manifestations, such as rash, swelling, and stinging at the affected skin site. Common skin irritants include cosmetics, dyes, and plants. Anesthetics and peanuts can also cause an allergic response, but usually the manifestations are systemic, such as anaphylaxis.
22. a. The standard initial dose for tetracycline is 125–250 mg q6h for 1–2 weeks; then the dose can be decreased to 125–500 mg daily or every other day.
23. d
24. a, b, d. The patient should be encouraged to report to the health care provider if she is pregnant or plans on becoming pregnant because tetracycline has possible teratogenic effects. Harsh cleansers may be irritating to skin that may already be sensitive. Tetracycline taken in combination with isotretinoin will increase the potential for adverse effects. Sunscreens with SPF15 and higher are recommended for all adults.
25. c. Hair loss or alopecia can be treated with minoxidil solution to stimulate hair growth. Acitretin and methotrexate are for psoriasis. Tretinoin can be used for acne and warts.
26. a, b, c. Contact dermatitis attributable to skin irritants can be treated with antiinflammatories or topical corticosteroids, such as triamcinolone and dexamethasone, and/or antihistamines, such as diphenhydramine. Fluconazole is an antifungal. Salicylic acid is used to treat acne, psoriasis, or verruca vulgaris.

Case Study

1. Full-thickness burns extend down and include the epidermis, the dermis, and the subcutaneous tissue. They have also been referred to as *third-degree burns*. Full-thickness burns may appear red, black, or white and are not painful because the nerve endings have been destroyed. Partial-thickness burns do not extend as deep; there may be blistering. Partial-thickness burns are very painful. Frequently partial-thickness (second-degree) burns surround a full-thickness burn.
2. Mafenide acetate is a broad-spectrum antibiotic that is applied topically (1.6 mm thick once or twice daily) to the burned area. Mafenide is a sulfonamide derivative, and it interferes with bacterial cell-wall synthesis and metabolism.
3. Another treatment option is silver sulfadiazine. It is also applied topically to the burned surface. Silver sulfadiazine acts on the cell membrane and cell wall. It is less likely to cause metabolic acidosis than mafenide.
4. Priority nursing interventions for this patient are adequate fluid resuscitation, pain control, and prevention of infection by providing sterile dressing changes. It will be easier for this patient to receive skin grafting when appropriate if there have been fewer to no infections.

CHAPTER 46: PITUITARY, THYROID, PARATHYROID, AND ADRENAL DISORDERS

1. f
2. h
3. i
4. a
5. m
6. b
7. l
8. n
9. c
10. g
11. d
12. k
13. l
14. e
15. Adrenal hyposecretion (hypocortisolism): anemia, hyponatremia, hyperkalemia, hypoglycemia, weight loss, fatigue, hypotension, tachycardia, diarrhea, hyperpigmentation. Adrenal hypersecretion (hypercortisolism): weight gain, hyperglycemia, buffalo hump, edema, delayed wound healing, hyperlipidemia, peptic ulcers, hirsutism, hypertension, hypernatremia, hypokalemia.
16. a
17. d
18. e
19. g
20. c
21. b
22. f
23. c. The normal dose is 25–50 mcg/day initially, with a maintenance dose of 50–200 mcg/day.
24. d. Manifestations from hypothyroidism are usually alleviated within 2 to 4 weeks without having symptoms of adverse reactions. Activity level

is usually improved within 4 weeks of thyroid treatment.

25. a, c, d. Symptoms of hyperthyroidism include palpitations, excessive perspiration, and tachycardia. Constipation is a symptom of hypothyroidism, not hyperthyroidism.

26. a. Levothyroxine should be taken on an empty stomach at least 30 to 60 min before breakfast.

27. a, e. Over-the-counter drugs are generally contraindicated in patients with hypothyroidism. Patients with thyroid disorders should be encouraged to wear a medical alert identification. Drugs for hypothyroidism should be taken on an empty stomach. Numbness and tingling of the hands occurs with hypoparathyroidism, not hypothyroidism. Hypothyroidism causes weight gain; it is not a priority to teach patients to increase food and fluid intake.

28. b

29. d. Prednisone is a glucocorticoid steroid. Long-term use can cause sodium and fluid retention.

30. b. Prednisone is a corticosteroid and should be taken with food to prevent irritation of gastric mucosa.

31. b, c, d, e. Concurrent use with NSAIDs including aspirin can increase the risk of GI bleed; phenytoin can decrease the effect of glucocorticoids; digitalis toxicity can occur and may cause dysrhythmias; and diuretics can increase potassium loss, increasing the risk of hypokalemia.

32. c, d, e. Obtaining a drug history is important before starting a patient on prednisone, because there are many drug interactions possible with glucocorticoids. Vital signs and daily weights should be monitored. Weight gain is a side effect of prednisone.

33. b. Glucocorticoids can lead to fluid retention. Adequate fluid intake should be ensured but not forced.

34. b. Corticosteroids can decrease serum potassium and cause hypokalemia. Herbal laxatives or diuretics taken concurrently with corticosteroids can worsen hypokalemia.

35. b. Corticosteroids increases metabolism and can cause insomnia; these effects can worsen when taken with herbal stimulants, such as ginseng.

36. a

37. a, b, c, d. Fresh fruit is not as high in potassium as dried fruit, although there are fresh fruit options, such as bananas and kiwi, that do provide a source of potassium.

38. a, b, e

39. b, c, d, e

Case Study

1. Signs and symptoms of adrenal insufficiency include muscle wasting, apathy, nausea, vomiting, electrolyte imbalances, hypovolemia, anemia, and cardiovascular collapse.

2. Hydrocortisone 20–240 mg/d in 2–4 divided doses can be given orally. This hydrocortisone, depending on its formulation, can be administered IV, IM, or subcut route; the dose and frequency may be different.

3. Priority teaching for this patient is to recognize and report symptoms of Cushing syndrome, which includes puffy eyelids, edematous feet, increased bruising, dizziness, and bleeding. Also, the patient should be advised against abruptly stopping the drug for adrenal insufficiency. Laboratory values will be monitored closely to watch for hypoglycemia, anemia, and electrolyte imbalances. The patient should be encouraged to carry a medical alert identification and a current list of drugs. Herbal preparations should be avoided unless discussed with the health care provider. Teach patient to weigh himself/herself daily.

CHAPTER 47: ANTIDIABETICS

1. d
2. f
3. h
4. c
5. g
6. e
7. a
8. b
9. 120 days, 3
10. obesity, stress, insulin resistance
11. abdomen
12. gastrointestinal secretions
13. lipodystrophy, rotating
14. insulin resistance, allergy
15. c
16. a
17. f
18. b
19. a
20. d
21. regular
22. Somogyi effect
23. Hyperglycemia, dawn
24. hypoglycemia
25. biguanide, glucose, absorption, receptor, peripheral
26. 48 hours, lactic acidosis
27. type 2, not
28. a, b, e. Three major symptoms of diabetes are characterized by the three p's that include polydipsia (increased thirst), polyphagia (increased hunger), and polyuria (increased urination).
29. a, b, d. Certain drugs increase serum glucose level (hyperglycemia), including cortisone, hydrochlorothiazide, and epinephrine. Doxepin is a tricyclic antidepressant that can lower blood glucose level. Thiazolidinediones are a class of oral antidiabetic drugs that lower blood glucose level.
30. b. Lipodystrophy, tissue atrophy or hypertrophy, can occur from frequent injections; insulin injec-

tions should be rotated to prevent lipodystrophy. Rotating injection sites does not prevent an allergic reaction, polyuria, or rejection of insulin.

31. d

32. b, c, d, e. The patient experiencing hypoglycemia can have headache, sweating, nervousness, and tremor. Abdominal pain and vomiting can occur because of a reaction to oral antidiabetic drugs.

33. b, c, d, e, f. Signs and symptoms of ketoacidosis include dry mucous membrane, fruity breath odor, Kussmaul respirations, polyuria, and thirst. The patient can also develop tachycardia, not bradycardia.

34. d. Tolazamide is a first-generation intermediate-acting oral antidiabetic drug. Oral drugs in this class should not be used by patients with type 1 diabetes; instead, insulin is used.

35. a, c, d, e, f. Insulin dose should be based on glucose testing and not how a patient is feeling. Compliance with the regimen is crucial.

36. a, b, c, d. Oral antidiabetic medications should be taken on a regular, prescribed basis and not adjusted by glucose testing results.

37. a. Lipoatrophy or tissue atrophy is a form of lipodystrophy involving a depression under the skin surface. Hypertrophy or lipohypertrophy, another form of lipodystrophy, is a raised lump or knot on the skin surface.

38. a. Unopened insulin vials should be kept in the refrigerator, and an opened vial can be kept in the refrigerator or kept at room temperature. They should not be stored in the freezer, exposed to direct sunlight, or left in a high-temperature area.

39. c. Cloudy insulin is mixed by rolling the vial. Shaking the vial can cause bubbles, which can lead to an inaccurate dose.

40. c. When giving both NPH and regular insulin at the same time, the regular insulin is drawn into the syringe first.

41. d. U100 syringes are used for U100 insulin.

42. a, c, e. The patient needs to develop a rotation pattern to prevent lipodystrophy and promote insulin absorption. Insulin is not administered IM. The ADA's suggested actions do not include injection into a different area of the body every day.

43. a. Regular insulin is short-acting, with an onset of 30 minutes to 1 hour.

44. c. NPH is an intermediate-acting insulin with a peak action in 4 to 12 hours.

45. b, d, e. Insulin glargine is a long-acting insulin that is evenly distributed over a 24-hour duration of action and is usually administered in the evening (bedtime). It is available in a prefilled cartridge, and some patients have complained of pain at the injection site. Hypoglycemia can still occur, but it is not as common as with other insulins. Some patients may need coverage with rapid-acting or short-acting insulins.

46. c

47. c. Insulin pumps are used for type 1 diabetics and they reduce the number of hypoglycemic reactions.

An insulin pump is not used with intermediate insulin, such as NPH, because of unpredictable glucose control. Insulin pumps use a needle to insert a cannula under the skin; the needle does not stay inserted.

48. a. Depending on the class of oral antidiabetic drugs, they can increase the insulin cell receptor sensitivity, increase insulin release from the pancreas, decrease hepatic production of glucose, decrease glucose absorption from the small intestine, and/or increase peripheral glucose uptake at the cellular level.

49. b. Repaglinide is a meglitinide, an oral antidiabetic drug, that stimulates beta cells of the pancreas to release insulin; there must be some beta cell function for this to occur. It is not insulin.

50. a, c, d. Metformin, a biguanide, increases tissue response and decreases glucose production by the liver.

51. b. Nonsulfonylureas include biguanides and alpha-glucosidase inhibitors that decrease glucose production by the liver. They can cause hypoglycemic reactions. Biguanides decrease, not increase, the absorption of glucose from the small intestine. Nonsulfonylureas are oral antidiabetic drugs that decrease serum glucose level, not increase it.

52. b. Pioglitazone is a thiazolidinedione that decreases insulin resistance, thereby increasing insulin cell receptor sensitivity.

53. b. Ginseng can lower blood glucose level; garlic may increase blood glucose level. Concomitant use of these complementary and alternative drugs may necessitate a change in the insulin or oral antidiabetic drug dose.

54. b, c, d

55. b, c, d, e. Aspirin, oral anticoagulants, and cimetidine can increase the action of sulfonylureas, especially with the first-generations, by binding to plasma proteins and displacing sulfonylureas. The action of sulfonylureas may be decreased by taking several different types of medications, including anticonvulsants such as phenytoin.

Case Study

1. Although there are a variety of causes for these symptoms, when a diabetic patient presents with a headache, confusion, slurred speech, and a glucometer reading of "low," a hypoglycemic reaction should be suspected. Although readings may vary depending on brand of glucometer, a reading of "low" may be in the 20 mg/dL range. This is an emergency and must be treated quickly.

2. As long as the patient is conscious, hard candy, sugar-sweetened fluids, or glucose paste may be given. Other options include fruit juice or peanut butter crackers.

3. Once the patient becomes unconscious, other options must be explored. The patient may receive

glucagon to stimulate glycogenolysis. A benefit of giving glucagon is that it may be administered IM, IV, or subcut. The blood glucose level begins to increase within 10 minutes after administration.

CHAPTER 48: URINARY DISORDERS

1. b
2. e
3. d
4. f
5. e
6. d
7. c
8. a
9. e
10.

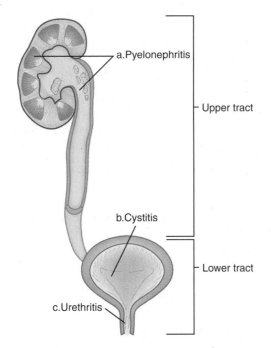

a. Pyelonephritis

Upper tract

b. Cystitis

Lower tract

c. Urethritis

11. c
12. b. Cranberry juice will help lower the pH and make the urine more acidic. Whole milk may make urine more alkaline and increase the pH. Although increased fluid intake is important when a patient has a urinary tract infection (UTI), simply increasing the amount of water alone will not decrease the urine pH. Prune juice will make the urine acidic, not alkalotic.
13. b. Flavoxate is an antispasmodic and is contraindicated in patients with glaucoma.
14. c, d, e. Ertapenem, an antiseptic, has side effects that include diarrhea, headache, and nausea. Other side effects include drowsiness, confusion, agitation, and elevated hepatic enzymes.
15. a, c, d, e
16. d. Tingling or numbness of extremities could be a sign of neuropathy, which can be irreversible and needs to be evaluated immediately. Brown- or rust-colored urine and diarrhea can be side effects of

nitrofurantoin, but they do not need to be immediately reported to the provider. Frequency in urination is common with UTIs.
17. a, b, e. Urinary analgesics, such as phenazopyridine, are used to relieve symptoms associated with cystitis (pain, burning, frequency, and urgency).
18. c. Phenazopyridine is a urinary analgesic. Bethanechol is a urinary stimulant, flavoxate is an antispasmodic, and trimethoprim is an antiinfective.
19. d. Bright reddish-orange urine is to be expected when taking phenazopyridine. This can be very startling to the patient if she is not told in advance to anticipate the change. Undergarments can also be stained orange while taking this medication.
20. b
21. a, c, d, e. Bethanechol is a urinary stimulant and would not benefit this patient who has overactive bladder. Nitrofurantoin is an antiinfective and, unless this patient has a UTI, there is no need for it. Oxybutynin and tolterodine tartrate, although beneficial to patients with overactive bladder, are contraindicated in patients with glaucoma.
22. b. Bethanechol chloride is a urinary stimulant that increases bladder tone. It is prescribed when bladder function is lost because of spinal cord injuries, such as with paralysis.

Case Study

1. Oxybutynin chloride is a urinary antispasmodic that has direct action on the smooth muscles of the urinary tract. By relaxing these muscles, the spasms are decreased.
2. Patients who have urinary or GI obstruction as well as those with narrow-angle glaucoma should not take oxybutynin. Oxybutynin blocks acetylcholine receptors that mediate parasympathetic function. Should the patient experience severe abdominal pain, constipation, or urinary retention, the health care provider should be contacted immediately.
3. Common side effects may include dry mouth, drowsiness, blurred vision, headache, insomnia, tachycardia, GI distress, and constipation. The patient should be encouraged not to participate in any activities where dizziness could be an issue (climbing, skateboarding, etc.). The patient should be warned not to drive or operate heavy machinery until he knows how the drug will affect him. If any of these symptoms are severe, his health care provider should be contacted.
4. No, the dosage range for adults and adolescents is 5 mg bid/qid, with a maximum of 20 mg/day.

CHAPTER 49: PREGNANCY AND PRETERM LABOR

1. g
2. f
3. j

Answer Key

4. i
5. a
6. b
7. d
8. e
9. h
10. c
11. a, b, c, d
12. a, c, d, g
13. c
14. c, d
15. g
16. e
17. f, h
18. h
19. a
20. c, d, e. Maternal physiologic changes seen during pregnancy affecting drug actions include increased maternal circulating volume, resulting in dilution of drugs; increased glomerular filtration rate and rapid elimination of drugs; and increased liver metabolism. Other changes are reduced GI motility and increased gastric pH, making the environment more alkaline; and the clearance of drugs is altered during late pregnancy, resulting in decreased serum concentration.
21. a
22. a, b, d. Timing, dose, and duration of drug exposure are crucial in determining the drug's teratogenicity. The teratogeni period begins 2 weeks after conception and exposure to teratogens can result in birth defects and/or death of the fetus.
23. b, d
24. b
25. b. Corticosteroids, such as betamethasone, accelerate lung maturity and surfactant development in the fetus in utero, thereby decreasing the incidence and severity of respiratory distress.
26. b, d, e. Gestational hypertension can have devastating maternal and fetal effects. Gestational hypertension can progress to preeclampsia and/or eclampsia, increasing the risk of HELLP syndrome and seizures. The goals for patients who develop gestational hypertension include prevention of HELLP syndrome, delivery of an uncompromised fetus, reduction of vasospasms, and prevention of seizures.
27. a, c, d. GI complaints are the most common during pregnancy, possibly resulting from elevated levels of progesterone, which causes decreased gut motility and relaxation of the cardiac sphincter.
28. c. In maternal iron deficiency anemia, iron supplements will show a modest reticulocyte count increase in 5 to 7 days; a rise in the hemoglobin level will be seen in 3 weeks.
29. b. Acetaminophen is generally considered safe in pregnancy. Combination cold medications, especially those that contain aspirin or ibuprofen, are not recommended. Mega doses of vitamins and any herbal preparations are not considered to be safe.
30. a, b. It is important to provide culturally competent care to all patients. All patients should receive information in the language in which they are most comfortable. Either obtaining a trained translator or using a service like a language line is crucial to show your respect for the patient and her culture. Family members should not be used to translate in the health care setting if at all possible. Allow the patient and family adequate time to ask questions and do not hurry since time frame of reference is different in the Hispanic culture.
31. a, c, d, e. Fluids should not necessarily be avoided before arising. Sometimes small sips of flat soda or apple juice may be beneficial.
32. a, b, c, e. Avoidance of spicy foods or foods known to cause heartburn is a mainstay in the nonpharmacologic treatment of heartburn. This includes citrus fruits and juices and tomato-based products. Smaller meals lead to less reflux of gastric contents, as does keeping the head slightly raised for a period of time after eating. Many pregnant women late in their third trimester find it more comfortable to sleep in a recliner to prevent reflux.
33. a, b, d. The patient should be instructed to lie on her left side to prevent supine hypotensive syndrome. Maintaining an adequate diet with proper amounts of fluids, protein, and sodium is important for the well-being of both mother and baby. Recording daily weights and looking for trends, as well as keeping track of symptoms such as headache, nausea, and extremity swelling, are important for the patient with gestational hypertension.
34. b, c, e. Iron supplements should be taken 2 hours before or 4 hours after antacids so the medication can be absorbed. Although best taken on an empty stomach, iron can be taken with food if necessary. Jaundice should be reported immediately to the health care provider. Vitamin C found in orange juice can enhance iron absorption.
35. a. Foods that are rich in iron include broccoli, red meat, nuts, spinach, and iron-fortified cereal.
36. b
37. a. Aspirin and ibuprofen use during pregnancy is contraindicated. Diphenhydramine is an antihistamine.
38. a. Breath sounds should be auscultated at least every 4 hours and assessed for the presence of wheezes, crackles, or coughing. Maternal myocardial ischemia and pulmonary edema can be an adverse reaction to beta-sympathomimetic agents, such as terbutaline.
39. b, d, e. The loading dose of magnesium sulfate 6 g is given over 20–30 minutes as an IVPB. It is administered via a pump. Too-rapid administration of magnesium sulfate can lead to cardiac arrest. Patients receiving magnesium sulfate are on bed rest while receiving therapy and should be monitored continuously. Calcium gluconate is the antidote for magnesium sulfate and should be at the bedside

for emergency. Decreased or loss of DTRs is an adverse reaction to magnesium sulfate.

40. a, d. Loss of DTRs and respiratory depression are manifestations for magnesium toxicity, and calcium gluconate should be administered. Tachycardia is an expected side effect and should be monitored.

41. d. Magnesium sulfate is used to halt contractions during preterm labor and should not be given for more than 5–7 days because of fetal harm.

42. a, b, c. NSAIDs, such as aspirin and ibuprofen, can cause maternal anemia and greater blood loss at delivery, and the overall homeostasis of the fetus can be compromised. Additionally, ibuprofen, when taken late in pregnancy, can prematurely close the ductus arteriosus.

43. a, b, d. Side effects and adverse reactions are generally dose related and include flushing, nausea, and slurred speech. Other side effects include feelings of increased warmth, perspiration, nasal congestion, lethargy, decreased gut motility, tachycardia, and hypotension.

44. d

45. b, d, e. Diuretics, such as furosemide, and ACE inhibitors, such as lisinopril, are contraindicated in pregnancy.

Case Study

1. Some priority questions to ask include if K.R. has been receiving regular prenatal care and the date of her last visit. The nurse should inquire if there are any known complications with this pregnancy such as gestational diabetes, gestational hypertension, or hyperemesis gravidarum. K.R. should also be questioned regarding membrane rupture and for any bleeding or changes in fetal movement. Other questions should include substance use, including herbals, caffeine, and tobacco use.

2. K.R. is at high risk because of her age, history of miscarriage, and previous PTL.

3. Nonpharmacologic measures that the nurse can suggest while K.R. is waiting to hear back from the health care provider include lying down on her left side, or if that is not possible, at least sitting down and putting her feet up. Dehydration may lead to PTL, so K.R. should drink several glasses of water. Having an empty bladder may also help, so the patient should be advised to void. If nonpharmacologic measures are not effective, the patient may require tocolytics. There are no FDA-approved drugs for PTL. But, beta sympathomimetics (terbutaline), magnesium sulfate, or prostaglandin inhibitors are used as "off label" to halt or delay labor. One of the major goals in tocolytic therapy is to interrupt or inhibit uterine contractions to create additional time for fetal maturation in utero.

4. Although the survival rate of a fetus at 33 weeks is fairly high, the baby is preterm and will require close observation. The mother may be given corticosteroids, such as betamethasone or dexamethasone, to accelerate fetal lung maturity and development of surfactant to decrease the incidence of respiratory distress syndrome in preterm infants.

CHAPTER 50—LABOR, DELIVERY, AND POSTPARTUM

1. a. spinal block; b. epidural block
2. b
3. d
4. e
5. a
6. c
7. b
8. d
9. a
10. c
11. latent, active, transition
12. neonatal
13. mu; kappa
14. should not
15. saddle block
16. oxytocin; also ergot alkaloids, prostaglandins
17. decreases
18. Rh$_0$(D) immunoglobulin
19. a
20. d. Postdural headaches are caused by leakage of cerebrospinal fluid through a puncture site. The decrease in pressure exerted by the CSF causes the headache.
21. a, b, c, d. Postural headaches can occur with regional anesthesia, such as epidural or spinal anesthesia. Patient should be advised that bed rest, oral analgesics, and/or caffeine can help relieve the headache. At times, an autologous blood patch may be needed.
22. a
23. d. Opioids can cause maternal or neonate respiratory depression. A reversal agent, naloxone, is given.
24. a. Before administering general anesthesia, antacids or other drugs that decrease gastric secretions are given to decrease gastric acidity. They may also prevent nausea and vomiting, but these are not the primary reasons for their administration just before general anesthesia.
25. a. A fluid bolus of 500–1000 mL should be given to prevent hypotension that frequently accompanies an epidural.
26. d. Patients with hypotension are positioned on their left side to facilitate placental perfusion.
27. c
28. d
29. a. Patients with hypertension should not receive methylergonovine. When this drug is given IV, dramatic increases in blood pressure can occur.

30. b. Naloxone is a narcotic antagonist and will reverse the effects of meperidine, leading to an increase in pain.

31. d. The choice of pain control is very individual. Each woman has an expectation of what she wants with regard to the labor experience.

32. d. Barbiturates provide rest and relaxation rather than pain relief. On the other hand, opioids affect the mu and kappa receptors for complete pain relief.

33. a, b, d, e. The time of delivery cannot be predicted, whether analgesics are utilized or not.

34. c. The patient should be placed flat immediately to ensure that the local anesthetic disperses evenly. The nurse must assess that the anesthetic is evenly dispersed. If this is not the case, the anesthesia provider should be made aware and the patient turned to the opposite side.

35. c

36. a, c

37. b, c, d, e. Deep tendon reflexes are usually assessed on a patient receiving magnesium sulfate, not oxytocin. A type and crossmatch should be obtained in the event that the patient will need an emergent cesarean section. The fetus may become hypoxic, and there is an increased risk for uterine rupture.

38. a, c, e. Signs of uterine rupture include FHR decelerations, sudden increased pain, loss of uterine contractions, hemorrhage, and hypovolemia leading to shock.

39. b, d, e

40. c, d. Somatic pain occurs during the transition phase and the second stage of labor. Pain is caused by the stretching of the perineum and vagina.

41. b, c, e. Anesthesia for cesarean delivery may be general, spinal, or epidural. General anesthesia allows for rapid anesthesia induction and control of the airway.

42. a, d. Topical agents used for pain relief for perineal wounds include benzocaine and witch hazel.

43. a

44. b

45. b

46. a

Case Study

1. Inductions are based on several factors, including intrauterine growth retardation. At 38 weeks' gestation, K.E. is considered full-term. There are several options to induce labor. Before delivery, the cervix must efface, or thin, and dilate. A mechanical device such as a Foley catheter can be placed through the cervical os, and then 30 mL of sterile saline instilled into the balloon. This will act similarly to manual stripping of the membranes to start labor. Another method is to place prostaglandin E_2 (PGE_2) either intracervically or intravaginally. It is usually left in place for approximately 12 hours and then synthetic

oxytocin is started intravenously to augment labor. Once the cervix has dilated to approximately 5 cm, an amniotomy ("breaking the bag") may be performed under sterile conditions. Labor will tend to get into an established pattern within a few hours of the amniotic sac being broken.

2. Priority teaching for this patient includes advising her to communicate her needs and desires to the health care team regarding analgesia and delivery. Ideally a "birth plan" will have been developed by the patient and her partner in advance. This plan is usually submitted to the health care provider and is brought with the patient to the hospital. As much as is possible and safe, the patient should be able to control her delivery.

3. Analgesia may be provided by intravenous narcotic agonists, mixed agonist-antagonists, and regional anesthesia (epidurals, blocks). The patient should also have the option of refraining from the use of analgesics if she desires ("natural childbirth").

CHAPTER 51: NEONATAL AND NEWBORN

1. Respiratory distress syndrome; surfactant
2. endotracheal
3. Hyperoxia; hypocarbia
4. newborn
5. ophthalmia neonatorum
6. d. Surfactant replacement, such as beractant, is given to premature newborns with immature lung development.
7. c. Exogenous surfactant must be warmed before administration by warming it in the hands for 8 minutes or at room temperature for 20 minutes. The vial should not be shaken.
8. b, d, e
9. a, b, d. Complications during and following administration of surfactant can cause bradycardia and hyperoxia. Desaturation can also occur because transient esophageal reflux an obstruct the ET tube. Cyanosis, not pallor, is another complication.
10. b. Generally, complications such as cyanosis and hypoxia after surfactant administration do not lead to severe complications when properly managed. The nurse should assist in repositioning the neonate to disperse the drug throughout the lung. Suctioning is appropriate if an obvious sign of airway obstruction is noted.
11. d. HBIG should be given to the newborn if the mother is hepatitis B positive. The first of three series doses of recombinant hepatitis B should be given as a separate injection and separate site. The HBIG provides passive protection while the newborn's body develops acquired immunity to the recombinant hepatitis B vaccine.
12. b
13. a. The swelling should decrease and disappear within 24–48 hours after administration of the ophthalmic medications.

Case Study

1. Hepatitis B virus transmission occurs vertically at the time of delivery when the neonate is exposed to the mother's blood and body fluids.
2. The nurse should acknowledge J.G.'s concerns and inform her that her baby will receive medications to decrease the risk of developing hepatitis B.
3. The nurse would anticipate administering hepatitis B immune globulin (HBIG) and the first dose of recombinant hepatitis B. HBIG should be administered within 12 hours of birth. HBIG provides immediate passive protection against liver damage. Recombinant hepatitis B stimulates the body to produce antibodies against hepatitis B viruses.
4. Recombinant hepatitis B vaccine is given in three series. The first one is given within 12 hours after birth. Subsequent doses are given at 1 month and again at 6 months of age.

CHAPTER 52—WOMEN'S REPRODUCTIVE HEALTH

1. b
2. e
3. d
4. c
5. a
6. menarche; menopause
7. estrogen
8. spironolactone; diuretic
9. 48
10. anovulation; amenorrhea
11. b
12. d
13. c
14. a
15. e
16. b, c, d
17. c. A woman with breast cancer should not take oral contraceptives because the hormones could accelerate tumor growth.
18. a, b, c. There are no contraindications for using combined hormone contraceptives (CHCs) in epilepsy, but other medications that the patient takes must be evaluated. There is no contraindication for a patient with depression taking CHCs. The 45-year-old patient is, in all likelihood, perimenopausal, so there may not be a need for CHCs, but they are not absolutely contraindicated. A person who smokes or has diabetes requires extra caution.
19. c. If only one dose has been missed, the patient should take the dose as soon as possible and then resume the regular schedule with the next dose.
20. a, b, c, d, e. Common side effects with conjugated estrogen include acne, breast tenderness, leg cramps, fluid retention, and nausea. Other common side effects are vomiting, breakthrough bleeding, and chloasma.

21. a, d, e. Aspirin toxicity can occur, increasing the anticoagulant effects. Barbiturates such as phenobarbital and topiramate, which can be used either for seizures or for migraines, are contraindicated in patients taking oral contraceptives. All women of childbearing age should take supplemental folic acid.
22. c. Potassium levels should be monitored closely. Drospirenone causes the body to retain potassium. Hyperkalemia is possible, especially in patients with undiagnosed kidney disease.
23. c. If the ring has been out less than 3 hours, it can be reinserted.
24. b. As part of the ACHES mnemonic [*A*bdominal pain (severe), *C*hest pain or shortness of breath, *H*eadache (severe), *E*ye disorders, *S*evere leg pain], severe headaches could be indicative of cardiovascular side effects and should be reported to the health care provider immediately.
25. c
26. a. The transdermal patch is convenient and does not require daily dosing. When applied to the skin, usually on the lower abdomen, estrogen is absorbed directly into the bloodstream.
27. b, e

Case Study

1. With these presenting symptoms and at her age, the patient is likely menopausal. Dyspareunia, frequency, urgency, thinning vaginal epithelium, and decreased elasticity on speculum exam are due to estrogen deficit. Frequency and urgency can also be associated with a urinary tract infection (UTI), so a urinalysis should be obtained; however, a UTI would not account for the findings on speculum exam. By definition, a lack of menstruation for 1 year is defined as menopause. Other symptoms associated with menopause may include hot flashes and night sweats.
2. Treatment may be symptomatic and include taking cool baths, using a fan, and sleeping in light clothing. Another option is hormone therapy (HT). HT should be administered at the lowest doses and for the shortest amount of time possible. HT improves vasomotor symptoms such as hot flashes, and it also improves vaginal dryness and irritation. It does, however, come with increased risks of cardiovascular events such as DVT, stroke, and MI and certain cancers (breast, ovarian, and lung). The health care provider should discuss the risk-to-benefit ratio with the patient to help her decide the best option.
3. HT also decreases the risk of osteoporosis. C.W. is thin and Caucasian, which are two risk factors for osteoporosis. Using HT, increasing vitamin D and calcium intake, and exercising (such as walking) may help prevent bone loss. The use of medications for osteoporosis includes bisphosphonates and SERMs. These medications help prevent the breakdown of bone.

CHAPTER 53—MEN'S REPRODUCTIVE HEALTH

1. g
2. h
3. j
4. f
5. e
6. i
7. b
8. c
9. a
10. d
11. d. Sildenafil is contraindicated in patients with significant cardiac disease.
12. d
13. c. The use of hormones to "bulk up" or improve performance occurs at all levels of sports competition. Side/adverse effects from the use of excessive intake of anabolic steroids include increased low-density lipoprotein cholesterol, decreased high-density lipoprotein cholesterol, acne, high blood pressure, liver damage, and dangerous changes in the left ventricle of the heart. Adverse effects may not be recognized until years later.
14. a. Blood glucose levels may be decreased in patients with diabetes when taking androgens. The patient should be instructed to carefully monitor blood glucose levels for changes so the insulin dose can be adjusted.
15. a, c. Androgens can be used to treat advanced breast cancer and endometriosis in women. Other uses include management of severe menopausal symptoms in women, refractory anemia in both genders, and tissue wasting associated with severe illness.
16. a, b, d
17. a, c, e

Case Study

1. Erectile dysfunction can occur in men at any stage of life. It occurs due to lack of sufficient blood flow to the penis. It may be seen in men with diabetes. Some of the medications used to treat hypertension, such as diuretics and beta blockers, may also cause erectile dysfunction.
2. One class of medications that the patient may be referring to is the phosphodiesterase (PDE-5) inhibitors, which includes sildenafil, tadalafil, and vardenafil. They work by increasing blood flow to the penis so the patient can maintain an erection.
3. Side effects may include upset stomach, blurred vision, flushing, and headache. The most serious side effect is a sustained erection (priapism) that lasts longer than 4 hours. Priapism is an emergency because a thrombosis may form in the corpora cavernosa, which can lead to permanent loss of function.

4. The nurse should teach the patient not to use any herbal preparations without discussing their side effects with his health care provider. The patient should also be advised to not use any nitroglycerin or nitrate-containing drugs while taking PDE-5 inhibitors because the combination can cause marked hypotension. PDE-5 inhibitors should also not be taken with grapefruit or grapefruit juice because it increases the amount of PDE-5 available. Side effects, such as headache and vision changes should be taught to the patient.

CHAPTER 54—SEXUALLY TRANSMITTED INFECTIONS

1. c
2. e
3. b
4. f
5. a
6. d
7. b
8. d
9. f
10. c
11. a
12. e
13. c
14. a. Abstaining from sexual activity is the safest practice to prevent any further transmission; however, if that is not an option, all partners should wear a condom during sex.
15. d. If the patient wants to participate in sexual activity, using a condom is the safest.
16. a
17. a, b, c, d

Case Study

1. The presumptive diagnosis is gonorrhea involving both her genitourinary and oral mucous membranes caused by *Neisseria gonorrhea*. Oral infections caused by *N. gonorrhea* cause pharyngitis and dysphagia. She may also have a fever, and if left untreated her infection can cause tubal scarring.
2. Dual drug therapy is recommended with ceftriaxone 250 mg IM *plus* azithromycin 1 g PO, both as a single dose. Dual therapy improves treatment efficacy and decreases the development of drug resistance.
3. K.E. should be informed that she is at risk for other infections, such as chlamydia, HPV, and HIV, and that she should be further tested. She should abstain from intercourse until therapy is completed and her partners should be treated. If she cannot abstain from intercourse, then instruct her to use condoms. Review how STIs are transmitted and how they could be avoided.

CHAPTER 55: ADULT AND PEDIATRIC EMERGENCY DRUGS

1. h
2. g
3. k
4. e
5. i
6. a
7. f
8. b
9. d
10. c
11. j
12. f
13. d
14. a
15. d
16. b
17. c
18. e
19. g
20. a. Nitroglycerin is a vasodilator and can cause a rapid drop in blood pressure, especially in first-time users. Tachycardia or bradycardia can also occur, but it is not as common as hypotension.
21. a. Morphine can cause respiratory depression so the patient's respiratory status must be monitored closely. Naloxone can be used to reverse respiratory depression if needed.
22. a. Atropine is the first-line treatment for symptomatic bradycardia. Although epinephrine can be used for bradycardia with hypotension, it is not the first-line treatment.
23. d. Myocardial ischemia can occur when a patient is receiving dobutamine. The nurse must monitor carefully for signs of myocardial ischemia, including chest pain and dysrhythmias. Dobutamine can cause tachycardia, not bradycardia.
24. b. Procainamide is an antiarrhythmic for ventricular dysrhythmias that are unresponsive to adenosine. Procainamide is discontinued if hypotension develops. Other end points to procainamide include when ECG changes occur (i.e., widening of the QRS complex by 50% or more), when the maximum dose has been given (17 mg/kg), or when the dysrhythmia is successfully treated.
25. b, e. Amiodarone is appropriate to treat ventricular tachyarrhythmia, such as ventricular fibrillation, and atrial fibrillation that is not controlled by other measures. The dose to administer is dependent on the presence or absence of a pulse. Amiodarone is not given in patients with bradycardia or atrioventricular blocks, such as second-degree block.
26. a
27. c. Mannitol is an osmotic diuretic to treat increased intracranial pressure.
28. c. This patient is exhibiting signs of an allergic reaction. Besides receiving epinephrine, the patient will receive diphenhydramine. Diphenhydramine reduces histamine-induced swelling and itching that occur in allergic reactions.
29. c. Naloxone is an opiate antagonist and naloxone 0.4 mg IVP is within the dose range to be administered. If this is an opioid overdose, the medication should reverse fairly rapidly, and the patient will become responsive. If this is not an opioid overdose, there will be no response. Benzodiazepines, such as diazepam, are also used for back spasms, but they do not produce pinpoint pupils. Flumazenil is the reversal agent for benzodiazepines.
30. a, d, e. Dopamine is a vasopressor and may be used to treat hypotension in cardiogenic, neurogenic, and septic shock after adequate fluid and/or blood product resuscitation, although norepinephrine may be preferred in neurogenic shock. Hypovolemic shock should be treated with fluids, either crystalloids or blood. *Insulin shock* is actually misnamed and refers to a hypoglycemic reaction. It should be treated with glucose, not vasopressors.
31. a
32. b. Norepinephrine is a catecholamine that acts on the alpha-adrenergic receptors and has potent vasoconstrictor actions, and as with other adrenergic agonists, abrupt discontinuation can cause a profound drop in the blood pressure.
33. d. D50 is used to treat severe hypoglycemia, most commonly attributable to insulin shock. Increased urine output and hyperglycemia can occur because of D50. D50 is highly irritating to the vein and should be administered through a large peripheral or central vein.
34. c. Adenosine is a first-line drug for supraventricular tachycardia. Adenosine 6 mg is given IV push as rapidly as possible followed by 20 mL of saline. If a second dose is needed, a 12-mg bolus is given 1 to 2 minutes after the initial dose.
35. a. Once the dysrhythmia has been suppressed, as long as a total of 3 mg/kg has not been exceeded, a maintenance drip of lidocaine at a rate of 1–4 mg/min is started.
36. b. The correct solution to utilize for IM injection is 1:1000 solution.
37. a. The standard concentration of 1 mg of 1:10,000 epinephrine is used in cardiac arrest.
38. a. Usual dosage for atropine in adults is 0.5 mg and may be repeated q3-5 min. Anything less than 0.5 mg can produce a paradoxical bradycardia.
39. b
40. c, d, e
41. d. Furosemide is a loop diuretic that inhibits reabsorption and promotes renal excretion of water, sodium, potassium, magnesium, calcium, and hydrogen. It also promotes vasodilation and diuresis, which can lower blood pressure.
42. b, d, e. Blue or brown color indicates the solution has degraded and should not be used. The bottle should be protected from light. Because this medication is a potent antihypertensive, the

patient will need to be monitored continuously in the critical care unit. As nitroprusside breaks down, the byproducts include thiocyanate or cyanide; therefore, levels must be monitored closely and the drug should be used for the shortest amount of time necessary.

43. a, c, d

Case Study

1. M.E. took three of his own nitroglycerin (NTG) tablets before calling EMS. NTG dilates the coronary arteries to improve blood flow and oxygenation to the ischemic myocardium. IV NTG infusion is reserved for chest pain related to unstable angina or acute myocardial infarction. BP and HR must be continuously monitored because hypotension is a common adverse effect.

2. An aspirin is given to patients having chest pain to decrease platelet aggregation in acute coronary syndrome and for acute myocardial infarction. Oxygen is given to provide adequate supply to the heart. It can be administered either by nasal cannula, nonrebreather mask, simple mask, or endotracheal intubation to maintain the oxygen saturation at >94%. This patient does not, at this point, require endotracheal intubation. Morphine is used to relieve pain, dilate venous vessels, and reduce the workload of the heart. IV nitroglycerin is reserved for patients with unstable angina or an AMI. A nitroglycerin drip is usually initiated at a rate of 5 mcg/min and increased by 5 mcg/min every 3–5 minutes, based on chest pain and blood pressure response.

3. The nurse would prepare to administer epinephrine 1 mg IV q3-5 minutes while continuing CPR and shocking any shockable rhythm. If the patient continues in ventricular tachycardia, then amiodarone 300 mg IV can be given and may be repeated once at a dose of 150 mg. The patient should be evaluated periodically for a pulse and/or change in rhythm.